Modern and Global Ayurveda

Modern and Global Ayurveda

Pluralism and Paradigms

Edited by

Dagmar Wujastyk and
Frederick M. Smith

SUNY
PRESS

Cover art: *Sage Sushruta, World's First Eye Surgeon*; painting by Raghupathi Bhatta

Published by
State University of New York Press, Albany

Printed in the United States of America

For information, contact State University of New York Press, Albany, NY
www.sunypress.edu

Production by Diane Ganeles
Marketing by Fran Keneston

Library of Congress Cataloging-in-Publication Data

Modern and global Ayurveda : pluralism and paradigms / edited by Dagmar Wujastyk, Frederick M. Smith
p. cm.
Includes bibliographical references and index.
ISBN 978-0-7914-7489-1 (hardcover : alk. paper)
ISBN 978-0-7914-7490-7 (pbk. : alk. paper)
1. Medicine, Ayurvedic. 2. Medicine, Ayurvedic—History. I. Wujastyk, Dagmar. II. Smith, Frederick M.
[DNLM: 1. Medicine, Ayurvedic—Europe. 2. Medicine, Ayurvedic—India. 3. Medicine, Ayurvedic—United States. 4. History, 20th Century—Europe. 5. History, 20th Century—India. 6. History, 20th Century—United States. 7. Medicine, Ayurvedic—history—Europe. 8. Medicine, Ayurvedic—history—India. 9. Medicine, Ayurvedic—history—United States. WB 50.1 M689 2008]

R605.M63 2008
610—dc22 2007036639

10 9 8 7 6 5 4 3 2 1

Contents

Tables

Foreword

It is with great joy and a deep sense of satisfaction that I set out to write this foreword for the volume on modern and global Ayurveda edited by Dagmar Wujastyk and Frederick M. Smith. The origins of this volume go back several years, to 2002, when I was director of the Dharam Hinduja Institute of Indic Research (DHIIR), a specialist research institution based at the Faculty of Divinity, University of Cambridge, United Kingdom (see http://www.divinity.cam.ac.uk/CARTS/dhiir). As part of its brief, the institute was committed to studying questions of multiculturalism, with special reference to issues of health and medical concerns, and with a focus on Indic (i.e., South Asian) traditions of knowledge. On this basis, we started our Indic Health and Medicine Research Programme, which ran from October 2000 to September 2004. For the first couple of years we concentrated on issues relating to the modernization of yoga, and in 2002 we added research work on Ayurveda.

In the same year the DHIIR was most fortunate in securing the cooperation of Dagmar Wujastyk (then Benner) as research assistant for the Ayurveda project, and she played a major role in organizing two DHIIR events on this topic: a specialist workshop that took place in December 2003 and the July 2004 public conference, on the proceedings of which the present collection is substantially based. Due to her involvement in the project, Wujastyk was the natural choice when we came to select an editor for the proceedings. The participation of Frederick M. Smith as coeditor also was secured early on, and from then onward the two editors have worked very hard to gather together the best possible expertise in the field. The excellent result of their work is in your hands: a unique, timely, useful, engaging volume that will be of great use to academics, to Ayurveda practitioners, patients, and students, and to other interested parties alike.

As will be apparent, our work at DHIIR focused on two of the aspects of Indic culture that are most popular in the English-speaking world and elsewhere across the developed world: yoga and Ayurveda.

We found, however, that while many people were interested, and often involved in the practice of these disciplines, there was very little awareness of their modern history, and of the social and ideological trends that drove their most recent developments.

Therefore, as in the case of yoga, our priority was to carry out work that would open up new areas of understanding and bring clarity to topics that, while well known at some level, were often misunderstood, or approached in simplistic fashion. Such considerations informed our decision to concentrate on the more modern and contemporary aspects of Ayurveda, and eventually a useful subdivision between "Modern" and "Global" Ayurveda emerged, the former a process taking place on South Asian soil from the nineteenth century onward, the latter a more recent phenomenon linked to transnational export trends and the commercialization and acculturation of this ancient medical science in places other than the subcontinent (for more details on these two aspects of Ayurveda, see the Introduction).

We also wanted our work to be relevant to as many people as possible. We were, for example, aware that efforts were afoot in the United Kingdom to put together a legal regulatory framework for the practice of Ayurveda. A publication such as this can be invaluable in this context: if used skillfully, it can truly help decision makers in their reflections, as it provides accurate and unbiased information on centrally relevant topics. In these cases the usefulness of academic research is immediately apparent: better information and contextualization of the topic is bound to create more informed and realistic discussions and to result in better laws and regulations in due course. Indeed, the usefulness of such efforts is demonstrated by the following anecdote. A number of key representatives of Ayurveda in the United Kingdom had been thinking of getting together to form a professional association. In 2004 they attended the DHIIR public conference on which the present publication is partly based. Hearing the presentations there brought home to them the urgency of the matter. They also got in touch with reliable experts and sympathizers with whom they have been collaborating since. They are now key players in UK ayurvedic circles and are well represented by the interest group they eventually set up, the Ayurvedic Practitioners Association (see http://www.apa.uk.com).

Other individuals directly involved in medical practice and studies, whether ayurvedic or otherwise, also will find this volume of great interest. Its mixture of firsthand, critical accounts from informed ayurvedic practitioners and full-fledged Ayurveda scholars is noteworthy. Such an engaged, "real life" scholarship (as it were) mirrors the work and concerns of an institution that matches—and surpasses—the DHIIR Ayurveda project's original aims, the International Association for the Study of Traditional Asian Medicine. The IASTAM was, and perhaps remains, "the only international organisation in the field of Asian medicine making a serious attempt to embrace both academics and practitioners" (see http://www.iastam.org). Indeed, many of the contributors to this volume are active members of the IASTAM, and it is good to know that now that the DHIIR no longer exists, alternative, lively, forums remain where such constructive discussions and activities can be carried forward.

Lastly, I would like to acknowledge the outstanding contribution of the coauthors of this collection. Many years of research and of medical, scientific, and institutional practice are distilled in these pages, from the four corners of the globe. We are privileged to be able to share in this communal pool of knowledge and scholarship. It is my heartfelt wish that this knowledge may be of help to further human happiness and well-being.

Elizabeth De Michelis
Oriel College, University of Oxford, United Kingdom

Acknowledgments

The editors wish to acknowledge generous support received from the Dharam Hindiya Institute of Indic Research, Cambridge, as well as from the office of the Vice President for Research at the University of Iowa.

CHAPTER ONE

Introduction

Frederick M. Smith and Dagmar Wujastyk

Ayurveda, the indigenous medical system of India, dates back at least 2,000 years in its codified form and has roots that are much deeper still. In the late twentieth and early twenty-first centuries, it is stretching well beyond the boundaries of its homeland. Because it is fast becoming a transnational and multicultural phenomenon, it is time to examine Ayurveda's interface with modernity and the pluralistic approaches and new paradigms it has developed to meet the challenges of its new diasporic presence.

Developments within Ayurveda during its long and varied history, the addition of new theories and practices to the established ones, their interrelations and the interweaving of medical thought with constantly mutating religious, political, and cultural climates, form a rich and complicated pattern of medical and social history. What we intend to present here is an account of recent developments in the long history of Ayurveda, which is to say its development in the face of three major challenges: (1) British colonialism and the dominance of allopathic medicine, (2) the pressures of modernization, and (3) Ayurveda's diaspora into the world beyond the boundaries of South Asia.

We will present the relatively recent history of modern and global Ayurveda from a number of perspectives that sometimes contrast and sometimes complement each other. The terms *modern Ayurveda* and *global Ayurveda* do not denote unified knowledge systems but rather serve as umbrella terms for a number of disciplines based on or concerned with ayurvedic knowledge. These include, for example, various forms of ayurvedic practice, ayurvedic pharmaceutical research, drug development and industrial production, and academic textual research (both for botanical and pharmaceutical research and for a broader understanding of ayurvedic theory).

"Modern Ayurveda" is here understood to be geographically set in the Indian subcontinent and to commence with the processes of professionalization and institutionalization brought about in India by what has been called the nineteenth-century revivalism of Ayurveda (Leslie 1998; Brass 1972; Jeffery 1988). Modern Ayurveda is characterized by a tendency toward the secularization of ayurvedic knowledge and its adaptation to biomedicine, and at the same time by attempts to formulate a unitary theory based on doctrines found in the classical ayurvedic texts.

"Global Ayurveda," on the other hand, refers to ayurvedic knowledge that has been transmitted to geographically widespread areas outside of India. Here we may differentiate three broad "lineages" of ayurvedic globalization: the first is characterized by a focus on the ayurvedic pharmacopoeia, beginning with the dissemination of ayurvedic botanical and pharmaceutical lore in the sixteenth century. The study of ayurvedic pharmacopoeia has developed into a full-blown scientific discipline as well as into a hugely profitable pharmaceutical industry in a global market. In line with the ideologies of modern Ayurveda, interest groups concerned with ayurvedic pharmacopoeia stress the "scientific" bases of Ayurveda and promote a secularized discipline stripped of its religious and spiritual connotations.

The second lineage of global Ayurveda is identified in the more recent trend of a globally popularized and acculturated Ayurveda, which tends to emphasize and reinterpret, if not reinvent, the philosophical and spiritual aspects of Ayurveda. This type of Ayurveda has been dubbed "New Age Ayurveda" (Zysk 2001; Reddy 2000). Zysk defines its characteristics as follows:

1. attributing a remote age to Ayurveda and making it the source of other medical systems
2. linking Ayurveda closely to Indian spirituality, especially Yoga
3. making Ayurveda the basis of mind-body medicine
4. claiming the "scientific" basis of Ayurveda and its intrinsic safety as a healing modality

Another important characteristic of New Age Ayurveda (which it shares with some forms of modern Ayurveda in urban settings) is a shift in self-representation from reactive medicine that cures ills to preventive medicine that offers a positive lifestyle index.

New Age Ayurveda is particularly prominent in the United States, and increasingly in Northern Europe. Furthermore, it has been reimported into India in the shape of "wellness" tourism that caters both to foreign tourists and urban, middle-class Indians. This has been described by Jean Langford (2002) and is examined further by Manasi Tirodkar in this volume. Thus paradoxically, despite its emphasis on spirituality, New Age Ayurveda has given rise to a new commercialized form of Ayurveda, emphasizing wellness and beauty as fundamental components of good health. Its commercial offerings encompass a range of cosmetic and massage treatments provided in beauty salons and spas, over-the-counter products (mostly cosmetics and nutritional supplements), and do-it-yourself or self-help literature (i.e., guides on beauty treatments, nutrition, and fitness). Selby (2005) describes how Ayurveda, twinned or even merged with yoga into "Ayuryoga," has become a branded commodity in North American spa culture. While the unprotected name "Ayurveda" is used freely in this context, it is not necessarily used to denote a real connection with premodern ayurvedic knowledge but often rather seems to stand for vague notions of "exotic" or "Eastern" self-cultivation. Thus we may find a spa offering a full-day treatment entitled "Ayurvedic Bliss," which in this case means "Luxury Spa Pedicure, Aromatherapy Salt Glow Body, Exfoliation and Hot Stone Back Massage,"[1] treatments that are not found in classical ayurvedic texts. As Sita Reddy (2004) has pointed out, images of the "exotic East" play a crucial role in certain sectors of the marketing of ayurvedic products or treatments.

A third, independent line of global Ayurveda originated in the context of the then-new scholarly discipline of Indic Studies in the early nineteenth century, when Orientalist scholars began to take interest in ayurvedic literature. While the first scholarly documentation on Indian medicine in the form of botanical encyclopedias was not concerned with the conceptual framework of Ayurveda, these scholars were interested in preserving, or even reviving, knowledge of Ayurveda as a historical and philological discipline. Spurred by the notion of a second renaissance inspired by an Indian antiquity, they set out to discover the roots of Indian medicine, printing and translating the medical texts and writing summaries of their contents. The scholars so involved—including Thomas Wise, Franciscus Hessler, Gustave Lietard, Palmyr Cordier, and Julius Jolly—were mostly medical men, trained in Western medical science.[2] Their work, however, seems never to have been directed at making practical use of the knowledge gained from the texts in regard to the more theoretical aspects underlying ayurvedic medicine. However, scholarly editions and translations of Sanskrit medical works have been important contributions to formalized ayurvedic education and research.

Indological textual research continues up to the present. From about the mid-1960s onward, the education and practice of Ayurveda as well as its political and social frameworks were studied from the perspective of medical anthropology, a new academic discipline pioneered by Charles Leslie and others. Academic work on Ayurveda has had some influence on the public perception of Ayurveda, due to literary output, on the one hand, and to its contribution to television or other media productions, on the other. However, scholarly publications on Ayurveda reach only a limited number of readers, much less than comparable publications from New Age and other public-oriented sectors. Television documentaries, popular periodical literature, and most Web sites can only provide reduced versions of scholarly research, as any production is necessarily guided by commercial considerations (i.e., broadcasting slots and viewing figures). It is interesting to note, for example, that parallel to rising interest in plastic surgery in the United States and Northern Europe, with serial documentaries or reality shows on modern plastic surgery regularly broadcast on television, a number of documentaries on ancient Indian surgery have been produced in recent years, presenting topics such as "the ancient Indian nose job."

Finally, Ayurveda has become the subject of interdisciplinary ethnopharmacological studies. Ethnopharmacology, a discipline that became prominent in the 1980s, aims to integrate the hard sciences (e.g., pharmacology or medicine) and the humanities (i.e., anthropology and other ethnographically based disciplines) in order to document and improve traditional pharmacopoeias.[3] Ethnopharmacological studies on Ayurveda ideally combine the various strands of modern and global Ayurveda. The work of the Foundation for the Revitalization of Local Health Traditions (FRLHT), as described by Payyappallimana Unnikrishnan in this volume, is an example of ethnopharmacological research within India.

THE ORIGINS AND HISTORY OF AYURVEDA

The term *Ayurveda* means "knowledge (*veda*) of longevity (*āyus*)," but it is often translated as "science of longevity" or "science of life," denoting an entire empirical system of healing. Ayurveda has antecedents in the medicine found in much earlier periods in India, and in texts as far back as the Atharva-Veda of around 1000 BCE (Zysk 1996; Bahulkar 1994). However, systematic medical theory began to be formulated only around the time of the Buddha (ca. 400 BCE). It is in early Buddhist texts that we first find explicit statements that disease arises from an imbalance of humoral substances, an idea that would become a cornerstone in Indian medical theory (Zysk 2000; Scharfe 1999; also see the various interpretations of humoral theory discussed in several chapters in this volume). Similarities with Greek humoral theory, and the fact that there is mention of Indian plants in Greek medical literature, suggest some form of exchange between Greek and Indian medicine at least at the level of pharmacopoeia. The exact nature of the contact between Indian and Greek medicine is, however, unclear and remains a subject of speculation, as there is no mention in either Greek or Sanskrit medical literature of contact or exchange with physicians from the other culture.

The first mention of Ayurveda as the name for the science of medicine occurs in the *Mahābhārata* (12.28.44, 12.328.9, 12.330.22), India's great epic, composed over a period of three to five centuries, most likely terminating in around the third century CE. The *Mahābhārata* also knows medicine as a science constituted of eight parts (*cikitsāyām aṣṭāṅgāyām*, 2.50.80 [Wujastyk 2003b: 394]), the same number that is found in the early ayurvedic compendia. These early texts, dated to the early centuries of the Common Era, are the *Caraka-Saṃhitā* (the compilation of Caraka) and the *Suśruta-Saṃhitā* (the compilation of Suśruta). These two texts, which contain a vast amount of information on areas of medical science, from diagnostics to clinical practice to pharmacopoeia, are generally followed today. They represent two of the three texts counted in the *bṛhat-trayī*, the "great-three" ayurvedic texts, the third being the *Aṣṭāṅgahṛdaya-Saṃhitā* (the "compilation of the heart of the eight limbs" of medical practice) composed by Vāgbhaṭa in the early seventh century.[4]

It is essential when thinking about Ayurveda to recognize that in India ancient knowledge is often regarded with great reverence. This does not mean—to take Ayurveda as an example—that all practitioners regard the recommendations or diagnoses in these ancient texts as more authoritative than recently discovered knowledge. While many of the recommendations of these ancient texts are in fact still followed to good effect thousands of years after their composition, the "tradition" of Ayurveda has remained dynamic for this entire period. New texts were continually being composed, new paradigms were explored, and influences from many other areas of Indian discourse were introduced into Ayurveda. Indeed, the practice of Ayurveda has been criticized unjustly by certain historians and members of competing medical systems for its rigorous adherence to antiquated prescriptions and paradigms. These critics are not aware of the vitality in the history of Ayurveda, largely because nearly all the textuality from about 900–1900 CE remains unknown and unstudied by a larger public.

Another criticism, emerging largely from within India, is that Ayurveda suffered a decline during the period of Mughal dominance, from the fourteenth to eighteenth centuries. Thanks now to the pioneering efforts of Jan Meulenbeld, whose five-volume *History of Indian Medical Literature* was completed in 2002, it is possible to effectively counter these criticisms. A current project focusing on Sanskrit knowledge systems on the eve of colonialism aims to shed further light on this gap in ayurvedic history,[5] and preliminary conclusions confirm that "production in no way diminished in the sixteenth, seventeenth and eighteenth centuries, which spawned rich and vitally important medical treatises of all kinds" (Wujastyk 2005b). While modern Ayurveda does in some respects resemble the Ayurveda found in the *bṛhat-trayī*, which is to say in the first half of the first millennium CE, in many ways it does not, and most of this is the result of internal developments and refinements in medical knowledge, a changing ecology, and the influence of ever-changing indigenous religious and cultural forms.

ENCOUNTERS AND EDUCATION

The history of global Ayurveda begins with the encounter between Indian and European practitioners of medicine through the spice trade.[6] These encounters were largely limited to the pharmaceutical and botanical sciences in the pursuit of two main objects: to provide the traders (and later the colonialists) with medical care adapted to the needs of their new situation, and to make commercial use of the newly acquired medical knowledge through the trading of Indian medical drugs. Indian medical knowledge had long before spread beyond India through the dissemination of texts and through oral transmission, but the export of Indian medicines (with a basic knowledge of their traditional use) had never before been organized—and *documented*—on such a large scale as part of commercial enterprise. The strong contemporary emphasis on ayurvedic pharmacology can trace its roots to these encounters, though its ideological background and scientific methodology emerged from later developments in both European medicine and British colonial politics in the nineteenth and twentieth centuries (see Bala 1991, especially pp. 48–57).

In the first third of the nineteenth century, British health and education policy in India began to emphasize support for the new medical knowledge and methodology that was then emerging in Europe. This resulted in the patronage of new medical colleges and hospitals and ultimately produced a number of practitioners with a medical reputation superior to that of traditional practitioners. The direct effects of British policy on indigenous medicine, however, date to a later period, when Indians were admitted to the biomedical colleges, and health services were extended to the Indian public. To meet the competition of the new system and to show the value of their science, traditional practitioners needed to articulate the theoretical foundations of their medical system and to establish their professional identity. In the case of Ayurveda this meant the birth of a new era, the beginnings of modern Ayurveda, as ayurvedic practitioners had never before organized themselves into one uniform body. The traditional education system—one that still can be found in practice in India today—had been that of pupilage, that is, a teacher passing his knowledge down to one or several pupils, often from father to son or uncle to nephew. This would lead to the formation of medical lineages or schools with individual emphases on specific teachings. One step toward a modernized Ayurveda therefore was a break with the educational tradition of pupilage and a compensatory movement toward an expanded college system. This proved to be the only way to keep up with the growing number of graduates and license holders that the modern medical colleges were producing. Another step was to present Ayurveda, at political and ideological levels, as a unified medical system that would then shape the curricula of the colleges. This proved to be one of the greatest challenges to modern Ayurveda. Modern Ayurvedists needed not only to overcome sectarian and regional differences (including language barriers and diverging religious identities) in search of a uniform identity but were also confronted with new educational methods and technologies for diagnosis and research introduced to India by the British. The dominant form of ayurvedic education that developed from this background at the end of the nineteenth century was an integrated or a concurrent education system, which included both Ayurveda and modern medical subjects in varying proportions. A brief passage from one of the model papers (see Table 1.1) for ayurvedic competitive examinations may give a glimpse of what knowledge such an education might provide.

Table 1.1. Questions 28–33 in Model Paper IV (Rao 1994)

Which of the following Srotas is not mentioned by Susruta A. Asthivaha srotas B. Majjavaha srotas C. Both D. None of the above	Islets of langhter hons [sic] present in A. Parotid gland B. Liver C. Kidney D. Pancreas
Vedhini is a variety of A. Kala B. Twak C. Dhamani D. Sira	Maximillary nerve is the branch of A. Trigeminal nerve B. Glasso pharyngeal [sic] nerve C. Vagus nerve D. None of the above
The extra asaya present in the female A. Mutrasaya B. Garbahasaya C. Raktasaya D. All the above	Function of the Risorius muscle A. Blinking B. Facial expression C. Dancing D. None of these

The basic education in modern biomedicine, as exemplified in the exam questions, was meant to enable students to play a role in public health programs. However, the debate on the educational system of Ayurveda (and of the other Indian systems of medicine) and its implementation into public health schemes is far from resolved, even today. The complicated history of government debate over the role of Ayurveda in national health schemes is discussed by Dominik Wujastyk in this volume.

The "biomedicalization" of Ayurveda is, however, not only a phenomenon that occurs within government institutions but also reaches into private practice, as Manasi Tirodkar shows in this volume.

Modern Ayurveda thus comes into being as a reaction to the introduction and patronage of a new medical system by the British colonialists. Ayurveda, not homogenous in itself to begin with, had always coexisted and even competed for patronage with other types of medicine. However, this was perhaps the first time that such a sharp distinction was made between one way of practicing medicine and another, one being given clear precedence over the other. The distinction made, however, was not one between modern medicine and Ayurveda: the British contrasted modern medicine (presumed to be a monolithic body of knowledge) with Indian indigenous medicine in general. Today, the Indian government distinguishes Ayurveda, Unani, and Siddha as separate medical systems and also acknowledges folk medical traditions as part of Indian medical heritage. While the distinction into separate medical systems is to some extent justified by identifiable textual traditions, the reality of medical practice does not necessarily fall in line with it. Nineteenth- and twentieth-century documents offer evidence that the boundaries between the different indigenous medical systems were far more fluid than they are represented today, and that the insistence on differences developed parallel to growing nationalism in India. The links between nationalism and the differentiation of the indigenous medical systems are addressed in this volume by Rachel Berger and Richard S. Weiss.[7]

Ayurvedic modernization and professionalization are thus marked by the ideological and formal separation of Ayurveda from other medical traditions. The establishment of the All-India Ayurveda Mahasammelan (Ayurvedic Congress) in 1907 was a landmark in this respect, though it originally understood itself as the representative body of all practitioners of indigenous medicine, including Unani and Siddha. The Bombay Medical Practitioners' Act of 1938, which established the first separate register for practitioners of Indian systems of medicine, was the first formal recognition of Ayurveda by the government of India. After Independence, further important formal structures were set up with the Central Institute of Research in Indigenous

Systems of Medicine in 1956, followed by the Central Council for Ayurvedic Research in 1959, the Central Council of Indian Medicine in 1971, and the Central Council for Research in Ayurveda and Siddha in 1978. In 1982, the Central Council of Indian Medicine issued the first comprehensive regulations regarding standards of professional conduct and etiquette and a code of ethics for practitioners of Indian medicine (see Benner 2005). In 1995, a Department of Indian Systems of Medicine was established, with a permanent secretary within the Indian Ministry of Health and Family Welfare. To date, there are more than 200,000 registered traditional medical practitioners in India and over 100 government-approved, degree-granting colleges of ayurvedic education.

The formalization and legal integration of Ayurveda in the twentieth century was complemented by what is described as its "pharmaceuticalization" by Madhulika Banerjee in this volume. Although, as Banerjee points out, this process has to some extent reduced Ayurveda to a mere supplier of pharmaceutical products, it has, on the other hand, contributed to its popularization: the growing ayurvedic pharmaceutical industry made ayurvedic medicine more accessible through its over-the-counter products and gave Ayurveda more presence in the public mind through advertising (see also Bode 2004 on Unani and Ayurveda industries). Other factors that were significant in the shaping of modern Ayurveda and its popularization were the introduction of the mass print press, along with growing literacy, the vernacularization of medical texts, and the growth of a new type of literature dealing with health issues. The new medical "self-help" literature not only brought specialist knowledge into Indian homes but also tackled a number of delicate issues that had not been publicly addressed before (see Alter in this volume). Ayurvedic self-help literature also became a domain in which women could participate and discuss women's health—and herein lies perhaps one of the most significant changes to Ayurveda in the twentieth century: the active participation of women in medicine as authors and as physicians.

GLOBAL AYURVEDA: THE DISEMBEDDING OF AN EXPERT SYSTEM

Ayurveda was first introduced to Europe and North America in the late 1970s and early 1980s, a period during which its formal regulatory structures and standards of education were being established and consolidated in India on a national level. Some of the challenges with which the pioneers of Ayurveda in the West were faced, in the context of setting up structures for ayurvedic practice and education, echo developments in India, while others are specific to the new cultural environment. The different approaches to these challenges are addressed in several chapters in this volume. Mike Saks gives an account of how Asian medicines have become part of Western medical pluralism as complementary and alternative medicine (CAM). Ananda Samir Chopra's description of his practice at a hospital in Kassel, Germany, provides a vivid depiction of the relationship of a modern practice with its Indian antecedents. Sebastian Pole, one of two founders of Pukka Herbs (a UK-based company that supplies organic medicinal herbs), writes about his experiences with the growing, harvesting, and marketing of ayurvedic herbal products. Chapters by Cynthia Ann Humes and Françoise Jeannotat discuss Maharishi Ayur-Ved(a) (MAV), a unique form of Ayurveda spawned by Maharishi Mahesh Yogi and his Transcendental Meditation (TM) movement. Suzanne Newcombe discusses a lawsuit involving two British MAV doctors in the early 1990s. Manasi Tirodkar discusses the practice of Ayurveda at a modern clinic in Pune, India, with its rising middle-class clientele and its issues in negotiating a place in the modern medical marketplace. Robert E. Svoboda, one of the most popular writers and lecturers on Ayurveda in the West, and Claudia Welch, an accomplished practitioner of both Ayurveda and Traditional Chinese Medicine (TCM), discuss some of the forces that have shaped contemporary Ayurveda in the United States. Both Svoboda, who was the first Westerner to be fully trained and licensed by an Indian college of Ayurveda (Tilak Ayurveda College, Pune, 1980), and Welch take India as their starting point in casting light on how global Ayurveda has emerged from local forces in India.

One of the most salient features of Ayurveda in the West is that it does not form part of the medical mainstream, nor does it participate in most of its formal structures. This has implications both for its legal status and its public acceptance. One of the most formidable problems here is that the predominant model of ayurvedic training in the West is lineage-based pupilage. As different lineages may offer quite different perspectives on ayurvedic theory and practice, and are resistant to standardization, they effectively disqualify themselves from entering the medical establishment, which requires strict standardization of practice and education. As Welch points out, several competing lineages have developed in the West, in which the teacher, rather than the teaching, is often paramount. Sometimes these lineages are headed by licensed ayurvedic physicians from India, such as Vasant Lad at the Ayurvedic Institute in Albuquerque, New Mexico. Sometimes, however, they are headed by individuals who are not accredited and do not have comparable theoretical or clinical experience. Overt competition with other schools seems to be the norm, as new ayurvedic lineages often construct their authority on Ayurveda with assertions of the superiority and exclusivity of their teachings. Many of the ayurvedic institutions teach topics historically regarded as peripheral to Ayurveda, creating a situation ironically like the Indian ayurvedic colleges that Svoboda criticizes for brazenly loading their ayurvedic syllabi with classes in allopathy. In the West, however, it is not allopathy that has tiptoed into the syllabus. Rather, it is Indian astrology (*jyotiṣa*) and yoga, the latter usually personalized to match the school of yoga practiced by local teachers (such as "Ayuryoga" at the Ayurvedic Institute).

FOUR PARADIGMS OF GLOBAL AYURVEDA

A brief examination of four paradigms of global Ayurveda should help set the stage for much of the material presented in the book. These are (1) New Age Ayurveda, (2) Ayurveda as mind-body medicine, (3) Maharishi Ayur-Ved, and (4) traditional Ayurveda in an urban world. The four paradigms partake in varying degrees of scientific fidelity, cultural accommodation, discourses of holism, and Hindu (or Vedic) practices. All of these paradigms embody lineage-based Ayurveda to one extent or another, though only one of them (the third) argues for its exclusivity and designs its practices in order to preserve this perceived exclusivity in the ayurvedic marketplace. The first paradigm—New Age Ayurveda—more openly than the others embraces an array of practices often labeled "New Age." It also is more preventative in its orientation than the others, though all of them emphasize that adopting an "ayurvedic lifestyle" will strengthen the immune system and help prevent disease. This has become an important discourse marker in modern and global Ayurveda. As it has become eclipsed by allopathic medicine, Ayurveda has increasingly identified itself as a kind of preventive medicine; indeed, it has become as much a positive lifestyle index as a system for curing illness.

The second paradigm—Ayurveda as mind-body medicine—is the most thorough in its attempt to translate the Indian discourse of Ayurveda into a Western one. The third—Maharishi Ayur-Ved—is the most strident in its assertions of its superiority to other forms of Ayurveda, yet it has increasingly moved away from the norms of Ayurveda as expressed in the canonical texts and the modalities of its clinical practice. The fourth paradigm—traditional Ayurveda in an urban world—is closest to a recognizable medical practice based on scientific and practice-based norms. Perhaps more accurately they are exemplars rather than paradigms, because they are representations of certain kinds of Ayurveda. Yet each of them abides in a paradigmatic approach to Ayurveda in its modernization.

The four paradigms are not closed categories; they are in many ways interconnected, as advocates of one paradigm often are teachers or students of practitioners of another paradigm. We must emphasize that these paradigms represent not just differences in style but in substance as well. By substance we mean that there may be substantial differences in the training and background of the practitioners, many of whom have undergone other kinds of bodywork training such as massage or nonbiomedical healing such as Reiki, and who bring elements of Ayurveda into an already flourishing practice. Among them, MAV is probably the most idiosyncratic, but it is paradigmatic because a number of other lineage-based ayurvedic teachers and institutions also assert the superiority and exclusivity of their teachings. Among the shared features of many of these groups and institutes is a view of the deep history of Ayurveda. It is axiomatic to find statements in nearly all institutional, lineage, and popular presentations of Ayurveda that it is 5,000 years old, with some claiming that it is 8,000 years old, that it is a direct descendant of the medicine of the *Atharva-Veda*, that it was always allied with Tantra, and that the increasingly popular diagnosis by pulse (*nāḍīvijñāna*), which is not mentioned in any classical text, is an ancient ayurvedic practice.[9]

The New Age paradigm

Consider, in this context, the following advertisement, titled "Introduction to Ayurveda and Panchakarma," which one of the editors came across while shopping in a health food store in the fall of 2005 in a small state in the American Northeast. The advertisement read, in part:

> This one-day workshop will give you an introduction to Ayurveda and Panchakarma. Originating in India, more than 5,000 years ago, Ayurveda, a sister-science to Yoga, is one of the oldest systems of health care in the world. It is an art of daily living that allows us to understand our unique nature and constitution, so we can prevent health disorders, correct present imbalances and maintain a high quality, long life. Panchakarma is a therapeutic Ayurvedic cleansing process that takes one on a deep, rejuvenating journey. It has been used in India for thousands of years to detoxify on a cellular level by cleansing deep seated toxins from the body. Panchakarma purifies at the physical, mental and emotional levels.

After listing the topics to be covered in the workshop, the practitioner lists her credentials: five years studying and working with a well-known Indian ayurvedic physician in America, completion of a yoga teacher training course in India, and licensing by a Swedish massage therapist in New York. The fee for the workshop was ninety-five dollars, which included a light vegetarian lunch. She "feels extremely blessed," she says toward the end of the advertisement, "to spread the knowledge of this beautiful science—Ayurveda."

This advertisement contains most of the discourse markers of the present state of Ayurveda in the West, particularly in the United States. The workshop was targeted at health food buyers, many of whom have an interest in complementary and alternative medicine, who distrust the impersonal and expensive mainstream allopathic medical system, and who search for alternative paradigms for living their lives. Such persons may read Eastern spiritual or New Age literature and may engage in practices taught by the purveyors of this literature, or otherwise consume its products in the form of short courses or products, including edible or nutritional substances, or dietary regimes. In other words, the advertisement is for consumers and practitioners of lifestyle paradigms generally considered "alternative," and is selling, in no small measure, not only the healing of physical diseases but a healing experience that is embedded in an ontological and epistemological paradigm that views itself as salvific.

Ayurveda as Mind-body Medicine

A second paradigm of modernization and adaptation is expressed in the writing of well-known ayurvedic practitioner John Douillard,[10] a doctor of chiropractic (DC) who also holds a PhD from the Open International Institute for Complementary Medicine in Sri Lanka.[11] His greatest claim to fame is not as a chiropractor or an ayurvedic practitioner but as a sports medicine doctor.[12] Nevertheless, ayurvedic categories appear to be among his basic explanatory tools. What is evident from Dr. Douillard's thorough and well-designed Web site is that basic approaches and definitions within Ayurveda are being reconsidered. This begins at the very outset. The site is introduced with the statement "Ayurveda is a universal system of health care that belongs to every culture." This serves notice that Dr. Douillard's Ayurveda will carve out a discursive and practical identity distinct from Ayurveda's cultural moorings in India, with an eye to its acceptance by the West. Dr. Douillard's ayurvedic educational offerings are limited to massage, in which he has apparently received training.

His approach operates in distinct opposition to certain other Western ayurvedic facilities, including the well-known institutes in Albuquerque, Dr. Vasant Lad's Ayurvedic Institute, and Dr. Sunil Joshi's Vinayak Institute, both vigorous if competing clinics and schools with facilities in India (Pune and Nagpur, respectively) for medical apprenticeships and advanced training. Dr. Douillard's site contains the following statement regarding the pharmacology of Ayurveda: "If adaptogenic herbs are botanical substances that help the body adapt to physiological and psychological stress, then Ayurveda is truly a system of adaptogenic medicine. Ayurveda identifies the cause of disease as the separation of mind, body and consciousness, due to the degenerative effects of mental, emotional and physical stress. This ancient premise for Ayurveda has been recently validated as researchers have identified stress as the cause of eighty percent of all disease" (http://www.lifespa.com/article.asp?art_id=23). Dr. Douillard does not attempt to provide a source of this statement in any ayurvedic text or lineage of ayurvedic practice. It is, however, quite consistent with the mind-body medicine espoused by well-known endocrinologist Dr. Deepak Chopra (for whom Dr. Douillard once worked) and Maharishi Ayur-Ved (where both Dr. Chopra and Dr. Douillard began their ayurvedic "careers" in the 1980s). Elsewhere, Douillard's Web site employs characteristic metaphors of detoxification.

Dr. Douillard thus represents a somewhat different school of thought about Ayurveda and a different sense of the way in which Ayurveda must be acculturated in the West than that represented in the health food store advertisement. While Dr. Douillard shares this concept with the health food store advertisement, he takes that idea in a different direction, toward a demystified engagement with Dr. Chopra's mind-body medicine. In this way, Dr. Douillard's paradigm illustrates the contestation within Ayurveda over basic approaches and definitions.

Maharishi Ayur-Ved

A third approach is embodied by Maharishi Ayur-Ved, which, as mentioned above, is discussed at length by Humes, Jeannotat, and Newcombe in this volume. MAV has now emerged as a single unit in a larger healing system with other ascendant modalities. These are the daily practice of TM, and, for the last few years, Maharishi Vedic Sound Therapy. One of the authors of this Introduction visited the main facility for Maharishi Ayurveda, more properly for "Maharishi Vedic Medicine," in Fairfield, Iowa, in July 2004, for an orientation to their clinical practices and a tour of the facility, called "The Raj: America's Premier Ayurveda Health Center."

The current treatment processes in Maharishi Vedic Medicine appear to take their inspiration from the work in the early 1990s of Tony Nader, an M.D. who also received a Ph.D. in neuroscience from MIT and who has dedicated himself to the TM movement since at least the early 1970s. His work that has provided this inspiration is the book *Human Physiology: Expression of Veda and the Vedic Literature.*[13] Nader's book is derived first from Maharishi's earlier ideas about the correlation of sound, physiology, and the Vedas; second, from Nader's study of brain physiology and structural aspects of Vedic and associated orthodox Hindu literature; and third, from a little-known (and wholly unattributed) book published in Bombay in 1931 by V. G. Rele called *Vedic Gods as Figures of Biology*. This book, in the scientific spirit of the time, tried to correlate brain structures with Vedic cosmogonic ideas and deities. For example, the Aśvins "appear to be the projections of efferent fibres on the interior surface of the medulla oblongata" (42) and Viṣṇu, known primarily for his three strides that take in the entire universe, "is comparable to the spinal cord which is long and supports the earthly matter" and the nerves that emerge from the vertebrae, which "cover and bind the whole earth together and all that is in earth and heaven" (71). Rele's book is part of a scientistic tradition going back to the nineteenth century of projecting contemporary anatomical categories onto premodern Indian concepts. Similar efforts are described by G. Jan Meulenbeld in this volume, using the example of the ancient Indian concept *"ojas."*

Nader updates Rele's "Vedic Science" considerably. His premise is that "human physiology (including the DNA at its core) has the same structure and function as the holistic- self-sufficient, self-referential reality expressed in the Ṛk [*sic*] Veda. The specialized components, organs, and organ systems of the human physiology, including all the various parts of the nervous system, match the 37 branches of the Vedic literature one to one, both in structure and in function" (vii). For example, Nader equates the sensory systems with the *Sāmaveda*, the hypothalamus with *vyākaraṇa*, pituitary gland with *nirukta*, the cerebellum with Vaiśeṣika, mesodermal tissues and organs with the *Caraka-Saṃhitā*, and voluntary motor and sensory projections with the *Mahābhārata*. As was Rele's volume, more than six decades earlier, Nader's book is dense with charts and detailed drawings of parts of the brain and nervous system. MAV practitioners need to know this, because the current practice at the Raj (and presumably other MAV facilities) is to evaluate the physical condition of the patient and determine which part of the brain or nervous system is associated with the afflicted body part. The nature of the affliction is in part discovered by resorting to ayurvedic analyses of *doṣa* imbalance, preferably through pulse diagnosis. The patient is then administered Maharishi Vedic Vibration Technology℠, about which the administrators are secretive. It appears, however, that once the source of the affliction is isolated in the brain or nervous system, mantras either from the Vedic or other orthodox texts associated with it are recited by Indian clinicians while they blow on or touch the afflicted body part.[14] This practice is clearly preferred at the Raj, though other ayurvedic therapies, including panchakarma, are also administered.

MAV literature contains some of the key terms of lineages that argue for their exclusivity, including "complete and authentic," which is pitted against all others, whose traditions and knowledge are "incomplete and diluted." Further, as a "revival of the authentic knowledge and practice," others are disbarred from legitimacy. One can argue that such claims to exclusivity were rarely present in the early Vedic and ayurvedic literature and go against a tradition of text and practice in which eclecticism and borrowing were the norm. In this way, MAV has isolated itself from other modern ayurvedic institutions, at least in the United States. Two other factors also have contributed to the current status of MAV. First, it has raised its prices stratospherically for both treatment and medicine. This has placed it out of reach to all but the most committed and enthusiastic (and wealthy) followers of the TM movement. Second, it has become stridently opposed to allopathic medicine. In the early decades of MAV, consistent with Maharishi's early advocacy of expressing his ideas in terms of Western science, one of the requirements for becoming an ayurvedic practitioner at an MAV clinic was that the practitioner had to first hold the M.D. degree. Not incidentally, this partially protected the TM movement from lawsuits (but see Newcombe in this volume). In 2005, however, all of the Western allopathic doctors who had received extensive ayurvedic training were dismissed from their positions and replaced with Indian ayurvedic practitioners. This is consistent with Maharishi's general movement away from an integrationist position in recent years, his increasingly venomous and discordant campaign against democracy as a viable form of government, and his embrace of the idea of the ultimate value of all things ancient in India. As such, MAV, which was so influential in bringing Ayurveda to public awareness in the 1980s and early 1990s, has practically disappeared from the map of global Ayurveda in the middle of the first decade of the twenty-first century.

Traditional Ayurveda in an Urban World

A fourth paradigm is modern practice in India, such as that described by Tirodkar in Pune. Before describing this, we should cite a statistic provided by Praful Patel, that 20 percent of BAMS (Bachelor of Ayurvedic Medicine and Surgery) graduates take hospital jobs, 10 percent go into private practice of Ayurveda, and 70 percent practice allopathic medicine.[15] This bears out the observations of Svoboda and Welch, who have had experience in the Ayurveda colleges in India. Though trained ayurvedic physicians who emigrate or travel in the West are trained in the same schools as those who not very surreptitiously practice allopathy, they are generally more committed to

Ayurveda (though see Svoboda on this) and thus find themselves preaching to a choir that has grown to distrust Western medicine, medical practice, and medical institutions. In opposition to this, they valorize the noninvasive diagnostic techniques of Ayurveda, the medicines themselves, which admittedly are often slower acting but have few if any negative side effects, and the individual attention of physicians who treat the body as a whole unit rather than looking at parts of it in isolation.

With this in mind, Tirodkar examines a modern medical practice in Pune. She divides contemporary ayurvedic practice into four areas of her own, rather different from the categories we are using here, though no less valid. These are "traditional," "modern," "commercial," and "self-help." She provides vivid descriptions of "urban traditional practitioners" who are modernizing their practices (as they are modernizing their lives) in order to compete with the now-dominant allopathic model. Examples of this in the urban West are Dr. Ananda Samir Chopra's practice in Kassel, Germany, and Dr. Vasant Lad's practice in Albuquerque, New Mexico. These two practices, however, differ from each other significantly. Many of these differences are due to the regulatory mechanisms in Germany and the United States. The topic of regulatory mechanisms—or their absence—in India and the West is a big one, and it is addressed here (in the chapters by Dominik Wujastyk, Mike Saks, and Sebastian Pole). Dr. Chopra's success derives in great measure from his ability to accommodate to the Western allopathic institutional model. Indeed, he practices in a hospital that also has a Department of Internal Medicine/Naturopathy, a Department of Oncology, and a Department of Psychosomatic Medicine. This is hardly possible in the United States. Regardless of this, it is clear from his chapter here that he resorts to both ayurvedic and allopathic descriptions.

AYURVEDIC LITERATURE IN THE WEST

In recent years, popular writing on Ayurveda has increasingly appeared in print and on the Internet. In comparison, a small amount is forthcoming from scholars and scientific researchers in technical publications.[16]

The contemporary literature of Ayurveda is an area of particular contestation. Ayurvedic literature written for a general audience usually contains a good deal of contextual information. This includes the lineage provenance of the authors, a feature that to a great extent is tied in with a targeted readership. For example, an author will typically consider it important to the reader of a book on Ayurveda to establish that he or she studied in the MAV system, or under Vasant Lad, Robert Svoboda, David Frawley, and others.

Many authors could be credited, at least in part, with the spread of Ayurveda outside its homeland in India.[17] It is beyond the scope of this Introduction to discuss and critique all the media through which this spread has occurred over the past three decades, but a few of the more notable trends and books should be mentioned. We can divide the material into three major categories. The first includes books that introduce the basic principles of Ayurveda to a largely Western, nonmedically trained readership. The second consists of authors who apply basic ayurvedic information to specific topics. The third consists of books intended for a more serious readership, including students of Ayurveda, scholars, and casual readers who are interested in deeper levels of ayurvedic knowledge.

The four names that dominate the first category, at least in the United States, are Vasant Lad, Robert Svoboda, Deepak Chopra, and David Frawley. Lad and Svoboda hold BAMS degrees from the Tilak Ayurveda College in Pune, Chopra is an M.D. endocrinologist, and Frawley has both studied with Lad in Albuquerque and Dr. B. L. Vashta of Mumbai and obtained a Doctor of Oriental Medicine degree through a correspondence course from the International Institute of Chinese Medicine, Santa Fe, New Mexico. Each has authored multiple books introducing Ayurveda to Western audiences.

Perhaps the first non-academic book to introduce Ayurveda to the West was Lad's *Ayurveda: The Science of Self-Healing* (1984). Though Lad has authored a number of books, this one gained such popularity that it has been translated into more than a dozen languages and has been distributed in at least twenty countries. Lad was trained in India both traditionally (by his gurus, Hambir Baba and Vimalandanda) and formally, receiving, in addition to a BAMS degree, an MASc (Master of Ayurvedic Science) degree from the Tilak Ayurveda College. He is thus qualified according to Indian government standards, but he also locates himself in a traditional lineage. In this book, Lad shows his dedication to traditional Ayurveda, but he also demonstrates some of his acumen at expanding or acculturating the repertoire of Ayurveda. For example, he includes iridology among ayurvedic diagnostic techniques. Though this is not mentioned in any ayurvedic text of any period, he stoutly defends it as a practice that fits ayurvedic thinking: it is natural and noninvasive, and it reflects the whole or macrocosm in the part or microcosm. In this way he reads the history of Ayurveda as one of innovation and empiricism rather than one of strict adherence to the first millennium CE classical texts.

Almost as popular as Lad's book is Svoboda's *Prakriti: Your Ayurvedic Constitution*. Translated into about a dozen languages, it was first published in 1988 and continues to sell steadily. It introduces readers to ayurvedic principles in an authoritative yet engaging manner. Like Lad, Svoboda's authority is based on both formal and traditional education in India. His other major introductory book, *Ayurveda: Life, Health, and Longevity* (1992), also has been well received in the community of practitioners. It is a straightforward account that limits itself to discussion of Ayurveda from within the boundaries of ayurvedic concepts, without reaching for Western or allopathic parallels in order to frame or acculturate the topic.

While Lad's and Svoboda's books have been popular with more serious students of Ayurveda, Deepak Chopra's books introducing Ayurveda to the West have been runaway best-sellers. Chopra has achieved considerable fame by appealing to large general audiences, to people who are not necessarily comfortable with or interested in Sanskrit vocabulary or technical ayurvedic terminology but who are attracted by "quality of life" issues and the idea that a few basic ayurvedic concepts can enhance their lives. Thus he avoids the pitfalls of New Age discourse, ayurvedic concepts beyond the most basic ones, and the technical language of biomedicine. In articulating accessible concepts of mind-body medicine, Chopra has attempted to create a bridge between Ayurveda and Western biomedicine. He has generated considerable interest in Ayurveda in spite of the fact that he is not trained in it, except to the extent that he was influenced by the *vaidyas* associated with Maharishi Mahesh Yogi in the mid- to late 1980s, when Chopra was a close disciple of the Maharishi. Indeed, his books reflect his lack of formal training in ayurvedic medicine within India, that he is trained in Western medicine (he is an M.D.), and that he is more concerned with drawing overarching conceptual connections between medical systems than he is with entering into the details of diagnostics and treatment modalities. Chopra's books have not proven to be as compelling for serious students of Ayurveda, and indeed they are not part of the syllabus of any Ayurveda college or institute. Other books present ayurvedic principles in a much deeper and more text-referenced way. Nevertheless, Chopra's personal insights on how Ayurveda relates to Western science and his manner of integrating these insights with a spiritual, feel-good format remain appealing to a wide audience and are not irrelevant to the present orientation of serious ayurvedic education in the West.

David Frawley, who has adopted the name Vamadeva Shastri, is the founder of the American Institute of Vedic Studies[18] and a prolific author of books on "Vedic" subjects, including various aspects of Ayurveda. Although his books cannot qualify as university-level scholarship, they have been influential in many ayurvedic institutions in America. Though largely an autodidact, for a period of about ten years he regularly visited and studied under Dr. B. L. Vashta of Mumbai. His books have reached a large number of students eager for secrets to be revealed by following deep, underlying threads present in Ayurveda. Part of Frawley's ayurvedic approach is to relate Ayurveda to Indian astrology, Hindu practice, and Vedānta. Though much of Frawley's writing is set within a context of an overwhelming concern with proving the deep antiquity (and therefore, in his view, superiority) of Vedic and Hindu history, methodological positions with which professional historians and Sanskrit scholars take serious issue, Frawley has gained considerable respect in popular ayurvedic circles. Throughout his books he offers thoughtful perspectives, though it is not often clear whether he is writing from his own intuition or from authoritative sources, because he almost never acknowledges his sources. Frawley's most popular books on Ayurveda have sold more than 50,000 copies and the more specialized ones less than 5,000 copies.

Although these authors are unquestionably the most influential in the introduction of Ayurveda to the anglophone West, they are not the only ones to have written on Ayurveda for either the popular or the specialized marketplace. The 1990s brought a wave of authors, each of whom introduced the basics of Ayurveda in formats that appealed to various tastes and proclivities, and that generally presented traditional, basic information mixed with the discourse of other modalities. These authors fall into the second of the three categories enumerated earlier, books that address specific topics. Among the most visible of the authors who fall into this category is Maya Tiwari, whose *Ayurveda: A Life of Balance* (1994) addresses diet in a comprehensive manner.[19] Tiwari has adopted another name, Sri Swamini Mayatitananda, since this book was written. She is now, according to her Web site, "a preeminent spiritual Mother who emanates silence and wisdom. A world renowned spiritual teacher, she has helped transform thousands of lives with her healing presence. Affectionately called Mother, she fills a significant void in the world culture as nurturer, healer, educator—transforming disease and despair into health and inner harmony. Mother belongs to India's prestigious Vedic lineage—Veda Vyasa" (http://www.wisearth.org/).[20]

A few other books in this category capitalize on the romance of both India and alternative therapies. The comparatively burgeoning genre of ayurvedic cookbooks usually begins with an assessment of what is digestible, and thus maximally efficient to physical maintenance, according to Ayurveda. Foods are broken down according to how they influence the three humors, *vāta*, *pitta*, and *kapha*, and how they build up the digestive *agni*, or fire. In nearly all cases the end result is rather toned-down Indian food, most of it regional Indian cuisines recast as "ayurvedic." Two of the common features of the general introductory books on Ayurveda, including Chopra's *Perfect Health*, Douillard's *Mind, Body, and Sport*, and many of the others, are, first, a self-test to determine one's own psycho-physical constitution (*prakṛti*) according to the relative predominance of *vāta*, *pitta*, and *kapha*, and a number of recipes for dishes congenial to different constitutions. Today, glossy advertising for prescription medicine is common, in which an aura of confident knowledge is extended from advertiser to patient, lobbying the patient to recommend that her or his doctor prescribe the advertiser's product. In comparison, such self-diagnosis and treatment as proffered by ayurvedic cookbooks, most of them not written by ayurvedic doctors, seem mild.

In addition to cookbooks, there are books on ayurvedic beauty care, Ayurveda for women, Ayurveda and yoga, Ayurveda and aromatherapy, ayurvedic weight loss plans, and so on.[21] It is important to note that these books are appearing in India as well as in the West. It also is important to note that nearly all books and Web sites on Ayurveda targeting the general modern public contain major chapters or sections on weight loss, yoga, meditation, the virtue of natural foods, and cures for menstrual cramps. Similarly, other features of first-millennium Ayurveda have been underplayed, including the use of animal products in both medicinals and diet, as well as therapies regarded as extreme, such as panchakarma in its original prescribed form. Zimmermann (1992) and Zysk (2001) comment on this in their accounts of the "flower power of Ayurveda" and New Age Ayurveda. These new directions in Ayurveda, part of a new paradigm, are understandable in terms of the concerns, lifestyles, available pharmacopoeia, and regulatory systems of the present day, just as the treatments and diet of the first-millennium texts were products of their times.

The first serious textbook of Ayurveda in English to be offered to the non-Indian and non-Indian language trained student was Lad's *Textbook of Ayurveda: Fundamental Principles* (2002). This is perhaps the first general book on Ayurveda in the West that is not targeted to a popular audience, although it is accessible to those educated in elementary biology and human physiology. Over the last few years, it has proven to be an invaluable resource for students of Ayurveda who are restricted to learning through English medium. It is the product of many years of clinical experience in the West and of introducing Western, mostly American, students to Ayurveda. It provides much reference material and generally adheres to traditional ayurvedic principles. In presenting his material, Lad never refers to Sanskrit text passages but presents his material as a personal distillation of the texts. As much as he references ayurvedic principles, he also references Western descriptive categories. For example, at the very outset he describes the three bodily humors, *vāta*, *pitta*, and *kapha*, as "the agents of DNA which form the blueprint for the physiology" (29). Elsewhere, he states that "prāṇa is located in the hypothalamus of the brain" (187), *ojas*, "the pure essence of all bodily tissues," is a "protoplasmic, biological substance that includes albumin, globulin, and many hormones" (212–13; on *ojas*, see Meulenbeld in this volume), that "soma is released in samādhi and . . . can be compared to serotonin" (214), and that the *Śiva-granthi* (knot of Śiva) is the pineal gland (ibid.). These and other speculative equations have been a part of ayurvedic discourse (cf. the extract from the ayurvedic examination cited earlier) and the discourse of "Vedic science" for a century (cf. Rele 1931, mentioned earlier) in its effort to legitimate itself in the face of European colonialism. Lad has evidently decided that the best way to present Ayurveda to serious students is to reformat it to a great extent in terms of Western categories. The volume, then, is pedagogical but not historically or textually referenced. This is the first of three such volumes that Lad proposes to write.

Finally, we should note that scholarly ayurvedic literature has not gained much of a foothold in the public culture of Ayurveda beyond academia. Even the briefest and clearest of academic books, such as Dominik Wujastyk's *The Roots of Ayurveda* (1998), are barely known outside of academic circles. Similarly, no scholarly or research journals dedicated to Ayurveda exist that have a general distribution among Western ayurvedic practitioners. Many ayurvedic institutions have in-house newsletters that are sent to their graduates and occasionally to other interested parties. The national ayurvedic organizations, such as the National Ayurvedic Medical Association (NAMA) in the United States and the Ayurvedic Practitioners Association (APA) in the United Kingdom, have limited mailing lists in which they advertise continuing education programs, including, in the United States, national conferences. These conferences have, so far, been held in the San Francisco Bay area and in Albuquerque and have not been heavily attended by people outside of California or the mountain west (except speakers and advertisers).

AYURVEDA ON THE INTERNET

Like almost everything else in the modern world, Ayurveda is being reinscribed on the Internet. And, like virtually every other topic known to mankind, there are too many Web sites to investigate. It is no exaggeration to say that they are increasing at a rate much too fast to monitor, even by the most assiduous researcher. A cursory search on Google in April 2006 found Ayurveda mentioned in nearly 16 million sites, an increase of 300,000 in two months. A survey of the first few hundred sites revealed a number of ayurvedic institutions, botanical companies, correspondence courses, books, attacks on Ayurveda as a dangerous cult or as unscientific, and so on. One thing immed comes to the fore: that the Internet is a great leveler. Whereas media is generally fairly local, Internet information is available ev where. One can easily locate ayurvedic institutions, panchakarma clinics, locally produced literature, and advertisements for rare or unusual pharmacopoeia. One also can relatively easily assess the provenance of material found on the Internet. For example, one can determine the local and regional lineages of ayurvedic institutions, evaluate the degree to which commodification is balanced with knowledge and education, and ascertain whether an ayurvedic spa does anything other than panchakarma.

Besides the Web sites mentioned in this Introduction, we should mention the sites of NAMA (http://www.ayurveda-nama.org/) and the APA (http://www.apa.uk.com/), useful for following the struggles regarding professionalization, conferences, and other events in the United States and the United Kingdom. NAMA is now circulating the draft "A Proposed Regulatory Model for Traditional Medicines: Guiding Assumptions and Key Components." This document presents "ideas for a new model for the regulation of traditional medicines in the United States" and is now subject to public review. NAMA welcomes any link to like-minded organizations that are involved with Ayurveda, Jyotisha, Sanskrit, and Yoga. It reserves the right to determine what organizations to list and reminds everyone that the NAMA does not endorse or specifically approve any site or its contents. Another similarly noteworthy site belongs to the Alternative Medicine Foundation (http://www.amfoundation.org/ayurveda.htm), a nonprofit organization founded in March 1998 "to provide responsible and reliable information about alternative medicine to the public and health professionals."

CONCLUSION

This volume introduces many of the important issues in the history of modern and global Ayurveda. No doubt the picture will change radically in the next twenty-five years. However, the present findings can help us assess recent developments in one of the world's most ancient and continuously practiced medical systems as it seeks a place in the modern world. From reports of contemporary practices in India and the West (Tirodkar, Chopra, Jeannotat, Humes), to issues and crises in ayurvedic education (Svoboda, Welch), to evolving physiological and medical concepts from classical sources (Meulenbeld, Alter), to questions of acculturation, professionalization, and identity (Wujastyk, Weiss, Berger, Newcombe, Saks), to issues over the identification and distribution of ayurvedic pharmacopoeia (Unnikrishnan, Pole) and the meaning of the pharmaceutical industry for the understanding of Ayurveda (Banerjee), we hope to convey the complexity and challenges of Ayurveda in its unexpected meeting with modernity and diaspora.

NOTES

We would like to thank all participants of the 2003 DHIIR Indic Health Workshop, and of the 2004 DHIIR Indic Health Conference, as their input at these events has been a valuable contribution to this volume.

1. Seen in a brochure of a spa in Cambridge, United Kingdom, in 2005.

2. See the introduction in Roşu (1989) and Appendix II in Zysk (1996) for a survey of academic work on Indian medicine.

3. See http://www.ethnopharma.free.fr/.

4. Some count the *Aṣṭāṅga-Saṃgraha*, a seventh-century text also ascribed to Vāgbhaṭa, as the third of the great three, and it is used in the Indian national syllabus for ayurvedic education. However, manuscript counts reveal much greater historical popularity of the *Aṣṭaṅga-Hṛdaya*. The concept of the "great three" may itself be fairly recent—no references can be found before the nineteenth century.

5. See http://www.dsal.uchicago.edu/sanskrit/papers/index.html.

6. A broad history of these encounters is sketched by Patterson (1987). Walker (2002) gives a detailed account of the Portuguese colonial spice and drug trade.

7. See also the monograph by Guy Attewell on the development of Unani in nineteenth- and twentieth-century India: *The Local and Beyond: The Shifting Terrains of Unani Tibb in India, c. 1890–1930* (Hyderabad: Orient Longman, 2007).

8. See Giddens (1997) and Horton (2003) on the concept of disembedding as a defining feature of globalization.

9. See, for example, the "Introduction to Ayurveda" at http://www.dhanvantri.com/#Ayurveda.

10. See http://www.lifespa.com.

11. This institute appears to be part of the Open University of Sri Lanka, a reputable institution that functions as an upper-level vocational and technical school. The Institute for Complementary Medicine is not a major part of the Open University, and upon inquiry we discovered that it is not recognized by any licensing or accreditation body in Sri Lanka or India. It was founded by an acupuncturist, Anton Jayasuriya, who bestowed upon himself the following title: Lord Pandit Raja-Guru Maha-Atma WHO Qualified Chinese Master-Acupuncturist Prof. Dr. Sir Holy Tibetian [*sic*] Lama Shaman Healer Anton Jayasuriya. The short form of this seems to be Lord Pandit Prof. Dr. Sir Anton Jayasuriya (http://www.home.swipnet.se/~w-63932/docs/biodaj.htm).

12. His book *Body, Mind, and Sport* has sold over 60,000 copies and has been translated into six languages.

13. Maharishi Vedic University Press, 4th ed., 2001.

14. See http://www.vedicvibration.com/techview.html: "The expert will administer specific Vedic vibrations that are traditionally held to restore order to the physiology by enlivening the inner intelligence of the body on the most fundamental level of sound." This is in some respects similar to the folk medical practice seen throughout India in Hindi called *jhārphūṁk* (sweeping and blowing).

15. Statement at the Punarnava Ayurveda conference in Mahabalipuram, January 2006. Patel, from London, is an Ayurveda activist and general secretary of an independent nongovernmental organization (NGO) in the United Kingdom, International Ayurveda Foundation.

16. Note Jan Meulenbeld's bibliography in volume 2B, pp. 783–1018 of his *A History of Indian Medical Literature* (2002). Though this bibliography of texts and scholarship is 235 pages in length and must contain in excess of 30,000 items, it pales in comparison to what is found on the Internet, in sheer bulk. This bibliography also is available at: http://www.ub.rug.nl/indianmedicine/.

17. The editors are grateful to Claudia Welch for providing the outline and first draft of this section.

18. See http://www.vedanet.com/Resources_Ayurveda.htm.

19. A few more specialized, but nontechnical, books geared to the popular market are John Douillard, *Body, Mind and Sport*; Svoboda, *Ayurveda for Women*; and Lad, *The Complete Book of Ayurvedic Home Remedies*, a useful reference book for the layperson and student of Ayurveda alike, as is his *Ayurvedic Cooking for Self-Healing*. Also see Frawley, *Ayurveda and the Mind* (1997), which discusses basic ayurvedic categories alongside simple concepts from popular psychology, and Frawley, *Yoga and Ayurveda* (1999), which connects Ayurveda to postural (*haṭha-*) yoga and *kuṇḍalinī* yoga. See also Mishra 1996, Mohan and Mohan 2004, and Verma 1999.

20. The Web site of her publisher, Inner Traditions of Rochester, VT, states: "Forced by cancer to reexamine and redirect her life, Maya Tiwari left a successful New York design career and returned to her native India to study Ayurvedic medicine. Now back in the U.S., she currently lectures and offers workshops on Ayurveda." See http://www.innertraditions.com/Contributor.jmdx?action=displayDetail&id=405.

21. For a practical guide to applying ayurvedic principles to diet and cooking, see Amadea Morningstar and Urmila Devi, *The Ayurvedic Cookbook* (1999); also see Amadea Morningstar, *Ayurvedic Cooking for Westerners* (1990), Usha Lad and Vasant Lad, *Ayurvedic Cooking for Self-Healing* (1997). See as well Melanie Sachs (1995), *Ayurvedic Beauty Care*, on natural, "ayurvedic" means of beautification. For weight loss, see, for example, http://www.naturalhealthweb.com/articles/lonsdorf3.html, an article titled "Maharishi Ayurveda Approach to Weight Loss," by Nancy Lonsdorf, one of the leading American Maharishi Ayur-Ved practitioners. Though in 2005 the Maharishi, then age eighty-eight, decided to replace all of the American ayurvedic practitioners with Indians, Dr. Lonsdorf, an advocate of the superiority and exclusivity of MAV to all other forms of Ayurveda, remains well known within the confines of the TM movement because of her books *A Woman's Best Medicine* (1995), which describes the MAV approach to major issues in women's health, and

A Woman's Best Medicine for Menopause (2002). For a book on Ayurveda and aromatherapy, see Miller and Miller 1995.

REFERENCES

Attewell, Guy. 2007. *The Local and Beyond: The Shifting Terrains of Unani Tibb in India, c. 1890–1930.* Hyderabad: Orient Longman.

Bahulkar, S. S. 1994. *Medical Ritual in the Atharvaveda Tradition.* Shri Balmukund Sanskrit Mahavidyalaya Research Series No. 8. Pune: Tilak Maharashtra Vidyapeeth.

Bala, Poonam. 1991. *Imperialism and Medicine in Bengal: A Socio-Historical Perspective.* New Delhi: Sage.

Benner, Dagmar. 2005. The medical ethics of professionalized Ayurveda. *Asian Medicine: Tradition and Modernity* 1 (1): 185–203.

Bode, Maarten. 2004. *Ayurvedic and Unani Health and Beauty Products: Reworking India's Medical Traditions.* PhD diss., Amsterdam University.

Brass, Paul R. 1972. The politics of ayurvedic education: A case study of revivalism and modernization in India. In *Education and Politics in India: Studies in Organization, Society, and Policy,* ed. S. Hoeber Rudolph and L. I. Rudolph, 342–75. Cambridge, MA: Harvard University Press.

Douillard, John. 1994. *Body, Mind, and Sport: The Mind-Body Guide to Lifelong Fitness and Your Personal Best.* New York: Harmony Books.

Frawley, David. 1997. *Ayurveda and the Mind: The Healing of Consciousness.* Twin Lakes, WI: Lotus Press.

———. 1999. *Yoga and Ayurveda: Self-Healing and Self-Realization.* Twin Lakes, WI: Lotus Press.

Giddens, Anthony. 1997 (reprint from 1991). *The Consequences of Modernity.* Cambridge, MA: Polity Press.

Horton, Richard. 2003. *Second Opinion. Doctors, Diseases, and Decisions in Modern Medicine.* London: Granta Books.

Jeffery, Roger. 1988. *The Politics of Health in India: Comparative Studies of Health Systems and Medical Care.* Berkeley: University of California Press.

Lad, Usha, and Vasant Lad. 1997. *Ayurvedic Cooking for Self-Healing.* Albuquerque, NM: The Ayurvedic Press.

Lad, Vasant. 1984. *Ayurveda: The Science of Self-Healing.* Santa Fe, NM: Lotus Press.

———. 1999. *The Complete Book of Ayurvedic Home Remedies.* New York: Harmony Books.

———. 2002. *Textbook of Ayurveda: Fundamental Principles.* Albuquerque, NM: The Ayurvedic Press.

Langford, Jean. 2002. *Fluent Bodies: Ayurvedic Remedies for Postcolonial Imbalance.* Durham, NC, London: Duke University Press.

Leslie, Charles. 1998. The ambiguities of medical revivalism in modern India. In *Asian Medical Systems: A Comparative Study,* ed. Charles Leslie, 356–67. Delhi: Motilal Banarsidass.

Lonsdorf, Nancy. 1995. *A Woman's Best Medicine.* Penguin/Putnam.

———. 2002. *A Woman's Best Medicine for Menopause.* Contemporary/McGraw Hill.

Meulenbeld, G. Jan. 1999–2002. *A History of Indian Medical Literature*, Volume IA Texts. Volume IB Annotations, Volume IIA Texts. Volume IIB Annotations, Volume III, Indexes. Groningen: Egbert Forsten.

Miller, Bryan, and Light Miller. 1995. *Ayurveda & Aromatherapy*. Santa Fe, NM: Lotus Press.

Mishra, Satyendra Prasad. 1996. *Yoga & Ayurveda: Their Alliedness and Scope as Positive Health Sciences*. Varanasi: Chaukhamba Sanskrit Sansthan.

Mohan, A. G., and Indra Mohan. 2004. *Yoga Therapy: A Guide to the Therapeutic Use of Yoga and Ayurveda for Health and Fitness*. Boston: Shambhala.

Morningstar, Amadea. 1990. *Ayurvedic Cooking for Westerners*. Santa Fe, NM: Lotus Press.

Morningstar, Amadea, and Urmila Devi. *The Ayurvedic Cookbook*. Delhi: Motilal Banarsidass.

Morrison, Judith. 1995. *The Book of Ayurveda*. London: Gaia.

Nader, Tony. 1995. *Human Physiology: Expression of Veda and the Vedic Literature*. Vlodrop: Maharishi Vedic University.

Patterson, T. J. S. 1987. Indian and European practitioners of medicine from the sixteenth century. In *Studies on Indian Medical History* II, ed. J. Meulenbeld and D. Wujastyk, 119–29. Groningen: Egbert Forsten.

Rao, P. G. 1994. *Model Papers for Ayurvedic Competetive Examinations*. Varanasi: Chaukhambha Sanskrit Bhawan.

Reddy, Sita. 2000. *Reinventing Medical Traditions: The Professionalization of Ayurveda in Contemporary America*. PhD diss., University of Pennsylvania. Unpublished.

———. 2004. The politics and poetics of "magazine medicine": New age Ayurveda in the print media. In *The Politics of Healing: A History of Alternative Medicine in Twentieth-Century North America*, ed. R. D. Johnston, 207–30. New York, London: Routledge.

Rele, V. G. 1931.*Vedic Gods as Figures of Biology*. Bombay: D. B. Taraporewala Sons & Co.

Roşu, Arion. 1989. *Travaux sur l'histoire de la médecine indienne: Un demi-siècle de recherches Ayurvédiques. Gustave Liétard et Palmyr Cordier; documents réunis et présentés par Arion Roşu*. Paris: Collège de France, Institut de civilisation indienne.

Sachs, Melanie. 1995. *Ayurvedic Beauty Care: Ageless Techniques to Invoke Natural Beauty*. Delhi: Motilal Banarsidass.

Scharfe, Hartmut. 1999. The doctrine of the three humors in traditional Indian medicine and the alleged antiquity of Tamil Siddha medicine. *Journal of the American Oriental Society* 119:4: 602–29.

Selby, Martha A. 2005. Sanskrit gynecologies in postmodernity: The commoditization of Indian medicine in alternative medical and new-age discourses on women's health. In *Asian Medicine and Globalization*, ed. Joseph S. Alter, 120–31. Philadelphia: University of Pennsylvania Press.

Svoboda, Robert. 1988. *Prakriti: Your Ayurvedic Constitution*. Santa Fe, NM: Lotus Press.

———. 1992. *Ayurveda: Life, Health, and Longevity*. London, New York: Arkana, Penguin.

———. 1999. *Ayurveda for Women*. Newton Abbot: David & Charles.

Tiwari, Maya. 1994. *Ayurveda: A Life of Balance*. Rochester, VT: Healing Arts Press.

Verma, Vinod. 1999. *Sixteen Minutes to a Better 9-To-5: Stress-Free Work with Yoga and Ayurveda*. Boston: Weiser.

Walker, Timothy. 2002. Evidence of the use of ayurvedic medicine in the medical institutions of Portuguese India, 1680–1830. In *Ayurveda at the Crossroads of Care and Cure. Proceedings of the Indo-European Seminar on Ayurveda held at Arrábida, Portugal, in November 2001*, ed. Ana Salema, 74–105. Lisbon: Centro de História de Além-Mar.

Wujastyk, Dominik. 1998. *The Roots of Ayurveda: Selections from Sanskrit Medical Writings*. New Delhi: Penguin Books.

———. 2003a. Indian medical thought on the eve of colonialism. *International Institute for Asian Studies Newsletter* 31: 21.

———. 2003b. The science of medicine. In *The Blackwell Companion to Hinduism*, ed. Gavin Flood, 393–409. Oxford: Blackwell.

———. 2005a. Change and creativity in early modern Indian medical thought. *Journal of Indian Philosophy* 33:1: 95–118.

———. 2005b. Policy formation and debate concerning the government regulation of Ayurveda in Great Britain in the twenty-first century. *Asian Medicine: Tradition and Modernity* 1:1: 162–84.

Zimmermann, Francis. 1992. Gentle purge: The flower power of Ayurveda. In *Paths to Asian Medical Knowledge*, ed. Charles Leslie and Allan Young, 209–23. Berkeley: University of California Press.

Zysk, Kenneth G. 1996. *Religious Healing in the Veda. With Translations and Annotations of Medical Hymns from the Ṛgveda and the Atharvaveda and Renderings from the Corresponding Texts* (Indian Medical Tradition I). Delhi: Motilal Banarsidass.

———. 2000. *Asceticism and Healing in Ancient India. Medicine in the Buddhist Monastery* (Indian Medical Tradition II). 1st ed. 1991. Delhi: Motilal Banarsidass.

———. 2001. New Age Ayurveda or what happens to Indian medicine when it comes to America. *Traditional South Asian Medicine* 6: 10–26.

CHAPTER 2

Plural Medicine and East-West Dialogue

MIKE SAKS

Medicine in Britain, Western Europe in general, and North America is currently becoming more plural. In particular, there is growing interest in a wide range of complementary and alternative medicine (CAM), including ayurvedic medicine and other practices that originated in Asia. These are increasingly coming to be used alongside more orthodox forms of medicine in Western societies, and multiple therapies are becoming available on an ever-more-level playing field (Cant and Sharma 1999). However, to understand the recent emergence of plural medicine in the West—of which Ayurveda is an important part—it is first necessary to define what is meant by the concepts "orthodox medicine" and "complementary and alternative medicine," which coexist in modern health care systems.

Orthodox medicine and complementary and alternative medicine are defined here by their level of political acceptability rather than the intrinsic characteristics of the practices they encompass. In these terms, orthodox medicine in Western countries covers those forms of health care that are officially underwritten by the state through research funding, inclusion in the orthodox health curriculum, and other mechanisms (Saks 1992). At present, these are based on biomedicine, which is centered primarily on the use of drugs and surgery. Complementary and alternative medicine, in contrast, is not typically supported by the state and to this extent is politically marginal—even if therapies used in a complementary manner to orthodox medicine are closer than the outright alternatives to the political mainstream. It includes a diverse range of practices spanning from aromatherapy and reflexology to herbalism and homoeopathy, many of which—such as acupuncture and meditation—have Asian roots (Saks

1997). In this sense, the nature of orthodoxy and unorthodoxy in the West currently differs from that of Asia, even if the orthodoxy of one period can readily become the unorthodoxy of another, and vice versa, according to the relativistic definitions employed here.

WESTERN HEALTH CARE IN THE HISTORIC PAST

The shifts that can occur in this regard are highlighted historically with reference to the development of Western health care. In Western countries in the immediate preindustrial era, an extremely diverse and undifferentiated health field existed with a broad range of therapies, from bonesetting and healing to bleeding and purging (Porter 2002). At this time there was no national system of legitimated medicine underwritten by the state. Indeed, it was very difficult to distinguish doctors from other health care practitioners in relation to the nature of their theories, the manner in which they were practiced, the amount and type of training they received, and their status or reputation in society in the fast-developing health care market. This was the case despite emerging attacks on "quackery." Even their language was similar—in Britain, for instance, references to magic by peddlers selling their wares in sideshows paralleled the use of obscure Latin mumbo jumbo in medicine (Porter 2001). As such, up to the nineteenth century the fields of orthodox medicine and complementary and alternative medicine could not really be said to exist in Western Europe and North America. Rather, health care at this time could be seen as pluralistic, in an age in which formal practitioner interventions were less common and self-help was more central than today.

However, all this was to change by the late nineteenth century and the first half of the twentieth century, when what is now accepted as orthodox medicine had established its dominance, as its achievements began to be demonstrated in a more scientifically oriented age—with an ever-expanding catalogue of innovations from the development of vaccines to the use of X-rays (Le Fanu 1999). By this time a legally underwritten state shelter for medicine had emerged in Western societies, with rising amounts of official funding support for practitioners. This was particularly highlighted by the professionalization of medicine in the Anglo-American context, based on the creation of enclaves of exclusionary social and political closure by doctors designed to give them market control. This resulted in the establishment on both sides of the Atlantic of legally restricted registers of medical practitioners with protection of title and self-regulatory powers over such matters as discipline and education in their fields (Saks 2003b). In these terms, professionalization helped differentiate orthodox medicine from rival practitioners in complementary and alternative medicine who were defined as being outside of the orthodox fold and attacked in the medical press as charlatans.

At the same time, medical unity had increasingly emerged throughout the West around the biomedical paradigm that developed following the seventeenth and eighteenth centuries. This paradigm was centered on the modernist separation of the mind and body, only the latter of which was seen as a symptom-bearing organism (Saks 2003a). As such, modern biomedicine superseded the predominantly person-centered "bedside medicine," in which clients as subjects were closely involved holistically through interactive dialogue in both their own diagnosis and treatment. Thereafter, biomedicine became based first on "hospital medicine," where increasing emphasis was placed on classificatory approaches to disease, and then on "laboratory medicine," where the patient was seen as a cluster of cells that could be diagnosed by tests conducted at a distance and became the object of ever-more-refined treatments (Jewson 1976). This philosophy, reflected in a range of procedures from the analysis of pathological specimens to the administration of radiotherapy, became increasingly embedded in the underlying knowledge base of medicine, the practice of which was supported by internal regulatory controls.

The establishment of biomedicine as orthodox medicine in the West was reinforced by further promising developments in medical knowledge such as the discovery of penicillin and advances in surgery that spawned an ever-increasing number of medical specialties as the body was divided conceptually into ever-more-fragmented parts (Le Fanu 1999). The rise of a range of limited or subordinated professions allied to medicine in the health care division of labor in this period, from nurses and midwives to pharmacists and dentists, also served to confirm the dominance of orthodox medicine, as its empire expanded (Saks 2001). The establishment of such dominance led to the creation for the first time of the category of complementary and alternative medicine as well as its growing marginalization, to the point where many unorthodox therapies in Western societies had suffered a serious decline in their credibility and status by the mid-twentieth century in the wake of its ongoing deprecation by orthodox biomedicine (Saks 1996). However, medical dominance was to be shaken by the development of a strong counterculture in the late 1960s and early 1970s.

THE COUNTERCULTURE AND PLURAL MEDICINE

The Western counterculture of the 1960s and 1970s developed from an attack on materialistic values, scientific progress, and the belief in tic solutions to problems and led to a mounting challenge to onal experts. It also was associated with a desire to explore ive lifestyles, leading to experimentation in everything from ns to drugs—with rising interest in Asian philosophies, spanning from meditation to mysticism (Roszak 1970; Saks 2000). In medicine specifically, the counterculture emerged in part as a result of an increasing awareness of the limits to the effectiveness and safety of technologically based orthodox medicine, as illustrated by its restricted impact on chronic illness, its counterproductive effects in cases such as thalidomide, and the positive influence of improved diet and sanitation on health (see, for example, Illich 1976). It also could be seen as a response to the depersonalization, fragmentation, and disempowerment of the client in biomedicine, coupled with a desire by patients to exercise greater control over their own health. Most importantly in this context, though, practices originating in Asia helped shape the new medical counterculture, particularly with the resurgence of complementary and alternative medicine based on more holistically oriented, integrative ideologies in which the mind, body, and spirit are seen as interdependent. Other attractive features of these complementary and alternative health practices were a greater client focus and a fuller link between health and the broader social and physical environments (Saks 2003a).

Cross-cultural influences in medicine and elsewhere have long existed in the West, not least through historic settlements of ethnic minorities from countries such as China and India. Knowledge of acupuncture reached Europe by the seventeenth century and North America by the nineteenth century, through China, Korea, and Japan (Saks 1995). What distinguished the counterculture of the 1960s and 1970s, however, was its pervasiveness and strength, propelled by near-universal literacy and modern methods of communication. Since the advent of this strong counterculture, members of the public have increasingly employed on a self-help and practitioner delivery basis forms of health care that complement and offer alternative models to orthodox biomedicine. This is indicated by the number of users of complementary and alternative medicine, including, among others, Ayurveda and Traditional Chinese Medicine (TCM). In Britain, over one-quarter of the population uses CAM each year, with one in seven visiting practitioners of these therapies (Thomas et al. 2001). In the United States, the proportion of the population that employs CAM has now risen to two-fifths annually, with almost one-fifth consulting practitioners directly (Eisenberg et al. 1998). There also is evidence of parallel growth in utilization in the rest of Europe and Canada (see Fisher and Ward 1994; Kelner and Wellman 1997). Given the politically marginal nature of CAM, much of this activity takes place outside the state sector in the private market, even if growing numbers of insurers are prepared to cover all or part of such expenditures (Fulder 1996; Bruce and McIlwain 1998).

An ever-greater span of health foods and complementary and alternative remedies has become available for purchase in the private sector in the West in recent years (Bakx 1991). At the same time, the growing popularity of CAM also has been reflected in increases in the numbers of its practitioners. In Britain, the number of such therapists had risen to close to 60,000 in 2000 (Mills and Budd 2000). In the United States, the scale of such practices is even greater, with some 50,000 chiropractors alone in operation, in addition to a fast-expanding range of practitioners from acupuncturists to herbalists (Wardwell 1994). Admittedly, there are variations in the West in the popularity of different forms of complementary and alternative practices. In the Netherlands, for example, spiritual healing is the most popular alternative practice, while reflexology is in Denmark (Fisher and Ward 1994). Indeed, there can be no doubt that the numbers of complementary and alternative therapists in the West are rising, whichever therapies they employ.

In this respect, one of the most striking recent trends on both sides of the Atlantic has been for orthodox health practitioners increasingly to embrace complementary and alternative practices, including aromatherapy, massage, and others linked to Asia. Although their professional bodies have not always been well disposed toward them, many doctors now actively employ such therapies themselves or delegate their use to allied health professionals in settings ranging from pain clinics to primary care. In Britain, for instance, it is now estimated that one in two general practices will offer some access to CAM (Thomas et al. 2003), while in the United States over one-third of physicians themselves will practice at least one complementary and alternative therapy, the most frequent being relaxation techniques, lifestyle diet, imagery, spiritual healing, biofeedback, and yoga (Cohen 1998). In countries such as France in Continental Europe, practices such as acupuncture and homoeopathy have long been exclusively restricted to medical practitioners (Fulder 1996).

CAM in the West also is increasingly being legitimated through other channels. Reference to it is now being included in medical courses, and membership of orthodox medical groupings in this area is expanding—from bodies focused on specific therapies such as the British Medical Acupuncture Society to the more generic American Holistic Medical Association (Saks 2003a). Added backing has been given by the state through the professionalization of various complementary and alternative therapies in the Anglo-American context, the most recent forms of which to be considered in Britain are acupuncture and herbalism (Saks 2003b). At the same time, there is now increasing research funding available for expansion in this area from governments, as illustrated by the National Center for Complementary and Alternative Medicine in the United States (Cohen 1998). In Europe, the five-year Cooperation in Science and Technology research project on unconventional medicine involving researchers from fourteen different European societies highlights the support for this area from the governments concerned (Monckton et al. 1998).

Clearly the position has moved a long way from the time when many forms of complementary and alternative therapies were rejected out of hand by the leaders of the medical profession in Britain and the United States in the 1970s and 1980s as "unscientific" quackery linked to primitive superstition (Saks 2003a). The improving evidence base for such therapies might help explain their increasing medical incorporation, although there is still a great distance to go in comparison to orthodox medicine (Ernst et al. 2001). Debate will continue to rage about the most appropriate methodologies for evaluating their effectiveness, given that they are, for the most part, individually rather than symptomatically oriented (Saks 1994; Callahan 2002). However, the more favorable recent medical response to CAM in Western societies is perhaps best accounted for by the interests of the medical profession in the face of rapidly growing public demand and political pressure. In these circumstances, it has come to be more in the interests of the profession to incorporate the most credible forms of complementary and alternative medicine into its repertoire, as long as this stops short of independently legitimating nonmedically qualified competitors (Saks 2003b).

EASTERN INFLUENCES ON COMPLEMENTARY AND ALTERNATIVE MEDICINE IN THE WEST

In this light, it is not surprising that the culmination of developments since the emergence of the counterculture of the 1960s and 1970s should be the publication of two positive high-level government reports on CAM. The report of the House of Lords Select Committee on Science and Technology (2000) in Britain and the White House Commission (2002) in the United States came to similar conclusions in that both recommended, among other things, that their respective health systems should ensure access to complementary and alternative medicine wherever there is evidence of efficacy and appropriate regulatory mechanisms that enhance public safety. The former committee, though, was somewhat controversial in this context—insofar as it placed acupuncture and herbalism in the top rank of therapies with the most credible evidence base and most organized groups of practitioners, while locating Ayurveda and TCM in the third rank, alongside crystal therapy, iridology, and radionics, as being less well organized and having the weakest foundation in research. This has been subject to strong criticism, not least in relation to ayurvedic medicine (see Wujastyk 2005).

However, in general terms, health care in the West seems to be coming full circle in that it is now beginning to return to the equivalent of the plural roots of its historic past, albeit in modernized guise with increasing acceptance by the state of more eclectic models of health care as manifested in, inter alia, increasing research support and legally underwritten regulation for complementary and alternative medicine (Cant and Sharma 1999). This is reflected in growing government interest in these areas in other Western countries such as Canada that are also making headway on the plural health agenda (Shearer and Simpson 2001). There is, though, one vital distinction from the medical pluralism of the past that should be highlighted here. This is that a number of currently used forms of complementary and alternative medicine have been shaped by contact with Asia. Some Asian medical traditions, such as Ayurveda, and, to a greater extent, TCM, have not only inspired Western indigenous medical practices and added to their techniques but have become an integral part of CAM as complete medical systems in their own right. While Ayurveda is a fairly recent addition to the ever-growing range of CAM therapies available in Europe and North America, TCM has long established itself successfully as both a complement and an alternative to biomedicine.

THE EAST-WEST DIALOGUE

Significant as they are, Ayurveda, with its Indian roots, and TCM are only illustrative of Eastern influences on Western health care. Other influences, including those from the Arab nations to Japan, have distinct but interlinked trajectories. Sometimes they have exerted a direct impact on Western health care, as in the case of early advances in Arabic medicine on surgery in the West (Duin and Sutcliffe 1992). However, influences from Asia have mostly fed into contemporary patterns of health care through CAM, as their traditional health philosophies have generally been at odds with orthodox biomedicine (Saks 1997). In this respect, though, it must be recognized that Western health care in general and CAM in particular have primarily been affected by indigenous rather than exogenous factors. The effect of indigenous influences on the development of CAM in the West can be exemplified by the impact of local herbal traditions. Parallel Western traditions are related to herbalism, including associated areas such as aromatherapy. In Europe contemporary herbal medicine certainly drew heavily on indigenous herbal folklore, as set out by well-known herbalists such as Culpeper (Woolley 2004). In the United States herbalism has been shaped by the use of Native American tribal medicines (Versluis 1993), as well as by the lineage of the populist Thomsonian movement in the nineteenth century, based on the employment of botanical medicines (Gevitz 1988). Other complementary and alternative medicines, including chiropractic and homoeopathy, unequivocally originated in the West. In this respect, it should also be noted that Western religious beliefs underpin still other complementary and alternative approaches, such as spiritual healing and faith healing (Fulder 1996).

Even the generic holistic basis of many CAM therapies cannot necessarily be seen to derive primarily from the interface with Asian systems of health, based on such influences as Ayurveda and TCM. Holism in the West stems at least as much from Hippocrates, the famous Greek physician from the fifth century BCE, who recognized the relationship between illness, environment, and the emotions, as well as the more general Greek philosophy of balancing the four humors of black bile, yellow bile, phlegm, and blood to achieve health (Duffin 1999). The theory of the humors, in fact, underpinned the practice of bloodletting that was so prevalent in the period immediately leading up to the Industrial Revolution and the associated rise of orthodox biomedicine (Porter 2002). While holism was central to the counterculture of the 1960s and 1970s, therefore, the extent to which it actually emerged as a result of Eastern influence, rather than simply being a flag of convenience in this heady period, is debatable.

It also should not be forgotten that Western medical thought has influenced health care in Asia. In some instances Western interference had a detrimental effect on health, not least during the period of Western imperialism in India and elsewhere that led to the importation of disease, the destruction of harvests, and colonial production methods that produced high morbidity and mortality rates among the local population (Saks 1997). A more positive recent feature of contact with the West, though, was that useful pharmaceuticals and other aspects of biomedicine became more widely available, even if Western medical practitioners tended to focus on the colonizers rather than the native population, unless there was a wider threat to the former, as in the case of mass insect-borne infections (Worboys 2000). The negative side of the influence of the West on Asia extended to the typical dismissal of indigenous health systems as backward superstition with little to teach Westerners. In spite of this and in some cases national efforts to one-sidedly modernize their health care infrastructure, India, China, and other Asian countries have developed plural health systems in which biomedicine constructively coexists with more traditional forms of medicine, including Ayurveda and TCM, that have received state recognition in these societies (Cant and Sharma 1999).

Regarding the more specific exchange of medical thought and its underlying philosophies, the depth of the influence of more holistic Eastern practices on complementary and alternative medicine in Western health care can sometimes be questionable. For various reasons, including the interplay of professional and other interests, such knowledge can be transmuted in different cultural contexts in such a way that practices are completely detached from their holistic origins and transformed into biomedical techniques (Saks 2000). Sometimes this pitfall is less apparent in the integration process, as exemplified by Deepak Chopra, who has achieved cult status in the West by linking Ayurveda to Western science. In his work relating health to energy levels, Chopra succeeds in creatively relating the three *doṣas* linked to individual body types to the control of movement, metabolism, digestion, physical structure, and fluid balance, even though some aspects of Ayurveda may have been lost in the process (Chopra 1995). This also is true of TCM in Western societies, where the classical practice of herbalism and acupuncture can be more fully maintained by practitioners operating in the private sector, despite being initially used for biomedically defined conditions (Fulder 1996). However, private medicine in itself does not guarantee protection from the "biomedicalization" (or "pharmaceuticalization," see Banerjee in this volume) of medical systems with differing theoretical foundations. This is clearly illustrated by the increasing sale of over-the-counter ayurvedic herbal remedies in commercial contexts for specific conditions without appropriate reference to individual constitution. This has been encouraged by the pharmaceutical industry, as it now increasingly cashes in on the mass market in complementary and alternative medicine (Cant and Sharma 1999). In the case of TCM in the West, the medical practice of acupuncture stands out as an even more obvious case where the transmutation of knowledge has occurred. When knowledge of acupuncture first arrived in medical circles in Europe and North America up to the end of the nineteenth century, its traditional philosophy was only dimly understood. By the 1960s and 1970s, though, far more was known about the classical theories that underpinned it. However, in medical hands today it tends to be used predominantly as a technique for pain and addictions justified by neurophysiological theorizing rather than being employed in its broader yin-yang application (Saks 1995). As indicated earlier, this type of stance has served not only to open up markets for the medical profession but also to limit the extent to which its unorthodox competitors are able to thrive by establishing the higher ground in this area.

CONCLUSION

If a more plural medical system is to develop in Western Europe and North America, there will be difficulties in reconciling fundamental clashes between the parameters of the biomedical paradigm and such classical Asian philosophies as are embedded in Ayurveda and TCM (Saks 1997). One way to resolve the position would be to allow such systems to operate alongside each other and let consumers select the one that they prefer. However, choosing health interventions is not the same as selecting philosophical standpoints in an abstract academic context, as there are significant—in some cases, life and death—implications for the well-being of clients, who are particularly vulnerable if they are insufficiently informed (Ernst et al. 2001). It is therefore vital that, at a minimum, sensitive methods are found for evaluating the relative efficacy, safety, and cost-effectiveness of CAM; for concluding which therapies may be practiced and in what context; for deciding which practitioners are allowed to practice in particular areas, and on what basis; and for agreeing on how consumers are to access each of the approaches concerned (Saks 2003a).

In arriving at a future position, it is helpful that neither traditional Asian medicine nor orthodox biomedicine has ossified in the West. Orthodox biomedicine has generally shown itself to be flexible, as witnessed by the shift from the initial outright rejection of CAM to its current limited incorporation. More significantly, orthodox biomedicine itself has recently become more holistic, with greater attention being paid, among other things, to the wider environment from a public health perspective and to relationships with other health and social workers in the delivery of care. At the same time practitioners of complementary and alternative medicine are not always as faithful in practice to the ideology of holism as they proclaim (Saks 2000). Despite this convergence, one major obstacle to meaningful integration is the continuing dominance of the ideology of biomedicine, even though the power of the medical profession has arguably declined in Western societies as a result of the rising influence of consumers and corporate bodies in health care (Cant and Sharma 1999). The form of plural medicine that exists in a number of Asian cultures, including India and China, may point the way forward in the West from the viewpoint of the public interest.

REFERENCES

Bakx, K. 1991. The "eclipse" of folk medicine in Western society. *Sociology of Health and Illness* 13: 20–38.

Benner, Dagmar. 2005. Healing and medicine in Ayurveda and South Asia. In *Encyclopedia of Religion*, 2nd ed., ed. James Lindsay, 3852–58. New York: Macmillan.

Bruce, D. F., and H. H. McIlwain. 1998. *The Unofficial Guide to Alternative Medicine*. New York: Macmillan.

Callahan, D., ed. 2002. *The Role of Complementary and Alternative Medicine: Accommodating Pluralism*. Washington, DC: Georgetown University Press.

Cant, S., and U. Sharma. 1999. *A New Medical Pluralism: Alternative Medicine, Doctors, Patients, and the State*. London: UCL Press.

Chopra, D. 1995. *Boundless Energy*. London: Ryder.

Cohen, M. 1998. *Complementary and Alternative Medicine: Legal Boundaries and Regulatory Perspectives*. Baltimore, MD: Johns Hopkins University Press.

Duffin, J. 1999. *History of Medicine*. Toronto: University of Toronto Press.

Duin, N., and J. Sutcliffe. 1992. *A History of Medicine: From Prehistory to the Year 2020*. London: Simon & Schuster.

Eisenberg, D., R. Davis, S. Ettner, S. Appel, S. Wilkey, M. Rompay, and R. Kessler. 1998. Trends in alternative medicine use in the United States, 1990–1997. *Journal of the American Medical Association* 280: 1569–75.

Ernst, E., M. Pittler, C. Stevinson, and A. White, eds. 2001. *The Desktop Guide to Complementary and Alternative Medicine: An Evidence-Based Approach*. London: Mosby.

Fisher, P. and A. Ward. 1994. "Complementary medicine in Europe." *British Medical Journal* 309: 107–11.

Fulder, S. 1996. *The Handbook of Alternative and Complementary Medicine*. 3rd. ed. Oxford: Oxford University Press.

Gevitz, N. 1988. Three perspectives on unorthodox medicine. *Other Healers: Unorthodox Medicine in America*, ed. N. Gevitz, 1–28. Baltimore, MD: Johns Hopkins University Press.

Hicks, A. 1996. *Principles of Chinese Medicine*. London: Thorsons.

House of Lords Select Committee on Science and Technology. 2000. *Report on Complementary and Alternative Medicine*. London: The Stationery Office.

Illich, I. 1976. *Limits to Medicine*. Harmondsworth: Penguin.

Jewson, N. 1976. The disappearance of the sick-man from medical cosmology 1770–1870. *Sociology* 10: 225–44.

Kaptchuk, T. J., and D. M. Eisenberg. 2005. A taxonomy of unconventional healing practices. In *Perspectives on Complementary and Alternative Medicine: A Reader*, ed. G. Lee-Treweek, T. Heller, S. Spurr, H. MacQueen, and J. Katz, 9–25. London: Routledge.

Kelner, M., and B. Wellman. 1997. Health care and consumer choice: Medical and alternative therapies. *Social Sciences and Medicine* 45: 203–12.

Low, J. 2004. *Using Alternative Therapies: A Qualitative Analysis*. Toronto: Canadian Scholars Press.

Le Fanu, J. 1999. *The Rise and Fall of Modern Medicine*. London: Abacus.

Mills, S., and S. Budd. 2000. *Professional Organization of Complementary and Alternative Medicine in the United Kingdom: A Second Report to the Department of Health*. Exeter: University of Exeter.

Monckton, J., B. Belicza,, W. Betz, H. Engelbart, and M. Van Wassenhoven, eds. 1998. *COST Action B4: Unconventional Medicine: Final Report of the*

Management Committee. Luxembourg: Office for Official Publications of the European Communities.
Porter, R. 2001. *Quacks: Fakers and Charlatans in English Medicine*. Stroud: Tempus Publishing.
———. 2002. *Blood and Guts: A Short History of Medicine*. London: Penguin Books.
Roszak, T. 1970. *The Making of a Counter Culture*. London: Faber and Faber.
Saks, M. 1992. Introduction. In *Alternative Medicine in Britain*, ed. M. Saks, 1–21. Oxford: Clarendon Press.
———. 1994. The alternatives to medicine. In *Challenging Medicine*, ed. J. Gabe, D. Kelleher, and G. Williams, 84–103. London: Routledge.
———. 1995. *Professions and the Public Interest: Professional Power, Altruism, and Alternative Medicine*. London: Routledge.
———. 1996. From quackery to complementary medicine: The shifting boundaries between orthodox and unorthodox medical knowledge. In *Complementary and Alternative Medicines: Knowledge in Practice*, ed. S. Cant and U. Sharma, 27–43. London: Free Association Books.
———. 1997. East meets West: The emergence of a holistic tradition. In *Medicine: A History of Healing*, ed. R. Porter, 196–219. London: Ivy Press.
———. 2000. Medicine and the counter culture. In *Medicine in the Twentieth Century*, ed. R. Cooter and J. Pickstone, 113–23. Amsterdam: Harwood Academic Publishers.
———. 2001. Alternative medicine and the health care division of labour: Present trends and future prospects. *Current Sociology* 49: 119–34.
———. 2003a. *Orthodox and Alternative Medicine: Politics, Professionalization, and Health Care*. London: Sage.
———. 2003b. Professionalization, politics, and CAM. In *Complementary and Alternative Medicine: Challenge and Change*, ed. ed. M. Kelner, B. Wellman, B. Pescosolido, and M. Saks, 223–38. London: Routledge.
Shearer, R., and J. Simpson, eds. 2001. *Perspectives on Complementary and Alternative Health Care*. Ottawa: Health Canada.
Thomas, K. J., P. Coleman, and J. P. Nicholl. 2003. Trends in access to complementary or alternative medicines via primary care in England: 1995–2001 results from a follow-up national survey. *Family Practice* 20: 575–77.
Thomas, K. J., J. P. Nicholl, and P. Coleman. 2001. Use and expenditure on complementary medicine in England: A population-based survey. *Complementary Therapies in Medicine* 9: 2–11.
Verma, V. 1995. *Ayurveda: A Way of Life*. Boston: Weiser Books.
Versluis, A. 1993. *The Elements of Native American Traditions*. Shaftesbury: Element Books.
Wardwell, W. 1994. Alternative medicine in the United States. *Social Science and Medicine* 38: 1061–68.
Warrier, G., H. Verma, and K. Sullivan. 2001. *Secrets of Ayurveda*. Lewes: Ivy Press.
White House Commission. 2002. *White House Commission on Complementary and Alternative Medicine Policy*. Washington, DC: The Commission.
Woolley, B. 2004. *The Herbalist: Nicholas Culpeper and the Fight for Medical Freedom*. London: HarperCollins.

Worboys, M. 2000. Colonial medicine. In *Medicine in the Twentieth Century*, ed. R. Cooter and J. Pickstone, 67–80. Amsterdam: Harwood Academic Publishers.

Wujastyk, D. 2005. Policy formation and debate concerning the government regulation of Ayurveda in Great Britain in the twenty-first century. *Asian Medicine: Tradition and Modernity* 1: 162–84.

CHAPTER 3

The Evolution of Indian Government Policy on Ayurveda in the Twentieth Century

Dominik Wujastyk

HEALTH REGULATION IN THE NINETEENTH AND EARLY TWENTIETH CENTURIES

The attempts by the British and Indian governments to regulate medical practice in India generated an outpouring of numerous, long, and scattered documents. In order to be able to grasp the outlines of these processes of attempted control, I offer here a framework for understanding this landslide of documentation. I shall also offer some perspectives concerning the relative importance of some of these documents, as well as a sense of their content and influence.

Broadly speaking, the documentation can be divided into two classes:

- reports into specific topics commissioned by governments
- government legislation in the form of acts

Documents in both of these categories have been generated both by

- individual Indian states
- the central government in Delhi (and Colombo)

Some regional reports (presidency or state) seem to have had as much authority as central government ones. For example, the Usman Report of 1923 was a regional Madras report but had national importance.

Regional reports predominated in the period up until Independence, after which central government reports become the norm.

As one might expect, in many cases the reports led to legislation in the form of bills and then acts. However, sometimes the findings of committees were politically or socially unacceptable in whole or in part, and it took several committees to produce a consensus that would satisfy the legislators at a given period. For example, the Chopra Report of 1948 can be seen as a direct reaction to the Bhore Report of 1946. However, this chapter does not primarily address the evolution of government acts but the discussions that preceded them, in which policy was formed prior to legislation.

I begin with a brief overview of the main documents that were relevant to health policy formation.

Government Reports

State government committees in the pre-Independence period that dealt specifically with indigenous medicine in South Asia include the following:[1]

1923 Madras: The Committee on Indigenous Systems of Medicine ("The Usman Report") [§§ 44–58]

1925 Bengal: The Ayurvedic and Tibbi Committees [§§ 59–69]

1926 United Provinces: Ayurvedic and Unani Committee [§§ 70–73]

1927 Ceylon: a Government Committee [§§ 104–106]

1928 Burma: Committee to Enquire into the Indigenous Systems of Medicine [§§ 74–75]

1939 Central Provinces and Berar: The Committee to Examine the Indigenous Systems of Medicine [§§ 76–83]

1942 Mysore: Committee "to go into the Question of Encouraging the Indigenous Systems of Medicine" [§§ 100–103]

1941 Punjab: The Indigenous Medicine Committee [§§ 84–92]

1947 Bombay: The Indian Systems of Medicine Enquiry Committee [§§ 93–95]

1947 Assam: The Scheme Committee to Report on Steps to be Taken for the Development of Ayurveda [§§ 96–97]

1947 Orissa: The Utkal Ayurvedic Committee [§§ 98–99]

1947 Ceylon: Commission on Indigenous Medicine, Ceylon [§§ 107–108]

In the period after Independence, the following reports on Ayurveda were published under the auspices of the Ministry of Health of the Government of India (Brass 1972: 454):

1948 Report of the Committee on Indigenous Systems of Medicine ("The Chopra Report")

1951 Report of the Committee Appointed by the Government of India to Advise Them on the Steps to be Taken to Establish a Research Centre in the Indigenous Systems of Medicine and Other Cognate Matters ("The Pandit Committee Report")

1956 Interim Report of the Committee Appointed by the Government of India to Study and Report on the Question of Establishing Uniform Standards in Respect of Education & Practice of Vaidyas, Hakims, and Homoeopaths ("The Dave Report")

1959 Report of the Committee to Assess and Evaluate the Present Status of Ayurvedic System of Medicine ("The Udupa Committee Report")

1963 Report of the Shuddha Ayurvedic Education Committee ("The Vyas Committee Report")

1981 Health for All: An Alternative Strategy ("The Ramalingaswami Report")

The last item was not in fact a government report but an independent document published by the Indian Institute of Education and distributed by the Voluntary Health Association of India. However, Ramalingaswami was a senior figure who contributed to many aspects of government health policy on other occasions, and the report was treated as an authoritative statement.

By far the most important health policy report was that produced by the Bhore Committee in 1946. This pre-Independence report did not primarily address indigenous medicine, although it expressed a disparaging view of it at various points. The Bhore Report can be said to be the main blueprint for the Indian government's post-Independence health system, which to this day adheres almost exclusively to the biomedical model.

Other government reports on health matters in general sometimes also refer to indigenous medicine in greater or lesser degree. Thus the strengthening of primary health centers was recommended by the Mudaliar Committee of 1961, while the Kartar Singh Committee of 1973 and the Srivastava Committee of 1975 both made recommendations for multipurpose health workers, for medical education, and for support of manpower, with an emphasis on community health workers.

Government Acts

Legal provisions regarding health matters preceding Indian Independence are to be found scattered over at least forty enactments dealing with diverse subjects. Some examples include the following:[2]

1825 The Quarantine Act

1859 The Indian Merchants' Shipping Act

1860 The Indian Penal Code

1880 The Vaccination Act

1886 The Medical Act

1890 The Indian Railways Act

1896 The Births, Deaths and Marriages Registration Act

1897 The Epidemic Diseases Act

1898 The Code of Criminal Procedure

1899 The Glanders and Farcy Act

1911 The Indian Factories Act

1912 The Indian Medical Act

1917 The Indian Steam Vessels Act

1922 The Indian Red Cross Act

1923 The Indian Mines Act

1924 The Cantonments Act

1933 The Indian Medicine Council Act

1938 The Bombay Medical Practitioners Act

Efforts to regulate teaching, practice, and research specifically in indigenous medicine continued after Independence with many more government acts, such as the following:[3]

1956 The Madras Registration of Practitioners of Integrated Medicine Act

1961 The Mysore Homoeopathic Practitioners Act

1962 The Mysore Ayurvedic and Unani Practitioners Registration Act

1970 The Indian Medicine Central Council Act[4]

1984 The Central Council reconstituted

1995 The Central Council reconstituted again

2002 The Central Council Amendment[5]

The most important of these acts, from the point of view of present-day ayurvedic practice, were those of 1938 and 1970. The former established the first professional register for ayurvedic (and Unani) practitioners, effectively creating a pan-national profession for the first time. The 1970 Act, with its later amendments, established the Central Council of Indian Medicine (CCIM), whose objects were as follows:

1. to prescribe minimum standards of education in Indian Systems of Medicine (i.e., Ayurveda, Siddha and Unani Tibb)
2. to advise central government in matters relating to recognition and withdrawal of recognition of medical qualifications in Indian Medicine
3. to maintain the Central register of Indian Medicine and revise the Register from time to time
4. to prescribe standards of professional conduct, etiquette, and code of ethics to be observed by the practitioners

The act included the following important "schedules," which are frequently referred to in later legislation and documentation, and which are regularly updated (at least sixty times between 1970 and 2002):[6]

The Second Schedule: "Recognised medical qualifications in Indian medicine [Ayurveda, Siddha, Unani] granted by Universities, Boards or other medical institutions in India."[7]

The Third Schedule: "Qualifications granted by certain medical institutions before 15th August, 1947, in areas which comprised within India as defined in the Government of India Act, 1935."[8]

The Fourth Schedule: "Qualifications granted by Medical Institutions in Countries with which there is a scheme of reciprocity [Only Sri Lanka]."[9]

In short, following the 1970 act, the CCIM became the main national and central regulatory body for overseeing indigenous medical education and for maintaining a register of recognized practitioners.

After these exercises, the central government of India formulated and adopted its new National Health Policy in 1983,[10] which was influenced by the Alma Ata Declaration (International Conference on Primary Health Care 1978). In 2002, the Department of Indian Systems of Medicine & Homoeopathy, part of the Indian Government's Ministry of Health & Family Welfare, published the National Policy on Indian Systems of Medicine & Homoeopathy—2002.[11]

Control of Drugs

Parallel to the reports and Acts discussed here, a mass of documentation and legislation exists concerning the control of drugs and poisons. This literature surrounds and intersects with that relating to medical registration and the practice of indigenous medical traditions. One of the Bhore Committee's members, Dr. R. A. Amesur, for example, made the following recommendation for legislation concerning the allowable use of the title "Doctor" based on the danger to the public of the illicit distribution of registered drugs (Bhore 1946: vol. 2, 459):

> (i) no medical practitioner shall be entitled to affix the designation "Doctor" before his name unless he is a registered medical practitioner in modern scientific medicine.
>
> (ii) no person shall be entitled to prescribe drugs which are in the British Pharmacopoeia, especially injections and poisonous preparations, unless he is a registered medical practitioner and
>
> (iii) those who practise the Unani or Ayurvedic system of medicine may style themselves as "Hakims" or "Vaidyas" as the case may be.

Three quite distinct issues are amalgamated in these recommendations: the use of professional titles, the right to prescribe certain medicines, and the exclusion of those styled "vaidyas" and "hakims" from such a right.[12] The possibility that "doctors" might style themselves "vaidya" or "hakim" is not addressed, which marks the social gradient implicit in Bhore's treatment.

Whether or not it is logically satisfying in particular instances to discuss such issues together, policies concerning drugs and poisons do intersect with the issues of how medical personnel are defined and regulated. Although interesting and important, the history of drug and poison control will not be further addressed in this chapter.

Individual Reports

I shall now turn to an examination of selected reports, chosen for their intrinsic interest and later importance and influence.

The Usman Report, 1923

Sir Mahomed Usman, K.C.S.I. (1884–1960), was born of a noble Muslim family from Madras.[13] His father was Mahomed Yakub Sahib Bahadur, and Usman himself married Shahzady Begam, daughter of Shifaulmulk Zynulabudeen Sahib Bahadur, also of Madras. He was educated in the Madras Christian College, and between 1916 and his retirement in the late 1940s he held a number of senior posts in the legal, civic, and educational establishments of Madras. Having served on the Executive Council of the government of Madras for nine years, he became Acting Governor of Madras in 1934. He was Vice-Chancellor of Madras University between 1940 and 1942, and he participated in the Governor General's Executive Council for India from 1942 to 1946. It was in 1921, at a relatively early point in his career, that he was invited to prepare a report on the indigenous systems of medicine practiced in India.

The Usman Report (Usman 1923) was the first major health report to be published in India. It appeared before 1947, and it was only a regional report, not a central government one, but already looked toward a time when India would be independent.

The government object of the inquiry was

> . . . to afford the exponents of the ayurvedic and Unani systems an opportunity to state their case fully in writing for scientific criticism and to justify State encouragement of these systems. (Usman 1923: i.154)

The report noted that experiments in state encouragement of these systems were already being tried in several Indian states, including Hyderabad, Mysore, Baroda, Indore, Jaipur, Travancore, Cochin, Gondal, Rewa, and Gwalior. The report also showed an awareness of a tension between practitioners of indigenous and Western systems of medicine. It noted that practitioners who had mastered both systems of medicine, such as Sir Bhalachandra Krishna and Dr Deshmukh of Bombay, or Mahamahopadhyaya Kaviraj Gananatha Sen and Kaviraj Yamini Bhushan Roy of Calcutta, could reasonably supply the "scientific criticism" called for in the government's objective (Usman 1923: i.154).

As reports go, it is long, containing four major parts. The report itself is fifty pages long, but the appendices and evidence take it into two long volumes, of almost 500 pages. It is organized as follows:

Part I: The Report with Appendices
1: Introductory
2: Medical Registration
3: Medical Relief and Medical Education
[4:] Appendices, including
- pp. 1–96 comprise "Appendix I: *A Memorandum on The Science and the Art of Indian Medicine,*" by G. Srinivasa Murti, Secretary to the Committee on the Indigenous Systems of Medicine, Madras
- pp. 135–53 comprise "A List of Indian Medical Works Extant (both Printed and Manuscript)"

Part II: Written and Oral Evidence
1. Evidence from outside the Presidency of Madras,
   a) Written in English: 26 vaidyas
   b) Written in Sanskrit: 5 vaidyas
   c) Urdu: 5 hakims
2. Evidence from Pres. of Madras:
   a) Written in English: 16 vaidyas
   b) Written in Sanskrit: 5 vaidyas
   c) Tamil: 10 hakims
   d) Telugu: 1
   e) Malayalam: 1
   f) Kanarese: 1
   g) Oriya: 1
3. Oral evidence: pp. 429–68

The Usman Report contains several interesting and important features. First, Appendix I, *A Memorandum on The Science and the Art of Indian Medicine*, by G. Srinivasa Murti, is a book-length study of traditional Indian medicine, old-fashioned in style but clearly written and still of value today. The tone of the work is defensive vis-à-vis Western medicine, with passages, for example, seeking to show that Ayurveda was aware of concepts parallel to the germ theory of infection. Second, the appendix giving "A List of Indian Medical Works Extant, Both Printed and Manuscript" is a valuable survey of the medical literatures in Sanskrit, Urdu, and Tamil were generally known in the 1920s.

But it is the evidence gathered in Part II of the Report that is of most unique interest. This comprises the testimonies of many vaidyas and hakims provided in their various original languages. They describe in their own words the ayurvedic and Unani medical traditions, their importance and value for their patients, and their basic tenets. The material is quite extensive, the oral evidence alone covering forty pages. A fuller study of these testimonials would be very interesting.

The committee prepared a detailed questionnaire (reproduced at Usman 1923: i.97–98), which was translated into Sanskrit, Urdu, and several vernaculars of the Madras presidency and was widely distributed. Written replies received total 183, from all over India, written in English, Sanskrit, Urdu, Tamil, Telugu, Malayalam, Kanarese, and Oriya. Forty representative witnesses were orally examined, and a three-member subcommittee toured all over India, visiting important centers and meeting with leading exponents and promoters of indigenous medicine. The report, therefore, represented an all-India survey, although it was commissioned and published specifically in Madras.

The Bhore Report, 1946

The next government committee of major importance, the Health Survey and Development Committee, was convened over twenty years later under the chairmanship of Sir Joseph Bhore (Bhore 1946).

Sir Joseph William Bhore, Knight Commander of the Order of the Star of India (1878–1960), was born in Nasik, the son of Rao Saheb R. G. Bhore.[14] In 1911 he married Margaret W. Stott, who herself received a number of honors including the Order of the British Empire. He was educated at Bishop's High School and Deccan College in Pune and at University College London. He entered the Indian civil service in 1902 and held a number of senior government offices in Madras and Cochin. He was the acting high commissioner for India in the United Kingdom from 1922 to 1923 and was an acting member of the Governor General's Executive Council from 1926 to 1927 and a full member from 1930 to 1932. His public service was predominantly in the Departments of Agriculture and Lands, Industries and Labor, and Commerce and Railways. In 1935 he represented India at the Silver Jubilee Celebrations in London.

Bhore was a slightly older but politically a considerably more senior figure than Usman. Both men were knights of the same two orders. They received their first knighthoods (Knight Commander of the Indian Empire) only three years apart (Bhore in 1930, Usman in 1933), but their second (Knight Commander of the Order of the Star of India) over ten years apart (1933, 1945). Both served on the Governor General's Executive Council, but Bhore served nearly twenty years before Usman. These facts highlight the more rapid promotion and more senior record of public service achieved by Bhore. Bhore's career was spent more in central government agencies, whereas Usman's was more specifically focused on Madras, the city and especially the university. It is true that Bhore had gained relevant experience in 1928 as secretary to an Indian Statutory Commission. Nevertheless, the fact that Bhore, rather than Usman, was invited in 1943 to provide a report on medical policy for the government suggests that the topic itself had, since the Usman Report, become more important, and therefore worthy of more senior representation from a central rather than a regional government figure.

It also suggests that central government sought committee leadership with a more political than academic color. Most important, it suggests a decisive swing in government opinion away from any recognition that indigenous medicine could make a contribution to the nation's health. It is impossible that Bhore did not know Usman personally, or that he was unaware of the Usman Report. Both men had worked at a senior level in the administration of Madras institutions at the same time, and both received knighthoods in 1933. However, Usman's name and his report receive no mention in Bhore's work.

Bhore's committee was the last but one to be convened before Independence. It was appointed in 1943 by the government of India to provide the following (Bhore 1946: vol. 1, 2):

- a broad survey of the present position in regard to health conditions and health organization in British India
- recommendations for future developments

The terms of the committee were sweeping, allowing it to examine all aspects of the nation's health and medical establishment.

Reading Bhore today, it should be remembered that at the time of the committee's work, modern medical facilities were restricted mostly to India's metropolitan and capital cities. Hospitals existed at the district and sometimes at the taluk levels, but these were generally ill equipped and did not provide any specialized services. Among its many final recommendations were two in particular that addressed issues at either end of the spectrum of the health and medical education system: the establishment of primary health centers and the creation of a major central institute for postgraduate medical education and research (Bhore 1946: vol. 2, ch. 20). After Independence, the new national government established the first primary health centers in 1952 and the All-India Institute of Medical Sciences (AIIMS) in 1956.

The Bhore Committee was a large group, consisting of twenty-four participants, predominantly from the world of British state medicine. The committee was a panel of the great and the good in establishment medicine, almost all of whom had trained in medicine in Britain. Several of the committee members had collaborated on previous government commissions. For example, Cotter, Paton, and Banerjea had worked together on the Jolly Committee of the Central Advisory

Board of Education, which produced the 1941 *Report on The Medical Inspection of School Children and the Teachings of Hygiene in Schools.*[15]

The report produced by this committee is an even longer, more detailed document than the Usman Report. It has four volumes:

Vol. 1: Survey (228 pp.)
Vol. 2: Recommendations (532 pp.)
Vol. 3: Appendices (351 pp.)
Vol. 4: Summary (90 pp.)

In the initial part of the report, the committee takes pains to locate itself within a particular history of medical work (Bhore 1946: vol. 1, 29) by listing a series of earlier legislative acts relating to medical administration (listed earlier). The Bhore Report's list is presented as a representative series of examples taken from forty earlier medical-related acts. The list itself is interesting for at least three reasons: First, it is informative at the factual level. Second, it amply exemplifies the scattered and disjointed nature of past efforts to regulate health. These efforts can be categorized as being in the states (i.e., at the periphery); buried as health adjuncts in legislation, primarily aimed at other issues; and temporally scattered over almost a century.

Third, and most important of all, it reveals the tradition of work and the medical belief system within which Bhore and his committee locate themselves. The report's list suggests that the committee itself is a successor to this series of earlier legislative acts. But its list is heavily edited. The acts it lists, which date up to 1924, are those that do not deal with indigenous medicine; subsequent acts that regulate indigenous medicine are omitted. No reference at all is made to acts or government efforts related to nonallopathic medicine.

There is no reference to professionalization efforts such as the formation of the All-India Ayurvedic Congress or the state-level work toward professionalization by P. S. Varier and others. There is no reference to the 1933 Indian Medicine Council Act or the even more important 1938 Bombay Medical Practitioners Act, which for the first time established a separate medical register for vaidyas and hakims, simultaneously legitimizing and controlling their practice.

The Bhore Report is robustly scientistic in its views and unreflective about the hegemonic nature of what it calls "scientific medicine." But being unreflective about its own preconceptions does not mean that it is not assertive about its views concerning indigenous medicine. It says:

> . . . no system of medical treatment which is static in conception and practice and does not keep pace with the discoveries

> and researches of scientific workers the world over can hope to give the best available ministration to those who seek its aid. (Bhore 1946: vol. 4, 74)

The committee's view that indigenous medicine was static was based on a common misconception of the nineteenth century, that Indian culture was ancient and unchanging.

The history of the emergence and uses of this view is complex and will not be discussed here.[16] However, it has been decisively demonstrated for Ayurveda that from its very earliest roots, the tradition of medical thought and practice was in constant flux and tension, with different schools vying for their own theories, different physicians using different therapies, and, in more recent times, traditionalists exchanging medical therapies and ideas with foreigners.[17]

The Bhore Report opens its principal statement on indigenous medicine in the following way:

> In considering the question of the place which the indigenous systems of medical treatment should occupy in any planned organisation of medical relief and public health in the country, we are faced with certain difficulties. We realise the hold that these systems exercise not merely over the illiterate masses but over considerable sections of the intelligentia [*sic*]. We have also to recognise that treatment by practitioners of these systems is said to be cheap, and it is claimed that the empirical knowledge, that has been accumulated over centuries, has resulted in a fund of experience of the properties and medicinal use of minerals, herbs and plants which is of some value. Further, the undoubted part that these systems have played in the long distant past in influencing the development of medicine and surgery in other countries of the world has naturally engendered a feeling of patriotic pride in the place they will always occupy in any world history of the rise and development of medicine. This feeling has not been without its effect on the value which is attached by some to the practice of these systems. (Bhore 1946: vol. 2, 455)

In this opening statement, we already see some of the attitudes that are played out more fully later in the report. The indigenous medical systems are associated with "illiterate masses," over which they have a "hold." The pejorative use of language here already discloses the report's presuppositions: other grammatical subjects that would more usually be said to "have a hold" over their predicates would typically include "superstitions" or "drugs" or any other force by which something or someone is affected or dominated through nonrational means. A note of supercilious incredulity may be detected in the statement that some of the intelligentsia are equally under the power of such medical systems. The knowledge of materia medica accumulated in the indigenous medical traditions, so highly valued in today's world of bio-piracy and patent protection, is reduced to a mere claim by unspecified persons that this knowledge may be only of "some" value. Indigenous medicine is projected into the historical past of medicine, where no doubt the authors of the report felt it rightly belonged. Indigenous medicine also is associated with patriotic pride, and this, rather than any intrinsic medical merit, is given to account for the value that some, perhaps otherwise intelligent, people find in these systems. Although identifying themselves with a scientific and progressive worldview, the authors of the Bhore Report offer no quantitative evidence for their criticism of indigenous medicine, offering instead only personal opinions and critical rhetoric.

The language and style of the Bhore Report's remarks on indigenous medicine reveal an impatience with the whole subject and a desire to dispatch it as soon as possible to some other realm where it need not trouble the makers of India's future health. The subtle use of metaphor and phraseology serves to undermine indigenous medicine without actually going to the trouble of presenting thought-out refutations or serious, factual, or research-based arguments for or against counterhegemonic medicine.[18]

The committee was clearly not prepared to engage in any serious consideration of the merits of indigenous medicine, and it roundly dismissed it on the grounds that it did not share the quality of progress, by which scientific medicine was characterized. The Bhore Committee believed that:

> It has, however, to be recognised that great improvements have taken place in the field of public health as the result of the many discoveries of science which are and can be implemented only through the scientific system of medicine and through personnel trained in such a system. It is also to be recognised frankly that the indigenous systems of medical treatment do not at present deal with such vital aspects of medicine as obstetrics, gynaecology, advanced surgery and some of the specialities. Above all it is necessary that we should keep prominently before our eyes the intimate relation between science and the advancement of medicine. No system of medical treatment, which is static in conception and practice and does not keep pace with the discoveries and researches

> of scientific workers the world over, can hope to give the best available ministration to those who seek its aid. (Bhore 1946: vol. 2, 455)

In this passage and most others, the report writer is careful to distinguish implicitly between indigenous medicine as practiced in the 1940s and as represented in the ancient literature of medicine. The ancient Sanskrit treatises do, of course, contain much material on obstetrics, gynecology, moderately advanced surgery, and other specialities.[19] That many of these practices had fallen out of use among indigenous physicians by the 1940s means that a distinction between ancient art and modern practice will implicitly devalue the tradition and preempt an argument for the value of indigenous medicine based on the rich tradition of the ancient texts.

Furthermore, the possibility of medical revival or the stimulation of growth from within the indigenous medical systems is not entertained. To be fair, however, the authors of the report did recommend the establishment of a professorial chair in medical history at the All-India Medical Institute, one of whose functions would be the study of the indigenous medical systems to discover "the extent to which they can contribute to the sum total of medical knowledge" (Bhore 1946: vol. 2, 457). Even here, however, what is proposed is not the stimulation of indigenous medical practice through fresh historical research but the expropriation of elements of traditional value by modern establishment medicine (henceforth MEM).

The Bhore Report's final summary recommendations relating to indigenous medicine follow:

> 281. We are unfortunately not in a position to assess the real value of these systems of medical treatment as practised today as we have been unable, with the time and opportunities at our disposal, to conduct such an investigation into this problem as would justify clear-cut recommendations. We do, however, say quite definitely that there are certain aspects of health protection which, in our opinion, can be secured wholly or at any rate largely, only through the scientific system of medicine. Thus public health or preventive medicine, which must play an essential part in the future of medical organisation, is not within the purview of the indigenous systems of medical treatment as they obtain at present. The indigenous systems of medical treatment do not also at present deal with such vital aspects of medicine as obstetrics, gynaecology, advanced surgery and some of the specialities. Further, no system of medical treatment which is static in conception and practice and

> does not keep pace with the discoveries and researches of scientific workers the world over can hope to give the best available ministration to those who seek its aid.
>
> 282. We feel that we need no justification in confining our proposals to the country-wide extension of a system of medicine which, in our view, must be regarded neither as Eastern nor Western but as a corpus of scientific knowledge and practice belonging to the whole world and to which every country has made its contribution.
>
> 283. We have been informed that, in China and Japan, a moratorium extending to a definite period of years was declared after which the practice of the indigenous systems in those countries would not be recognised. We were further told by Dr. Ognev, the Soviet Representative, that indigenous systems of medical treatment were nowhere recognised in the Soviet Union.
>
> 284. We consider that it should be left to the Provincial Governments to decide what part, if any, should be played by the indigenous systems in the organisation of Public Health and Medical Relief. It is for them to consider, after such investigation as may be found necessary, under what conditions the practice of these systems should be permitted and whether it is necessary, either during some interim period or as a permanent measure, to utilise them in their schemes of medical relief.
>
> What we have said in regard to the indigenous systems applies generally to Homeopathy also. (Bhore 1946, vol. 4, 73 f.)

There are several interesting points in this statement, and some disingenuousness. At face value, the report states that it did not have the time and resources to investigate the matter of indigenous medicine. But it appears to be more truthful to say that the committee had no wish to engage with the community of indigenous practitioners, because it was ideologically committed to a form of medicine that denied the value and efficacy and, more importantly, the epistemological basis of indigenous medical practice. For example, the report makes no mention of the Usman Report, which provided a great deal of relevant material in a readily accessible form, and which was, moreover, a government-sponsored report of only twenty years earlier. Had the committee had even a slight wish to consider indigenous medicine seriously, it could have begun by looking at the copious materials made available by Usman.

A footnote to the last paragraph, § 284, printed in the report, registers the dissent that existed on the committee regarding licensing medical practitioners:

> Drs. Butt, Vishwa Nath and Narayanrao do not accept this view. They desire to see that the services of persons trained in the indigenous systems of medicine are freely utilised for developing medical relief and public health work in the country.

The voices of Drs. Butt, Vishwa Nath, and U. B. Narayan Rao appear as footnotes at various other parts of the report too. They regularly disagree with Bhore and the rest of the committee in matters relating to indigenous systems of medicine. For example, they want vaidyas and hakims to be brought into a legislative framework within which they could be licensed to function as physicians. Bhore, however, wants to exclude them firmly. In the fuller recommendations relating to indigenous medicine, for example, the Bhore Report states:

> Three of our colleagues (Drs. Butt, Narayan Rao, and Vishwa Nath) desire to make a definite recommendation suggesting the free utilisation of the services of persons trained in indigenous systems for promoting public health and medical relief in India. Their note will be found at the end of the next chapter. (Bhore 1946: vol. 2, 457)

The note in question is reported as follows (Bhore 1946, vol. 2, 461 § 13):

> Three of our colleagues (Drs. Butt, Narayan Rao, and Vishwa Nath) desire to make more positive recommendation than that indicated in paragraph 11 above regarding the training of practitioners in the indigenous systems of medicine and their utilisation for promoting public health and medical relief activities in the country." They state, "We are of the opinion that the teaching of indigenous systems of medicine should be regulated by the State. The Bombay Medical Practitioners Act, 1938, represents in regard to registration, the medical curriculum and examinations preliminary to registration, a step in the right direction. Practitioners trained and registered under the requirements of the above Act, or similar legislation, should be freely utilised for promoting public health and medical relief in India.

Ultimately, it was the position argued for by these three physicians that prevailed in India after Independence.

The impression one gains is that the Bhore Committee refused to engage intellectually with indigenous medicine not, as it claims, out of a lack of time or resources but as a result of ideological preconceptions that prevented it from engaging with the relevant issues in a meaningful way and that betray an aversion to all that indigenous medicine represented to the committee members. This impression is reinforced when we read what the report has to say elsewhere about the relationship between "scientific medicine" and indigenous medicine. In its *Recommendations*, the report cites with strong approbation an article from the *Indian Medical Gazette* (Bhore 1946: vol. 2, 455–56).[20] The article is a startlingly brazen example of the Whig interpretation of history.[21]

> The science of medicine is a very ancient one. It progressed slowly throughout the earlier ages of history—such slow advance, as there was, being arrested from time to time by religious prejudice or by undue reverence for alleged authority. . . . It was not until the middle of the 19th century that medical science became firmly established on a secure foundation. The invention of the compound microscope, the rapid development of Organic Chemistry and latterly of Bio-Chemistry and Bio-Physics have led to such an advance that we can say with truth that 95 per cent of the total corpus of knowledge with regard to the working of the human body has been obtained within the life time of men who are still with us. . . . Science is one and indivisible. No advance is possible with one subdivision of knowledge without its reflection in all other sub-divisions, and rejoicing over a discovery is not to be confined to the members of the particular scientific band immediately concerned.

The metaphor of progress that is used in this anonymous citation perfectly illustrates Butterfield's classic characterization of the immature historian who "tends in the first place to adopt the Whig or Protestant view of the subject, and very quickly busies himself with dividing the world into the friends and enemies of progress" (1931, Introduction). Butterfield notes that this attitude is characteristic of historians who know too little of their subject. The Whig interpretation is almost always corrected when further research takes place, and when the historian gains fuller knowledge of the historical sources. Perhaps this would have happened if the Bhore Committee had indeed had more time, or had included professional historians on its staff. It is ironic that the most famous and widely cited example of Whiggish historians is Thomas Babbington Macauley (1800–1859), also the author of the famous *Minute on Education* of 1835, which so decisively changed the course of Indian education away from the study of India's own traditions and toward the wholesale adoption of British educational models in language and content. Macauley's reforms ultimately led to the inevitability of a body such as the Bhore Committee, so unsympathetic to India's own historic cultural heritage, being given charge, a century later, of the medical services of India.

The most forceful statement in Macauley's *Minute* begins with a declaration of his own complete ignorance in the matter upon which he is expressing an opinion: "I have no knowledge of either Sanscrit or Arabic." This absence of knowledge did not prevent him from asserting famously that "a single shelf of a good European library was worth the whole native literature of India and Arabia" (Macaulay 1957). The remarks on indigenous medicine found in the Bhore Report are stamped with the same mixture of ignorance and rejection, under the guise of a metaphorical interpretation of history as a wagon in motion, whose wheel hits sometimes a stone of religion, or sometimes one of false authority.

Ultimately, we should read the Bhore Report's view on indigenous medicine stripped of its historical pretensions, as a simple assertion by one hegemonic group over another, couched in social and epistemological terms. The Bhore Committee consisted almost entirely of British-trained physicians who had reached high positions in the government medical establishment of British India. They were interested in diagnosing India's medical ills according to the criteria with which they were familiar from their own tradition of medicine, and in designing treatments for those ills using solutions they had been taught by their teachers and colleagues in professional British medicine. Their assertions are power claims.

Center and Periphery

After a number of inconclusive, yet strongly worded comments on the regulation of vaidyas and hakims, the authors of the report decided to transfer the consideration of all such matters to the provincial governments, from the center to the periphery.[22] This might sound plausible at first hearing, but it was in fact an oblique way of halting any movement toward the registration of indigenous practitioners. For elsewhere in the report it is argued forcefully that the provincial governments should have no power over the registration or licensing of physicians, and that all such powers should be centralized as soon as possible.

> 3. In India the Indian Medical Council was established by the Medical Council Act of 1933, but its functions differ materially from those of the General Medical Council in the United King-

> dom. It has not been authorised by law to maintain an All-India Medical Register. Moreover, the basic qualifications for medical registration are those of medical licentiates, a body of practitioners who are the concern of the Provincial Medical Councils. The maintenance of Medical Registers and the supervision of the basic qualifications required for entry into them are, at present, responsibilities entrusted to Provincial Medical Councils and Faculties. The supervision of the Indian Medical Council is, as yet, restricted to certain medical qualifications which are granted by Indian Universities and which are incorporated in the First Schedule of the Indian Medical Council Act.
>
> 4. We consider this position unsatisfactory. We are recommending that, for the future, there should only be one basic medical qualification for entry into the profession throughout India and that the portal of entry should be a University degree. . . . the Medical Council of India should be empowered to maintain an All-India Register when the training of licentiates ceases throughout the country. One of us (Dr. Vishwanath) considers that, in such a register, all the existing graduates and licentiates should be eligible for inclusion. With the creation of the All-India Medical Register the functions of the Medical Council of India would approximate closely to those of the General Council of Medical Education and Registration of the United Kingdom. (Bhore 1946, vol. 2, 458–59)

A footnote (ibid.) to this passage once again raises the familiar voices of dissent:

> Two of our colleagues (Dr. Vishwa Nath and Dr. A. H. Butt) are not in agreement with the recommendations set out above. They state, "In our opinion the functions as at present exercised by the Provincial Medical Councils and the All-India Medical Council are properly discharged and there is no need for any change."

Since it was clearly the Bhore Committee's aim to centralize control of medical education and licensing, its suggestion of devolving decision making regarding indigenous physicians to the provinces can only be read as a disingenuous attempt to disenfranchise these physicians by stealth.

Medical Licentiates and the Society of Apothecaries

When reading the Bhore Report it is important to remember that the committee was writing at a time before any central national medical authority existed. Thus large parts of it show Bhore and his committee wrestling with the issues of the relationship between center and periphery. As shown in the earlier citation, the Bhore Committee wants to bring control of finance and policy into the center, to replace a plural and decentralized system of medical licensing with a unified and centralized one that recognizes only university-trained physicians. The model presented for this is the United Kingdom. In particular, the General Council of Medical Education and Registration of the United Kingdom ("General Medical Council" or GMC) is held up as an example to be followed.

However, in contrasting a plural and disorganized Indian situation with a centralized and controlled British one, the Bhore Committee misrepresents the situation in the United Kingdom. In fact, a system of medical licensing quite separate from that administered by the GMC existed in Britain at the time the Bhore Report was written. Indeed, it exists today.

The Worshipful Society of Apothecaries was incorporated as a City Livery Company by royal charter from James I in London in 1617 in recognition of apothecaries' specialist skills in compounding and dispensing medicines. The Apothecaries' Act of 1815 empowered the society to institute a Court of Examiners to examine and to grant licences to successful candidates to practice as an apothecary in England and Wales. It also gave the society the duty of regulating such practice. The title of the original medical qualification was "Licentiate of the Society of Apothecaries" (LSA).

Following the establishment of the General Medical Council by statute in 1858 the LSA became a registrable qualification. In 1907 the title was altered by parliamentary act to LMSSA to indicate the inclusion of surgery in the examination, a subject required by law following the Medical Act of 1886.

Today the society continues to award its license as a member of the United Examining Board, which is the only non-university medical licensing body in the United Kingdom.[23]

It is impossible that all of the members of the Bhore Committee were unaware of the Society of Apothecaries and its licentiate. But it is not mentioned, and it would seem likely that information about the Worshipful Society was suppressed because it would have greatly strengthened the argument of those who wished to maintain a separate professional licensing system for vaidyas and hakims.

The Bhore Report was in many ways a successful and an influential document, especially in forming the policy foundation of the allopathic establishment in India. But it created an immediate reaction among those who wished the indigenous systems of Indian medicine to have a place in India's national health care scheme. As a result, Sir Ram Nath Chopra was commissioned to chair a committee in 1946 and to produce a report to redress this balance (Chopra 1948).

The Chopra Report, 1948

Sir Ram Nath Chopra (1882–1973) was a distinguished Indian pharmacologist.[24] Born in the Punjab in 1882, he was educated at the universities of the Punjab and Cambridge, and at St. Bartholomew's Hospital in London. After service in the war, he spent the majority of his professional career at the Calcutta School of Tropical Medicine, retiring as its director in 1941. He held a number of other senior posts and chairmanships, and he published extensively. In particular, his famous *Indigenous Drugs of India* (1933, reprinted often) testifies to a lifelong professional engagement with Ayurveda and the other indigenous health systems of India. In his 1941 presidential address at the Annual Meeting of the National Institute of Sciences of India, held at Benares Hindu University, Chopra gave his own overview of the history and prospects for public health organization and medical service in India (Chopra 1941). This wide-ranging and well-informed survey provided a preliminary blueprint for an Indian national health service. Given Chopra's professional eminence in the early 1940s, and his prominent and substantial public statements on health reform, it is surprising that he was not invited to join the Bhore Committee. It is tempting to conjecture that Chopra's interest in indigenous medicine disqualified him in Bhore's eyes.

Drs. A. H. Butt, Vishwa Nath, and U. B. Narayan Rao, the dissident members of the Bhore Committee, joined the Chopra Committee, which supported their views.

One of the other members of the Chopra Committee, Mazhar H. Shah, later gave the following description of the committee's purposes and activity, which is worth citing as a fair account of matters:

> In 1946 the Government of India appointed the Indigenous Systems Inquiry Committee, under Sir Ramnath Chopra as Chairman, and three Hakims, three Vaids, Dr. B. N. Ghosh Professor of Pharmacology and myself [Mazhar H. Shah] as members. The committee was required to make recommendations on:
>
> (a) the provision for research in Ayurveda and Unani Tibb,
> (b) Improvement of facilities for training,

(c) desirability of state control,
(d) increasing usefulness of these systems, and
(e) holding enquiry as to whether the three systems—Ayurveda, Unani, and Modern—could be combined into one comprehensive system.

In their report the committee expressed the view that "if the aim of all (systems) was the maintenance of health and prevention and cure of disease, they should all be properly investigated and integrated in the form of a single system which should be capable of suitable alteration and adaptation in accordance with the time and other conditions." . . . the sudden partitioning of India brought the inquiry prematurely to a close (Shah 1966: vii).

The Chopra Report consisted of the following chapters:[25]

1: Introductory. The history and development of Ayurveda and Unani or Arabian systems of medicine—Their past achievements—The cause of decline and their present position—Attempts at their revival

2: The appointment and personnel of the committee and the procedure adopted by it

3: Progress of work of the committee

4: Previous committees on indigenous systems of medicine set up by provincial and other governments Madras (1923) . . . Ceylon (1927 and 1947)

5: Existing conditions of medical relief

6: Integration of Indian and Western medicine leading to their ultimate synthesis

7: Education and medical institutions

8: The organisation of rural medical relief

9: State control of medical practice and education

10: Research

11: Drugs and medicinal preparations

12: Administration and finance

13: Summary of the recommendations

14: Conclusions

The Chopra Report is often cited in later works, and it has several interesting features. Chapter 4 gives a useful overview of the work of previous committees between 1923 and 1947 (just cited).

The report's apparent aim is to give indigenous medical systems a proper place in India's health care structure—however, this aim is undermined in an insidious way in Chapter 6. This chapter argues that a careful study of ayurvedic principles, for example, will show that the various humors and other traditional and nonallopathic parts of the body will eventually be found to coincide with modern medical categories as revealed by science. Thus the report's aim is not to integrate traditional and modern sciences but rather for modern medicine to absorb traditional medicine by reinterpreting its principal categories. Ultimately, all traditional practices and explanations will be subsumed by scientific medical ones.

Nevertheless, Chapters 10 and 11 of the report do emphasize the importance of investigating India's flora and fauna for medical uses. Again, this shows the report's orientation toward traditional medicine as a source of potential therapies that can be absorbed and taken over by modern medicine. Following his work on the committee, R. N. Chopra himself engaged energetically in this ethnopharmacological activity and produced a series of important and influential publications on the Indian materia medica (see, e.g., Chopra et al. 1956, 1958, 1965).

The Aftermath of Chopra: The 1950s and 1960s

The Chopra Report, which ultimately proposed complete equality in training and practice between indigenous and establishment physicians, was in fact rejected by the government of India (Shankar 1992: 146), but a number of committees were convened in the 1950s with the aim of completing, or advising on, the implementation of aspects of Chopra's recommendations. The need for these continuing efforts highlights the difficulty and controversy surrounding these issues.[26] A series of committees was appointed to "cherry pick" acceptable themes from Chopra.

One of the issues that repeatedly occupied these committees was whether Ayurveda should be integrated with MEM, or whether it should be kept "pure" (*śuddha*) and be taught and practiced solely in accordance with tradition.

The Pandit Report, 1951

The Pandit Committee was established to finalize just those recommendations of the Chopra Report regarding "Education and Medical Institutions" and "Research." The idea was that a common integrated syllabus for all medical colleges would be rejected, but that research should be undertaken into the validity of indigenous medicine from the point of view of contemporary establishment medical science. One early outcome of the Pandit Report was the establishment of the Central Institute of Research in Indigenous Systems of Medicine in and the Postgraduate Training Centre for Ayurveda, both in Jamnagar in 1952 (Jaggi 2000: 312; Shankar 1992: 146).

The Dave Report, 1956

The Dave Report presented a model-integrated syllabus to be used in colleges that would teach only physicians of indigenous systems of medicine (ISM). At the outset, this report positioned itself as a corrective to the Bhore Report. It stated:

> The Bhore Committee . . . was not in a position to assess the value of the various systems on account of paucity of time and opportunity to conduct such investigation into the problem. (Dave 1956: 1)

This is a notably tolerant response to the Bhore Report's hostility regarding indigenous medicine. After this nod to Bhore, the Dave Committee articulated its work specifically as carrying forward or "finalizing" the proposals of the Chopra Report relating to the state control of medical practice and education, and to come to a practical solution to the issue of the Chopra Report's recommendations relating to education and medical institutions.

> The present committee has been entrusted with the work of recommending the ways and methods and rules to bring about uniformity as regards legislation, medical education, and practice of Vaidyas, Hakims, and Homoeopaths. (Dave 1956: 2)

The report cites Sanskrit sources (in Devangarī script), including Suśruta, Śukra (*Śukranīti*), Caraka, Kauṭilya, and so on. The main thrust of these quotations is to show that the Sanskrit tradition was aware of the problem of medical quackery and disapproved of it strongly.

The report made sixteen recommendations about the regulation of practice, postponing issues of education to a second part of the committee's report (Dave 1956: 11), which apparently never appeared.

The Udupa Report, 1959

K. N. Udupa was invited by the government of India to chair the "Committee to Assess and Evaluate the Present Status of Indian Systems of Medicine" (Udupa et al. 1958). The committee's task, undertaken between 1957 and 1958, was nothing less than to review the entire situation relating to ayurvedic medicine in India (Jaggi 2000: 312). The chief recommendation of the committee was that the government should establish a Council of Indian Medicine (to regulate educational standards) and a Council of Ayurvedic Research. The latter council was soon established and itself sponsored further committees to investigate the question of ayurvedic medicine. It arrived at the conclusion that an integrated training was appropriate (Jaggi 2000: 312–13). Udupa himself was later to participate as a member of the Ramalingaswami Committee.[27]

The Mudaliar Report, 1962

The report prepared by Dr. Arcot Lakshmanaswami Mudaliar and his committee took the opposite approach, rejecting integrated medical education. Instead it recommended that systems of indigenous medicine should be taught and practiced in a purely classical form, with due attention to language skills and access to original sources (Jaggi 2000: 313–17; Shankar 1992: 146). Once fully trained, indigenous physicians could be separately trained in MEM. The final practical effect would be the withering away of indigenous medical practice in the face of superior MEM, which would absorb its best features, although this was not stated quite so baldly as this. But this view is perhaps less surprising when we remember that Dr. A. L. Mudaliar had formerly been a member of the Bhore Committee.

The Mudaliar Committee's recommendations were accepted by the government and proved influential, laying the foundation for the administrative and regulatory systems in place today (Mudaliar 1962). The Central Council for Research in Indian Medicine and Homoeopathy was founded in 1969 to promote various research agendas defined by Mudaliar.

The Vyas Report, 1963

The chairman of this report, Mohanlal P. Vyas, was the Minister for Health and Labour, Ahmedabad, Gujarat. One of the most prominent among the committee members was Pandit Shiv Sharma. Pt. Sharma was educated in medicine and Sanskrit by his father, the court physician to the Maharaja of Patiala. When Mahatma Gandhi was dying and his wife called for an ayurvedic physician, it was Pt. Sharma who was summoned. An articulate, scholarly person with a commanding presence, equally at home among Sanskrit pandits or at the golf club joking in English, Pt. Sharma became the renowned champion of "pure"

(Sanskrit *śuddha*) Ayurveda, that is, the practice of Ayurveda without any addition of allopathic concepts or therapies.[28] The report, in its opening statement, said the purpose of the committee was

> to draw up a curriculum and syllabus of study in pure (unmixed) Ayurveda extending to over four years, which should not include any subject of modern medicine or allied sciences in any form or language.

Indeed, the main part of this report (the fifty-six pages of chapter 7 that give the curriculum and syllabus) were written entirely in the Sanskrit language (Vyas 1963: 31–86). The report's title, "Report of the Shuddha Ayurvedic Education Committee," emphasized its dedication to the ideal of Shuddha, or fundamentalist ayurvedic doctrine and practice.

The Ramalingaswami Report, 1981

Professor V. Ramalingaswami (1921–2001), Fellow of the Indian National Science Academy, Fellow of the Royal Society, and former president of the Indian National Science Academy, was considered one of the most illustrious Indian scientists of his day. His major scientific work consisted of studies on nutritional pathology, especially protein-calorie malnutrition, iodine deficiency disorders, and nutritional anemia. He served as director of the All-India Institute of Medical Sciences and as director-general of the Indian Council of Medical Research, and he contributed to the work of international bodies such as World Health Organization, United Nations Children's Fund, and International Development Research Council.

The committee he chaired included in its final recommendations that the existing model of health care in India should be replaced by one that combined "the best elements in the tradition and culture of the people with modern science and technology" (Ramalingaswami 1981: 14ff.). In this it differed subtly from the Chopra Report, which recommended not a combination of systems but an absorption of the best elements of tradition by modern medical science.

The Ramalingaswami Report makes bold statements, for example, on the connection between health and social and educational development, particularly the connection between political development and health status. It says:

> In most developing countries, oligarchies of the upper and middle classes are in power. Their health status is very good and they derive the largest benefit from the public health ser-

> vices. On the other hand, the poor in these countries who form the large majority and are deprived of effective political power, have a low health status and receive only marginal benefits from the public health services. The situation is very different in countries where the democratic process is taken to the community level and the common people are involved actively in planning and implementing programmes for their welfare. . . . It will thus be seen that the political system does exercise considerable influence over the health system.
>
> It is also true that the health system can influence political development. For instance, primacy health care can be organised on a community basis and the people can be actively involved in studying their problems, deciding upon feasible solutions and implementing them. This is an essentially political experience which enables them to organise themselves and fight their battles in other fields as well.
>
> . . . The greatest weakness of Indian society today is poverty which compels the majority of its population to live subhuman lives and the great inequality between the small privileged classes at the top and the bulk of the underprivileged people at the bottom. (Ramalingaswami 1981: 19–22)

These hard-hitting remarks on the linkage between health and politics exemplify the sophistication of the Ramalingaswami Report and raise the question of whether it was considered too radical in some political circles. It is noteworthy in this connection that the report was not published by the government of India but by an independent educational institute in Pune.

The Ramalingaswami Report's "Alternative Model" of health provision starts by attributing India's present health dilemma squarely to British colonial myopia:

> These [health] services were first organised by the British administrators who totally ignored the indigenous belief systems, life-styles and health care institutions and practices which formed an organic unity. Instead of building on these foundations and evolving a new system more suited to the life and needs of the people with the help of modern science and technology, they decided to make an abrupt and total change by introducing the Western system of medicine in toto. This decision created a wide gulf between the culture and traditions of the people on the one hand and the health services on the

> other. It also deprived the latter of several valuable contributions which the Indian tradition could have made. (Ramalingaswami 1981: 81 ff.)

While there is much truth in this claim, there also is some oversimplification. The report underestimates the extent to which the British administrators in some cases continued the medical funding patterns established by the earlier Mughal administration (Brimnes, unpublished). Nevertheless, the report's attribution of the dominance of the "urban-biased, top-down, and elite-oriented" medical provision to its origins in the British establishment of such institutions is convincing (Ramalingaswami 1981: 82). It certainly applies to the efforts from Bhore onward. The main aim of the Ramalingaswami Report's "Alternative Model" (ch. 6) is that health provision should be founded on a strong community base, and that it should integrate promotive, preventive, and curative services. Health provision should be focused on community efforts and interventions, with a radical redefinition of the position of the doctor and drugs.

It explicitly distances itself from the recommendations of the Bhore Committee which, it says, "tried to move away from the exclusively curative model [. . . but still] placed too heavy an emphasis on doctors" (Ramalingaswami 1981: 91). The Ramalingaswami Report notes further that the Bhore Report was silent on the subject of India's indigenous culture and medical traditions, and in contrast it recommends that the health care system of India should be given a national orientation by the incorporation of the culture and traditions of the people (Ramalingaswami 1981: 95).

The report recognizes the following five broad elements of traditional Indian culture that it feels are relevant to its recommendations: (1) the *varṇāśrama* concept of the stages of Hindu life, which inculcates "the right attitudes to pain, to growing old, and to death," (2) a nonconsumerist approach to life, (3) a devolved and distributed attitude to health service provision, and a withdrawal of centralized state intervention, (4) the use of yoga as an instrument for physical and mental health, and (5) an emphasis on "simple but effective things" such as naturopathy, the use of simple medicines, and homegrown herbs for day-to-day illnesses, games and sports that require little equipment, and similar practices that oppose "a profit-motivated capitalist civilization [that] tries to encourage consumerism" (Ramalingaswami 1981: 96f.).

The central messages of the Ramalingaswami Report are about decentralization and the devolution and integration of health services, and these messages are normally delivered in a rational and sociopolitically sophisticated manner. Unfortunately for this report, the World Health Organization's slogan "Health for All by the Year 2000" became increasingly jaded and untenable as the end of the second millennium actually approached. Inspired by the justifiable euphoria surrounding the eradication of smallpox in the 1970s, the WHO believed that other major disease groups also could be conquered. But by the 1990s, it was already plain to all that such a goal was beyond reasonable reach. This was not only because of a general loss of faith in medical science and technology, when faced, for example, by the kinds of challenges articulated by Illich (1990 [1976], 1986), including the dramatic rise of iatrogenic disease and various other structural failures in scientific medicine.[29]

The absurdity of the concept of total world health by 2000 also was shattered permanently by the appearance of the human immunodeficiency virus (HIV), which taught the world what epidemiologists and medical historians had always known, that diseases evolve, and that an ever-changing balance exists between human populations and their viral and bacteriological environments, a balance that shifts in response to random mutations, evolution, and the advances of medical science.[30] The Ramalingaswami Report, by necessarily situating itself within the discredited WHO "Health for All" agenda, now shares the fate of that agenda, being ignored for all practical purposes. This is regrettable, since this report is the most sociologically astute of any of the Indian reports on health.[31]

CONCLUSIONS

In this chapter I have surveyed some of the twentieth-century attempts by the governments of India, both before and after Independence, to control and regulate health policy and practice, especially in relation to indigenous types of medicine such as Ayurveda. The initiatives by the British and Indian governments to regulate medical practice in India generated large quantities of documentation. I have investigated some of this material and discussed the contents and purposes of the more important government committee reports that addressed the issue of indigenous medicine. I have also offered a framework for understanding the meaning of these processes of attempted control and a critique of their purposes, which often are more political and hegemonic than medical. I have offered as well some perspectives concerning the relative importance of these documents and a sense of their content and influence.

The unjustly neglected Usman Report certainly deserves further study, especially for the account it provides of indigenous medicine in India at the beginning of the twentieth century, given in the practitioners' own voices. The Bhore and Mudaliar reports were the chief influences in forming the administrative and organizational establishment of national health care in India today, with their principal support given to MEM, and secondary support (Mudaliar) for indigenous health systems in an integrated form. The Chopra Committee and its sequels attempted to give a more prominent place to indigenous health traditions but only achieved a limited influence, mainly in establishing institutions to undertake ethnopharmacological study, in designing integrated curricula for colleges of indigenous medicine, and in setting up regulatory bodies for indigenous medical professionals. Finally, the Ramalingaswami Report showed a quantum leap in sophistication in studying the medical situation in India with a modern socio-medical awareness. While perhaps open to criticism in some areas, it is unfortunate that it did not have the influence it undoubtedly deserved.

NOTES

1. The paragraph numbers (§) refer to discussions of reports by Chopra (1948: 25–67).

2. The acts up until 1924 are cited from Bhore (1946: survey, 29).

3. The acts up until 1962 are cited from Stepan (1983: 302).

4. Government of India (1970).

5. Government of India (2002).

6. The First Schedule deals with bureaucratic matters concerning regional representation on the council.

7. See http://www.ccimindia.org/1_10.htm.

8. See http://www.ccimindia.org/1_11.htm.

9. See http://www.ccimindia.org/1_12.htm.

10. The full text is available at http://www.mohfw.nic.in/kk/95/ii/95ii0101.htm.

11. Government of India, Dept. ISMH 2002.

12. The discussion of these recommendations makes reference to Rule 65(9) of the Drugs Rules, 1945, under the Drugs Act, 1940, which provides that a number of poisons shall not be sold in retail except on and in accordance with a prescription of a registered medical practitioner. Major government reports had already addressed issues of drug use and control in the nineteenth century, for example, the Indian Hemp Drugs Commission 1893–94 report (Mackworth Young 1894–1895).

13. In his report, he gives his name as Khan Bahadur Muhammad Usman Sahib Bahadur. Details from Anon. (1964, 1967: 1110).

14. Details from Anon. (1964, 1967: 100).

15. See http://www.shikshanic.nic.in/cd50years/g/52/4W/Toc.htm.

16. Pollock (1989) is a valuable point of entry into the large literature on this topic.

17. Meulenbeld (1999–2002) documents these changes extensively. See also Wujastyk (2005a).

18. Ramsey (1999: 286–91) gives a valuable discussion of terminology and introduces the term *counterhegemonic medicine*.

19. For surveys of these topics, see, for example, Rây and Gupta (1980), Rây et al. (1980); Wujastyk (2003).

20. The authorship of this article is not stated, and this raises the possibility that it is by a member of the committee itself.

21. Whiggish history demonstrates "the tendency in many historians . . . to emphasize certain principles of progress in the past and to produce a story which is the ratification if not the glorification of the present" (Butterfield 1931: Preface).

22. The theorization of the distinction is owed to Shils (1982 [1961]), who described how actors close to the center of society carry or express its main ("core") values, ideas, and beliefs. On the other hand, those who belong to the periphery do not accept or promote such values, ideas, and beliefs to the same extent. He also outlined various processes of dissemination or diffusion from the center, and various forms of tensions between the center and periphery.

23. The Worshipful Society of Apothecaries of London (2003).

24. See the *British Medical Journal* obituary (P.N.C. & G.R.McR. 1973).

25. The Chopra Report's title page states that it is Vol. 1: Report and Recommendations. This is all that is available in the British Library's copy.

26. Some of the key issues arising out of this period have been insightfully explored in a series of studies by Charles Leslie (1972, 1975, 1983, 1992, 1998a [1976]).

27. Dr Udupa subsequently met medical anthropologist Prof. Charles Leslie, and their detailed conversations informed some of Prof. Leslie's later writings on medical professionalization and modernization in India (Leslie 2004).

28. The career and medical and political views of Pt. Sharma are discussed by Leslie (1992: 179–85, et passim), who also reproduces a photograph of him.

29. Further discussion is given in Wujastyk (2005b).

30. For a classic evocation of this balance, see McNeill (1976).

31. Carl E. Taylor, the medical sociologist and anthropologist and colleague of Charles Leslie (see, e.g., Taylor 1998 [1976]), is specifically thanked in the Foreword of the Ramalingaswami Report for his "immense help" in the committee's deliberations and the finalization of the Report (Ramalingaswami 1981: ii).

REFERENCES

Anon. 1964, 1967. *Who Was Who 1951–60: A Companion to Who's Who, Containing the Biographies of Those Who Died during the Decade 1951–60, Who Was Who*, vol. V. London: Adam & Charles Black.

Bannerman, Robert H., John Burton, and Ch'en Wen-Chieh. 1983. *Traditional Medicine and Health Care Coverage: A Reader for Health Administrators and Practitioners*. Geneva: WHO.

Bhore, Joseph. 1946. Report of the health survey and development committee. 4 vols. Technical report. Delhi: Government of India. The Bhore Report.

Brass, Paul. 1972. The politics of ayurvedic education. In *Education and Politics in India*, ed. L. H. Rudolph and S. I Rudolph, 342–71, 452–59. New Delhi: Oxford University Press.

Brimnes, Niels. Unpublished. Coming to terms with the native practitioner: Indigenous doctors in colonial service in South India 1800–1825. Paper delivered at the conference Imperialism, medicine, and South Asia: A socio-political perspective, 1800–1980, Wolfson College, Cambridge, June 15–16, 2001.

Butterfield, Herbert. 1931. *The Whig Interpretation of History*. London: G. Bell. Online edition: http://www.eliohs.unifi.it/testi/900/butterfield/.

Chopra, R. N. 1948. Report of the committee on indigenous systems of medicine. Technical report. New Delhi: Ministry of Health, Government of India. The Chopra Report. Vol. 1: Report and Recommendations (further vols. not available).

Chopra, R. N., I. C. Chopra, K. L. Handa, and L. D. Kapur. 1958. *Chopra's Indigenous Drugs of India*. Calcutta: Dhur & Sons.

Chopra, R. N., R. L. Badhwar, and S. Ghosh. 1965. *Poisonous Plants of India*. New Delhi: Indian Council of Agricultural Research.

Chopra, R. N., S. L. Nayar, and I. C. Chopra. 1956. *Glossary of Indian Medicinal Plants*. New Delhi: Council of Scientific and Industrial Research. 3rd reprint, 1992. Vol. 2, *Supplement to Glossary of Indian Medicinal Plants*, first published in 1969 New Delhi: Publications and Information Directorate, reprinted 1986.

Chopra, Ram Nath. 1941. Organization of public health and medical service in India. *Current Science* (Supplement) 10:2: 109–16. Available at http://www.ias.ac.in/j_archive/currsci/10/vol10contents.html.

Dave, Dayashanker Trikamji. 1956. Interim report of the committee appointed by the government of India to study and report on the question of establishing uniform standards in respect of education & practice of vaidyas, hakims, and homoeopaths. Report. New Delhi: Government of India, Ministry of Health. The Dave Report.

Government of India. 1970. The Indian Medicine Central Council Act, 1970. Technical report. The Hindi text of the act was published in the *Gazette of India, Extraordinary*, Part II, Section 1A, no.33, vol.VII, dated September 9, 1971, pp. 285–318. See http://www.ccimindia.org/1.htm.

Government of India. 2002. The Indian medicine central council (Amendment Act), 2002. Technical report. See http://www.ccimindia.org/ccim_1.htm.

Government of India, Dept. ISMH 2002. National policy on Indian systems of medicine and homoeopathy—2002. See http://www.indianmedicine.nic.in/html/news/draftnat.pdf. Author of PDF file given as "Opey A." Date of PDF file 12/12/2002.

Illich, Ivan. 1986. Body history. *The Lancet*, 328:8519: 1325–27.

———. 1990 [1976]. *Limits to Medicine: Medical Nemesis: The Expropriation of Health*. 3rd ed. London: Penguin. First published 1976.

International Conference on Primary Health Care, Alma-Ata, USSR 1978. *Primary Health Care = Report of the International Conference on Primary Health Care, Alma-Ata, USSR, 6–12 September 1978 / Jointly Sponsored by the*

World Health Organization and the United Nations Children's Fund. Geneva: World Health Organization.

Jaggi, O. P. 2000. Revival of Ayurveda. In *Medicine in India*, ed. O. P. Jaggi. *Modern Period, History of Science, Philosophy, and Culture in Indian Civilization*, series ed. D. P. Chattopadhyaya, vol. 9, pt. 1, chap. 23, 311–18. New Delhi: Oxford University Press.

Kleinman, Arthur, Peter Kunstadter, E. Russell Alexander, and James L. Gale, eds. 1975. *Medicine in Chinese Cultures: Comparative Studies of Health Care in Chinese and Other Societies. Papers and Discussions from a Conference held in Seattle, Washington, U.S.A., February 1974*. Washington, DC: John E. Fogarty International Center for Advanced Study in the Health Sciences.

Leslie, Charles. 1972. The professionalization of ayurvedic and unani medicine. In *Medical Men and Their Work*, ed. Eliot Freidson and Judith Lorber, 39–54. Chicago, New York: Aldine-Atherton. Repr. from *Transactions of the New York Academy of Sciences* 30 (1968): 559–72.

———. 1975. Pluralism and integration in the Indian and Chinese medical systems. In *Medicine in Chinese Cultures*, ed. Kleinman, Kunstadter, Alexander and Gale, chap. 24, 401–17. Commented on in Obeyesekere.

———. 1983. Legal aspects: Policy options regulating the practice of traditional medicine. In *Traditional Medicine and Health Care Coverage*, ed. Bannerman, Burton & Wen-Chieh, 314–17.

———. 1992. Interpretations of illness: Syncretism in modern Ayurveda. In *Paths to Asian Medical Knowledge*, ed. Charles Leslie and Allan Young, 177–208. Berkeley, Oxford: University of California Press. Repr. Munshiram Manoharlal, Delhi.

Leslie, Charles, ed. 1998b [1976]. *Asian Medical Systems: A Comparative Study*, Indian Medical Tradition. Vol. 3. Delhi: Motilal Banarsidass. First published Berkeley, London: University of California Press, 1976.

———. 2004. Personal communication.

Macaulay, Thomas Babington. 1957. Minute of February 2, 1835, on Indian education. In *Macaulay, Prose and Poetry*, ed. G. M. Young, 721–24, 729. Cambridge, MA: Harvard University Press.

Mackworth Young, William. 1894–1895. Indian Hemp Drugs (Mackworth Young) Commission 1893–1894. Report, Simla, Calcutta.

McNeill, William H. 1976. *Plagues and Peoples*. Harmondsworth: Penguin.

Meulenbeld, Gerrit Jan. 1999–2002. *A History of Indian Medical Literature*. 5 vols. Groningen: E. Forsten.

Mudaliar, Arcot Lakshmanaswami. 1962. Report of the health survey and planning committee. Technical report. Delhi: Government of India, Ministry of Health.

Obeyesekere, Gananath. 1975. Some comments on the nature of traditional medical systems. In *Medicine in Chinese Cultures*, chap. 25, 419–25.

P. N. C. and G. R. McR. 1973. Brevet-Colonel Sir Ram Nath Chopra. *British Medical Journal* 5879:3: 547.

Pollock, Sheldon. 1989. Mīmāṃsā and the problem of history in traditional India. *Journal of the American Oriental Society* 109:4: 603--10.

Ramalingaswami, Vulimi. 1981. *Health for All: An Alternative Strategy*. Pune: Indian Institute of Education (distributed by the Voluntary Health Association of India). The Ramalingaswami Report.

Ramsey, Matthew. 1999. Alternative medicine in modern France. *Medical History* 43:3: 286–322.

Rây, Priyadaranjan, and Hirendra Nath Gupta. 1980. *Caraka saṃhita (A scientific synopsis)*. 2d ed. New Delhi: Indian National Science Academy.

Rây, Priyadaranjan, Hirendra Nath Gupta, and Mira Roy. 1980. *Suruta saṃhita (A scientific synopsis)*. New Delhi: Indian National Science Academy.

Shah, Mazhar H. 1966. *The General Principles of Avicenna's Canon of Medicine*. Karachi: Naveed Clinic.

Shankar, Darshan. 1992. Indigenous health services: The state of the art. In *State of India's Health*, ed. Alok Mukhopadhyay, 129–61. New Delhi: Voluntary Health Association of India.

Shils, Edward A. 1982 [1961]. Center and periphery. In *The Constitution of Society*, 2d ed., ed. Edward A. Shils, chap. 4. Chicago: University of Chicago Press. First published in 1961.

Stepan, J. 1983. Legal aspects: Patterns of legislation concerning traditional medicine. In *Traditional Medicine and Health Care Coverage*, ed. Bannerman, Burton, and Wen-Chieh, 290–313.

Taylor, Carl E. 1998 [1976]. The place of indigenous medical practitioners in the modernization of health services. In *Asian Medical Systems: A Comparative Study*, 285–99. First published Berkeley, London: University of California Press, 1976.

The Worshipful Society of Apothecaries of London. 2003. http://www.apothecaries.org/.

Udupa, K. N. et al. 1958. Report of the committee to assess and evaluate the present status of Indian systems of medicine. Technical report. New Delhi: Ministry of Health, Government of India.

Usman, Muhammad. 1923. The report of the committee on the indigenous systems of medicine, Madras [1921–1923]. 2 vols. Technical report. Madras: Government of Madras, Ministry of Local Self-Government, Committee on the Indigenous Systems of Medicine.

Vyas, Mohanlal P. 1963. Report of the shuddha ayurvedic education committee. Technical report. Delhi: Government of India, Ministry of Health. The Vyas Report.

Wujastyk, Dominik. 2003. *The Roots of Ayurveda: Selections from Sanskrit Medical Writings*. 3rd updated ed. London, New York: Penguin Group.

———. 2005a. Change and creativity in early modern Indian medical thought. *Journal of Indian Philosophy* 33: 95–118.

———. 2005b. Policy formation and debate concerning the government regulation of Ayurveda in Great Britain in the 21st century. *Asian Medicine: Tradition and Modernity* 1:1: 162–84.

CHAPTER 4

Divorcing Ayurveda

Siddha Medicine and the Quest for Uniqueness

RICHARD S. WEISS

Practitioners of the three generally recognized traditional Indian systems of medicine—Sanskrit Ayurveda, Tamil Siddha, and Islamic Unani—have often affirmed their solidarity when putting up a united front in their opposition to biomedicine.[1] In other contexts, however, many traditional specialists, *vaidyas* (ayurvedic and Siddha practitioners) and *hakims* (Unani), have drawn, redrawn, and exploited lines of separation, distinguishing branches of indigenous knowledge in order to promote certain practices over others.

These lines closely parallel the political divisions that grew with Indian nationalism. Hindu/Muslim tensions are reflected in Ayurveda/Unani formulations, while an emergent Tamil separatism has encouraged characterizations of Siddha medicine as absolutely distinct from Ayurveda. Siddha *vaidyas*, fearing that their practices will be sacrificed by biomedicine on the altar of reason, or appropriated by Ayurveda in the name of a united India, argue for the separate treatment of Siddha medicine, or, more hopefully, for the absorption of all medicine into Siddha. In doing so, they draw on, and contribute to, broader Tamil utopian imaginings of a pure and unique Tamil tradition.

While the sustainability of Siddha medicine is threatened by the specter of a future that might see it eclipsed by biomedicine, the challenge to the unique identity of Siddha from other indigenous medicines reaches both into the future and the past. In asserting a distinct historical trajectory for their knowledge, Siddha practitioners overwrite a past in which the lines between two discrete medical systems, Ayurveda and Siddha, were not clearly, and rarely even faintly, drawn. Scholars, practitioners, and patients too often assume the durability of these lines that distinguish South Asian medical systems. By examining some of the motivations and strategies by which Siddha *vaidyas* have articulated a distinct medical system, I will suggest a genealogy in Foucault's sense: "The search for descent is not the erecting of foundations: on the contrary, it disturbs what was previously considered immobile; it fragments what was thought unified; it shows the heterogeneity of what was imagined consistent with itself" (Foucault 1984: 82). As genealogies reveal the dispersed nature of origins, a genealogical approach to history likewise reveals "the heterogeneous systems which, masked by the self, inhibit the formation of any form of identity" (Foucault 1984: 95). I argue that the practice of traditional medical knowledge in South Asia is as much a matter of community identity as it is a matter of science.

TAMIL MEDICINE AND AYURVEDA

While today most medical practitioners and scholars in India assume a clear distinction between Siddha and Ayurveda, in the early decades of the twentieth century, many *vaidyas* of these "two" systems of medicine did not clearly define their practices as either Siddha or Ayurveda. As part of *The Report of the Committee on Indigenous Systems of Medicines,* published in 1923, a questionnaire was distributed to practitioners of indigenous medicines and 183 replies were received in several Indian languages and in English. The responses of many practitioners to the question "Which system do you practice?" suggest that the division of traditional practices into three distinct indigenous medical "systems" was not clear. Veluswami Pillai, a non-Brahman *vaidya* responding in Tamil, declared that he practices "Tamil Ayurveda," which Shiva taught to Devi, who taught Nandi, who taught the devas (gods), the munis (sages), and the siddhars (yogis), expressing one of the origin myths claimed by contemporary Siddha practitioners (*The Report of the Committee on the Indigenous Systems of Medicine, Part 2* 1923: 366). Another Tamil practitioner, Shanmukanandaswami, wrote: "I will speak about Siddha medicine, Tamil medicine, or Tamil Ayurveda medicine, which has been practiced in Tamil Nadu from ancient times" (ibid.).

The key distinction highlighted by these practitioners was not that of medical technique, theory, or medicinal preparations but of the language of the texts that serve as an authoritative corpus of medical knowledge. To call one's practice "*Tamil* Ayurveda" or "*Tamil* medicine" was to emphasize that one follows a medical tradition that is transmitted through Tamil manuscripts rather than Sanskrit manuscripts. Yet to call one's practice "Tamil *Ayurveda*" was also to assert an overlap between the medical practices and theories contained in Tamil and Sanskrit texts. V. Ponnuswami Pillai,[2] from Kumbakonam, spoke of traditional medicine as primarily distinguished along linguistic lines yet similar in their methods.

> The three fields of medical knowledge, generally called "Ayurveda," meaning the path to bodily health, were bestowed by the eighteen great siddhars for the benefit of the human world. Though there are no differences in their general principles, and only small differences in their methods of treatment, they are called by the names ayurveda, unani, and Siddha (Tamil) medicine, as they are written in the three important languages of our country, Sanskrit, Hindustani, and Tamil. I will speak of Siddha medicine, preeminent in the South and born in the Tamil country. (*The Report of the Committee on the Indigenous Systems of Medicine, Part* 2 1923: 354)

Pillai was correct to describe the basic principles of these systems as similar, and also to link the most significant difference to language. However, he was wrong in attributing the authorship of all three to the eighteen *siddhars,* since the tradition of Siddha authorship is unique to Tamil manuscripts. *Siddhars,* who in Tamil mythological texts are yogis with supernatural powers, are the purported authors of Tamil medical texts, texts that have come to serve as the ancient canon of a Siddha medical system. When I was doing my research in 1998–1999, practitioners always clearly affirmed their medical affiliation as Siddha, Ayurveda, or Unani, and they generally asserted these as discrete *systems* of practice. I never heard anyone mistake the siddhars as the authors of Ayurveda or Unani. In 1923, while there was a clear sense that medical texts were written in Sanskrit, Tamil, and Urdu, *vaidyas* were less insistent that these different literary traditions reflected distinct medical practices or histories.

In the first half of the twentieth century, the cultural forms generally associated with the emerging Indian national community were Sanskritic, and medicine was no exception. Many Indian nationalists celebrated a coherent ayurvedic system of texts and practices as the medical system of an independent India. An article in the *New India,* August 15, 1919, stated, "Ayurveda is the National system of medicine. . . . There can be no doubt whatever that it is a veritable science, superior to the Western system in its curative value in relation to certain diseases, and indubitably well-adapted to Indian bodies and to Indian constitutions" (Hausman 1996: 182). In line with Gandhi's formulations of an Indian nation that placed classical Hindu texts and idioms at the center of a unified Indian culture, nationalists most often promoted a corpus of Sanskrit medical texts as the basis of an original medical system of a homogenous Indian people. They emphasized the natural differences between Indian and British bodily constitutions as primary criteria of medical and more generally social differentiation in order to mask the linguistic, ethnic, cultural, and racial disparity within India, a move they hoped would unify the diversity of South Asian societies and histories in their opposition to colonial domination.

Sanskrit sources, therefore, would set the agenda for the future of all Indian traditional medicine, and medical texts in other Indian languages were often viewed as flawed translations of Sanskrit originals. M. R. Pandit Narayana writes, "The classification . . . in the Ayurveda, Unani or Siddha is not quite correct; strictly speaking, both Ayurveda and Siddha are comprised in what may conveniently be described as the Sanskrit system of medicine dealt with in the ancient Sanskrit books" (*The Report of the Committee on the Indigenous Systems of Medicine, Part 2* 1923: 247). The other authors of the *Report* present a similar opinion, identifying Siddha as a branch of Ayurveda and thus proposing to examine only Ayurveda.

> All our general observations and recommendations are meant to be equally applicable to all schools of Indian medicine . . . having regard to the views of our experts as to the common foundations of all these three schools [Ayurveda, Siddha, Unani], we have thought it best to consider them all as one triune whole, rather than as so many isolated and independent entities; for we have it on the high authority of Janab Hakim Ajmal Khan of Delhi that Arabian medicine was founded on Ayurveda; and it is well-known that the Siddha and the Ayurveda have very many things in common. (*The Report of the Committee on the Indigenous Systems of Medicine, Part 1* 1923: 1)

Ayurveda is the common term that links all traditional medicine, and throughout the rest of the report, indigenous medicine is solely equated with Sanskrit Ayurveda. The threat to Tamil practitioners since the early decades of the twentieth century has not been simply that their practice will be superseded by Western medicine, but also that they will be viewed as practicing a secondary, inferior form of Ayurveda, a vernacular approximation of the Sanskrit original.[3] Just as Tamil separatist leaders lobbied for an autonomous Tamil state, *vaidyas* who trace their lineages from the siddhars through texts composed in Tamil argue for an autonomous medical space predicated on their formulations of a unique Siddha medical tradition.

NARRATING A UNIQUE HISTORY OF SIDDHA MEDICINE

If Indian nationalists exploited the lack of rigid distinctions in traditional medical practices in early-twentieth-century South Asia in order to articulate and shape a homogenous medical system Sanskritic in character, practitioners who looked to Tamil texts for medical authority felt threatened by this very same contiguity of practices. These Tamil non-Brahman *vaidyas* strove to clarify the fuzzy lines that distinguish indigenous medical practices in India, asserting a radical distance from Brahman ayurvedic practitioners. They did this by narrating a distinctive history and unique character of their knowledge and practices. Paralleling, drawing from, and contributing to a political discourse of difference that was gaining momentum in the early decades of the twentieth century, these *vaidyas* tell a story of an original, perfect medical system that was corrupted with Aryan influence. They try to "untangle" this history of Tamil/Sanskrit interaction by locating their medical history in Tamil revivalist narratives that imagined a Tamil origin of all civilization and society (Thirunarayanan 1993: 2–3).

As early as 1923, Siddha *vaidyas* began to blame the confusion between Siddha and Ayurveda for the decay of Tamil medicine. In response to the question "What, in your opinion, are the causes of decay of the indigenous systems of medicine?" Shanmukanandaswami writes:

> Because both medical texts in Tamil and medical texts in Sanskrit are generally called "Ayurveda." Because even though brahmans are a minority, many of them are educated and they have most government jobs. They support only their own texts and their own language, without allowing Tamil and Tamil medicine to flourish. Tamil doctors have experience but no education. Our Aryan brothers in South India deceptively practice Tamil medicine but call themselves Ayurveda practitioners. [Tamil medicine] is not supported by local chiefs, wealthy people, or merchants, who are confused by their [the brahmans'] deception. (*The Report of the Committee on the Indigenous Systems of Medicine, Part 2* 1923: 341)

This Tamil *vaidya* traces the lack of distinction between Siddha and Ayurveda, the result of intertwined histories of Tamil and Sanskrit medical texts and practices in South India, to deception perpetrated by ayurvedic practitioners, who he feels have no unique medicine of their own. His basis for medical difference is not only language but also race and caste, the Aryan/Dravidian and non-Brahman/Brahman distinctions that were becoming so important in South Indian politics also being played out in medical arenas.

The historical narratives that frame many Tamil *vaidyas'* accounts of the origins of Siddha medicine are a complex mix of European science, Orientalist theories of Aryan migration, and Tamil revivalism. In the last half of the nineteenth century, European geologists extrapolated from new theories of continental movement to posit an ancient South Asian continent. German Darwinian biologist Ernst Heinrich Haeckel picked up on this theory to explain the distribution of lemurs and other species in India, Africa, and Malaysia, calling this land mass "Lemuria" (de Camp 1970: 51–52). Tamil revivalists asserted that Lemuria was the original site of human development and as such contained the seeds of all future human civilization. They further claimed that the original human society was a Tamil society, that Tamil culture is the oldest in the world, and that subsequent human history developed away from an original, utopian Tamil community.[4]

Siddha practitioners have drawn from this revivalist history in formulating a history of Siddha medicine. In 1968, the Tamil government organized the Second World Tamil Conference, a forum to celebrate Tamil traditions. In the proceedings of an auxiliary conference on Siddha medicine, Es. Kē. Es. Kāḷimuttup Piḷḷai, a registered practitioner of Indian medicine, wrote "Our ancestors enjoyed and utilized a medical system that establishes the way to live a life without death. This medicine, called Siddha medicine and Tamil medicine, has been in practice from time immemorial, from the time that the earth first appeared" (Es. Kē. Es. Kāḷimuttup Piḷḷai 1968: 64). Piḷḷai argues that because the Tamil language is the primary language of the world, and because Siddha medicine is Tamil medicine, that Siddha medicine also was the first medical system in the world. "Just as other languages operate taking Tamil as their basis, other medical systems and medical fields function taking Siddha medicine as their basis" (Es. Kē. Es. Kāḷimuttup Piḷḷai 1968: 66).

He imagines a time in which all language was Tamil, all civilization was Tamil, and all medicine was Siddha medicine, a time of ethnic and racial purity. The "time" of which Piḷḷai speaks, even as the Lemurian narratives that claim particular dates for Tamil utopia, is more of the "once upon a time" sort than it is a part of history. This is a time in which anything is possible because being beyond history it is imagined.

Extending Orientalist scholarship, Tamil revivalists tell a history of an Aryan invasion and the subsequent subjection of the Tamil people. They draw on nineteenth-century philologists, most importantly Robert Caldwell, according to whom Aryan Brahmans imposed the caste system on indigenous Dravidians and relegated them to the lower rungs of caste (Caldwell 1998: 112). Tamil non-Brahman leaders employed this history to justify the unification of diverse non-Brahman communities, and to distinguish this group historically and racially from Tamil-speaking Brahmans. This history not only serves to formulate and distinguish communities but also to assert a relationship between these designated communities, specific practices, and particular tracts of land.

> Ayurveda, unani, allopathy, and homeopathy, though practiced in our country at present, are medical systems that entered our country [from elsewhere]. The Aryans came to our country, and over a thousand years later, they created the ayurvedic system, written in Sanskrit. Then the Muslims defeated our country and after establishing their rule, they introduced the unani system, written in Arabic and Urdu. Then the Europeans came and took control, bringing with them allopathic medicine, written in English and in other European languages. (Kastūri 1970)

Kastūri depicts a natural and historical relationship between Tamil medical traditions, non-Brahmans, and the Tamil land. The later arrival of other medical systems, and their introduction by "foreigners," attests that their presence in South India is not only unnatural but threatens the sustained vitality of Siddha medicine.

Tamil scholars tell a tale of blatant Aryan and Muslim plagiarism of Tamil medicine, a plundering of the intellectual and practical wealth of Tamils that led to the dilution of the purity of Siddha medicine and the subsequent loss of its extraordinary effectiveness. In his review of Tamil literature, M. S. Purnalingam Pillai narrates a history in which the practice of North Indian, Aryan ayurvedic medicine began in 500 CE, long after the origin of Siddha medicine. According to Pillai, early authors of ayurvedic texts wrote their treatises based on "borrowed knowledge" after learning medical techniques from treatises written by the Siddhars. However, they claimed this knowledge as their own.

"Now that the Aryans have in course of time enriched their medical science in the way pointed out above [borrowing from Tamil science], they have come forward to assert the Ayul Vaithiam [medicine of longevity] as their own and to look upon their ancient Tamil masters with contempt. The followers of the Siddha School have begun to expose the Aryan indebtedness and prove its comparative modernness to the vexation of the ungrateful" (S. Purnalingam Pillai 1929: 265–66). T. V. Sambasivam Pillai's *Tamil-English Dictionary of Medicine, Chemistry, Botany, and Allied Sciences*, in five volumes, first published in 1931 by the Research Institute of Siddhar's Science in Madras, is a landmark in the modern formulation of a Siddha medical system. Pillai describes Sanskrit medical texts as "literary forgeries [of Tamil manuscripts] mingled with the ideas of Ayurveda in Sanskrit translation" (T. V. Sambasivam Pillai 1931, vol. 3: 2104). Sambasivam Pillai also assigns Siddha origins to Unani medicine, characterizing Muslims as "avowed borrowers of science" and noting the opinion of a "Prof. Wilson" that "the Arabs followed the Siddha works on medicine more closely rather than of the early Greeks" (ibid.).[5]

More than fifty years later, V. R. Madhavan, a Siddha medical manuscript scholar, repeats this narrative of Aryan invasion and pillaging of the "greatness of Tamil culture in all its branches" in order to "enrich their culture by the assimilation of the highly civilized culture of the Tamilians." He blames Aryan theft of Tamil medicine for "causing heavy damages to the independent development of Siddha" (Madhavan 1984: 34). In spite of the harm this plagiarism has caused Siddha, however, Madhavan credits Ayurveda for its "great service to the medical world in collecting, preserving, arranging and incorporating in a marvellous method all the facts then available about the Siddha medicine" (Madhavan 1984: 35). The origins of Siddha medicine that have been obscured by history can be recovered, then, by looking at the best parts of Ayurveda. Indeed, because of its contemporaneity with "Egyptian, Mesopotomian, Chinese and Grecian medicines," Madhavan reasons that literary research into the origins of Siddha medicine, to be "scientific and useful, should commence with a comparative study of the medicines of those ancient civilizations, which will illuminate many of the dark corners of our system" (Madhavan 1984: 52). Reversing the view that Siddha medicine developed out of Ayurveda, Siddha *vaidyas* emphasize the primacy of their knowledge, following the logic of tradition according to which older is better because it is closer to the origin of things.

Siddha *vaidyas* describe a history of degeneration from a prior, utopian time, when Siddha medicine was at its most effective because it most closely reflected the essence of the Tamil people. Indigenous medical practitioners often emphasize this organic connection between an essence of a people and a medical practice. In 1923, Siddha *vaidya* Ponnuswami Pillai writes from Kumbakonam: "Just as each country naturally has a particular type of civilization, education, and religious practice, likewise medicine is appropriate for each country's natural environment, climate, and culture" (*The Report of the Committee on the Indigenous Systems of Medicine, Part 2* 1923: 356). In his opening address of the 1935 "Exhibition of Indian Medicines," Siddha practitioner A. J. Pandian declares that the founders of Indian medical knowledge, the *siddhars* or "Saints, Rishis, or Angels," developed "the subtle treatment that has been prescribed for the very many diseases of our land, particularly suited to the physical and mental constitution of our people" (Pandian 1935: 32). The narrative of the autochthonous essence of Siddha medicine and other components of Tamil tradition justifies an inalienable, organic relationship between Tamils, their land, and their medicine. Kastūri, a Tamil scholar and member of the Coimbatore District Agastya Siddha Medical Association, argues that Siddha medicine is different from all other medical systems practiced in the world.

> Siddha medicine is ours. Just as the Tamil language, the culture (*paṇpāṉu*) of the Tamil people, and the Tamil land (*tamiḻakam*) are ours, in the same way the techniques of siddha medicine are ours. The art of siddha medicine is an enduring treasure which was discovered and passed on by our ancestors. Its excellence suits the Tamil race. Siddha medicine is the method of our country. (Kastūri 1970)

Here Kastūri uses an essentialist argument to claim that Siddha medicine is particularly suited to the culture, language, and racial constitution of the Tamil people. It is a cultural possession, distinguished from other systems currently practiced in Tamil Nadu because of its status as the original medical system of the land and people. By implication, all other medicines are alien to the Tamil region.

The relativistic logic of these assertions that Siddha medicine is uniquely suited to the Tamil people would seem to compel a more general view that there can be no universal medicine. If Siddha medicine is the most effective for Tamil bodies, then the same should be the case for Ayurveda on Aryan, Brahman bodies, and biomedicine for the British. However, Tamil *vaidyas* often juxtapose their claims to relative uniqueness with aspirations for medical imperialism. Virudal Sivagnanayogigal, writing from rural Koilpatti in 1923, questions the desirability of integrating indigenous and Western medicine.

> According to Tamil medical texts, there are 112 mineral substances, 9 metals, 25 types of salt, 64 types of arsenic, . . . and thousands of other medicines. These are not suited for the Sanskrit, Unani, or English medical systems, only for Tamil medicine. Therefore, there is no need for Tamil doctors to learn Western medicines. But if Western doctors learn and use siddha medicines, the differences between the two will disappear, I think. (*The Report of the Committee on the Indigenous Systems of Medicine, Part 2* 1923: 337).

What Sivagnanayogigal prescribes is that integration should not be an absorption of Siddha into other Indian medical systems nor into

Western medicine but of all medicines currently practiced in India into Siddha. As Tamil revivalists trace all rational civilization of India to Tamil civilization, Siddha practitioners promote Tamil or sometimes Dravidian medicine as the original medicine of India, a history that is at the same time an argument that Siddha medicine serves as the "national" medicine of India. As Madhavan argues, "Siddhars were Dravidian in their origin and they were the greatest intellectuals of ancient time [*sic*]. The science of medicine expounded by them, viz., 'Siddha system of medicine,' comprehends the entire system of Indian Medicine" (Madhavan 1984: v).

While *vaidyas* narrate the decay of Siddha medicine, they also assert its contemporary relevance. They finesse this contradiction by positing an ideal space in which a pure Tamil medical tradition bides its time, ready for revival. The knowledge of Siddha medicine is only submerged, not destroyed. B. Āṉantarāmaṉ, a registered Indian Medical Practitioner, writes:

> The eminent siddha medical art has continued for ages (*yukam yukamāka*) in the Tamil land, passed from guru to student in the proper manner (*muṟaippaṭi*). Even though the conclusions set out in [medical] texts have been clouded by history, by the cruelty of foreign governments, by ignorance, and by poverty, the life breath (*uyir mūccu*) of siddha medicine lives on even today among the Tamil people. Thus it is clear that siddha medicine has divine features and stable theories (Āṉantarāmaṉ 1983).

P. Muttukkaruppa Piḷḷai laments the loss of Siddha medical knowledge, destroyed "when the Lemurian continent was submerged in the Indian Ocean," yet he also confirms that traces of ancient medical glory have survived.

> Even though we know of countless texts that were written at the time of the last academy, only a few of those are still available to us. Through those few texts which have survived all these sorts of destruction and which we have in our hands, it is clear that our ancestors attained great expertise in wisdom, clarity, research and service, and rose to the foremost position as the greatest race in the world. With all the great texts written by the siddhars which we still have, is there any limit to the benefits we can obtain? (P. Muttukkaruppa Piḷḷai 1968: 37)

Tamil medicine, like the pure Tamil society of Lemuria, can be purified and revived. Like the utopian homeland of Lemuria, the essence of Siddha medicine has been submerged by history yet remains unchanged. This submerged core of tradition is both behind history and beyond history, testified in its timelessness by its ancientness, its present relevance, and its future potential.

G. Sreenivasamurthi, one of the original forces behind the founding of the Government School of Indian Medicine in Madras and its first principal, gives voice to the hopes of many Siddha practitioners.

> The recent excavations in the North West India had shown that learning and culture had, in very ancient times, gone from South India to many parts of the world, and a day will soon come when through translations from the original difficult Tamil, people all over the world could understand the wonderful Siddha literature which is still mostly a closed book. Then the value of the Baspams and Chendoorams and other preparations would come to be realized.[6] In my vision of the future, I have the picture of students from all over the civilised world coming here, to South India, to learn what only this land could teach. (Subramanian and Madhavan 1983: vii)

Drawing from narratives of Tamil identity that celebrate Tamil civilization as the point of origin of all civilization, Siddha practitioners locate their practice at the pinnacle of human achievement. In narrating a history of Siddha medicine distinct from that of other medical traditions of India, and a future distinct from that of biomedicine, Siddha practitioners strive to establish that their knowledge and techniques have a unique character, an essence that does not derive from any other source and that cannot be absorbed into any other framework. In generating a utopian narrative of the glory of Siddha medicine, Tamil *vaidyas* claim a market for their knowledge beyond the narrow confines of their particular tradition.

THE DISTINCTIVE SCIENCE OF SIDDHA MEDICINE

Throughout the twentieth century, proponents of Tamil tradition have celebrated Siddha medicine as a central part of a story of the rational and scientific nature of the Tamil people. Since the late eighteenth century, defenders of South Asian traditions have sought to establish the scientific character of these traditions. Both Siddha and Ayurveda *vaidyas* have defended their practices as rational when faced with biomedical critiques. Siddha *vaidyas* have often further distinguished their medicine from other traditional practices by arguing that Siddha is the only truly scientific medicine in India.[7] In formulating a character and a history of Siddha medicine, these *vaidyas* draw from broader discourses of Tamil identity and tradition. In turn, Tamil revivalists have celebrated Siddha medicine as an ancient and indigenous Tamil science distinct from Ayurveda, which they describe as "Sanskrit medicine" and thus as false, misleading, and superstitious.

According to the most influential Tamil revivalist histories, Aryan Brahmans subjugated Tamils by propagating Hindu caste ideologies. For one of the early leaders of the non-Brahman movement, E. V. Ramasami, Hinduism is a Brahman "scheme" (*cūḻcci*) to "make Aryans superior, to put other people in the dark so that they could be ruled for the benefit of the Aryan" (Ramasami 1996: 45–46). Its central texts, especially the epics and *dharmashastra*, are instruments of oppression. In 1930, he writes, "The Ramayana and the Mahabharata are the foremost of the Aryan propaganda fictions that were created to capture the Dravidians in the Aryan net and to degrade them, to make them people without self-respect or rationality (*pakuttaṟivu*), and to destroy their humanity" (Ramasami 1972: 11). In a book on Lemurian civilization, Irāma Tarumanīti speaks of an Aryan invasion of South India. He claims that the Aryans first destroyed the great Indus Valley civilization and then set their sights on destroying the Tamil culture of the south (Tarumanīti 1987: 219–20).

> With the change of the times, foreigners entered the Tamil country, attained a high social place, made the Tamils slaves, dug a hole and buried the Tamil language and Tamil civilization. Tamils, seeing the magic and illusions demonstrated by the foreigners, were mentally corrupted (*putti keṭṭa tamiḻarkaḷ*), and bit by bit they lost the four good qualities and became arrogant like animals. No longer knowing the incomparable greatness of Tamil, Tamils, like beggars grasping onto spit, took an interest in the poison [foreign] language. They regarded Tamil as insignificant, and forgot it, rejected it, despised it. (Tarumanīti 1987: 16–17)

It was the loss of rationality (*pakuttaṟivu*), more literally "analytic thought," that led to the loss of the other qualities and the downfall of Tamil civilization. The Aryans blinded the rational nature of the Tamils with their "magic and illusions." These Aryan superstitions, which the more polemical revivalist authors equate with Sanskritic, Brahmanic Hinduism, seeped into the bodies and minds of Tamils. Their original purity tainted, Tamils lost sight of their original scientific nature. The recovery of rationality will put Tamils back in touch with their real selves, will unify the Tamil race, reveal to them the greatness of their language and culture, and set them on the path to a new, ideal Tamil society, envisioned as the revival of the greatness of Lemuria. Siddha *vaidyas* and Tamil revivalists see patronage of Siddha medicine by Tamils and the rejection of medical practices deemed foreign to be an essential part of this return to tradition.

Tamil texts, both medical and classical literature, are the main sources for these reconstructions of tradition. Thousands of palm leaf medical manuscripts, attributed to the *siddhars* and probably authored sometime around the fifteenth century, have been collected into several libraries and archives throughout Tamil Nadu state.[8] Much older literature is also cited as testifying to the ancientness of Siddha medicine and to the scientific nature of the Tamil literary corpus. The *Tirukkuṟaḷ*, or simply the *Kuṟaḷ*, occupies pride of place in this regard. The *Kuṟaḷ* is a collection of 1,330 aphorisms, written around 400–500 CE, probably by a Jain (Zvelebil 1974: 119). It has characteristics that make it well suited to the project to reconstruct a nonreligious Tamil tradition: it contains almost no references to divine beings, is considered to be authored by humans, and is primarily concerned with ethical rather than devotional conduct. The *Kuṟaḷ* appealed to Ramasami, for whom it "is impelled by ideas that are in accordance with practical knowledge, and in tune with Nature and Science. . . . The author of the Kural did not accept God, Heaven and Hell. You could find only virtue, wealth and love in the Kural" (Ramasami 1985: 50–51). Madhavan sees the essence of Siddha medicine contained in the text, which "addresses itself without regard to caste, people or beliefs, to the whole community of mankind. It formulates sovereign morality based on reason. . . . The important and fundamental principles of the Siddha system of medicine are embedded in the Tirukkural" (Madhavan 1984: 10).

Es. Kē. Es. Kāḷimuttup Piḷḷai, a registered practitioner of Indian medicine, sees the rational character of Tamil traditions emerging from the nature of the Tamil language. Piḷḷai claims that Tamil is both the oldest and the only natural language in the world, coinciding precisely with the natural world and therefore being the best language for a science that describes nature.

> It is known through research that what is natural to people—the Tamil language and siddha medicine which is Tamil medicine—must have been prevalent throughout the [ancient] world. The evidence for this is that Tamil is the language which resounds with nature. The best of all animals is the cow. . . . Calves of cows which are abundant in Tamil Nadu today, and calves of cows of foreign countries, think of their mothers and cry only "ammā"! They don't cry "mother" in English which is the language of foreign countries, nor do

> they cry "mātā" in Hindi, the North Indian language which is now stirring up language controversy. Therefore, that Tamil is the mother tongue that resounds with nature is not just something I say but a fact that everyone can agree with. . . . Because Tamil was the only language that corresponded to original nature at the time of the world's creation, all the people of the world must have taken it as their mother tongue. After that, with changes due to the grip (*vacam*) of time, other languages must have emerged, taking the sounds of eminent Tamil as their basis. I say this with authority based on the conclusions of my research. (Es. Kē. Es. Kāḷimuttup Piḷḷai 1968: 64–65)

The natural language of people is Tamil, and the natural medicine of people is Siddha, Piḷḷai argues, because both emerge from "original nature" (*mutal mutal iyaṟkai*) and correspond absolutely to it. Like the Tamil language, Tamil tradition is *the* natural tradition, not just one tradition among many. In this narrative of degeneration from pure origins, Tamil tradition and Siddha medicine are not only unique and original but they also possess universal value.

Madhavan holds that the language itself has healing qualities. "Tamil means Amiltam (Ambrosia) and if one takes amiltam it will bring bliss to oneself. Amiltam or Nectar is also a restorative and reviving medicine towards diseases. Logically the language itself is a medicine" (Madhavan 1984: 2–3).[9] Maraimalai Adikal, the leading proponent of Tamil Shaiva Siddhanta in the twentieth century and a major figure in formulations of Tamil tradition, recounts a story that contrasts the healing nature of Tamil with the injurious effects of Sanskrit.

> In my youth, I would recite the [Sanskrit] Vedas. After reciting, blood would flow from my mouth. I went to many doctors to discover what the reason was for the bleeding. The doctors gave many different answers. For every doctor there was a different answer. I didn't understand it at all. When I'd recite Sanskrit shlokas in the morning, I would become depressed. As soon as I would wake up and recite them, my body would become very weak. After a half an hour, I would recite Tamil songs. Then my sadness would disappear, and I would be happy. One doctor told me to stop reciting the Upanishads and Vedas for fifteen days. I stopped reciting the Upanishads and the Vedas and only sang Tamil. Then the blood stopped! From that time, I decided that Sanskrit is the "blood language." I did some research into the reasons for this difference. Tamil is the language of the great ascetics. Tamil words are constructed in such a way that the strength of our bodies will not dissipate. (Maṟaimalaiyaṭikaḷ 1959: 23-24)

As Tamil is a natural language, the use of Tamil is not antagonistic to the body. So Adikal does not speak metaphorically when he proclaims that "Mother Tamil (*Tamiḻttāy*) protects us. Mother Tamil is not seduced by others. Tamil ceaselessly protects us!" (Maṟaimalaiyaṭikaḷ 1959: 21). He means this literally, that the physical well-being of the Tamils depends on the continuation of their relationship with Tamil. In addition to being the language of science and social unity, Tamil is also the language of health, a view that is expressed by Siddha *vaidyas* in promoting their practices.

In line with these assertions of the rational essence of the Tamil language, *vaidyas* cite the scientific inclinations and natural intelligence of the Tamil people. In his article for the "Siddha Medicine Seminar Special Souvenir," presented at the Second World Tamil Conference in 1968, Ṭāktar Ciṟcapai writes, "Characteristically, Tamils are lively researchers. They are eminent thinkers. Their hypotheses, abilities, and knowledge are amazing. One can even call them the brain of the world" (Ciṟcapai 1968: 78). Most *vaidyas* consider the *siddhars* themselves to best embody this Tamil propensity for rational activity. T. V. Sambasivam Pillai attributes perfect knowledge of nature to the Siddhars, calling them "the greatest scientists in ancient times. Their works in Tamil are supposed to be more valuable than many that have been written in Sanskrit; and they are said to be works less shackled by the mythological doctrines of the original Ayurveda" (T. V. Sambasivam Pillai 1931, vol. 3: 2083). The celebration of the *siddhars* as scientists not only meets the competition of biomedicine, then, but also responds to the challenge posed by ayurvedic practitioners. Indeed, it is the particularly *Tamil* science of the *siddhars* that makes their extraordinary accomplishments possible.

> The said animated mercurial pills according to Siddhar's process would, if retained in the throat, not only enable one to travel in the aerial regions, but also neutralize the action of fire, dematerialize the body, lead one to the path of wisdom, throws [*sic*] the Astral light and serve for various other purposes. No books so far, either in Sanskrit or in any other language except in Tamil Siddha works could be found treating on such a subject; and no nation in the whole world except Tamilians, was aware of this wonderful art. This in itself is a sufficient proof that the highest attainments of the Siddhars in spiritual science are marvelous and awe inspiring. (T. V. Sambasivam Pillai 1931, vol. 3: 2090)

More interesting than the simple claim *that* Siddha medicine has the potential to master the natural world are the *ways* by which it is said to have conquered the world, and the *characteristics* given to the world. In line with the demands of revivalist formulations of tradition, recent accounts of the *siddhars'* mastery of nature stress the scientific and Tamil character of this mastery. Already in their superior control of nature, the *siddhars* have laid the groundwork for the hope of all Siddha *vaidyas*, that their knowledge will eventually master today's global medical world as well. That is to say, while Siddha *vaidyas* claim the essential "Tamil-ness" of their knowledge and its appropriateness for the Tamil people, the criteria through which they judge their knowledge to be specifically Tamil are qualities that also justify its universal application: its durability, its rationality, and its adherence to natural laws.

Tamil revivalists assign particular qualities to various groups: Tamils are rational, Aryans deceitful, the British materialistic, and Muslims carnivorous. *Vaidyas* read these characteristics into medical practice. I. Kastūri speaks of the treatment of damaged organs. Biomedical doctors do transplants, or use artificial organs, corresponding to the propensity of the West to discard the old (i.e., tradition) in favor of the new (i.e., innovation). These British doctors focus only on material realities, believing that if the damaged material is replaced by new material, health will be restored. The ayurvedic doctor, on the other hand, applies medicine that misleadingly appears to effect a cure, while the organs remain damaged. Again, medicine imitates culture, ethnic character, and history, as many *vaidyas* inscribe illusion and superstition at the heart of the character of Aryans. "According to ayurveda, the reasons for the occurrence of disease are god's will, fate, the anger of the gods, or sins committed in past lives" (Kastūri 1970).

Unani (Islamic) practitioners give medicine made from animal organs, reflecting a common stereotype of Muslims as carnivores due to their consumption of beef. "Therefore, these other medical systems do not give the final, true causes [of disease]. The causes given in Siddha medicine are in accordance with reason" (Kastūri 1970). Siddha medicine, therefore, effects permanent relief, because it is a medicine that strives for durability by salvaging old things, whether traditions or organs, rather than discarding them. "Once a patient is cured according to the Siddha medical system, that disease will never return. Siddha medicine cuts disease at its root" (Kastūri 1970).

Siddha medicine cuts disease at its root is because it is the root of all medicines. Ilā Kiruṭṭiṇamūrtti, in language similar to Kastūri's, asserts that Siddha medicine has certain features that make it both unique and highly effective. Of the medicines currently practiced in the world, "English medicine (allopathy) and German medicine (homeopathy) are the most influential and are used by common people. But do these medicines cut at the root all diseases that appear in the body? Do they destroy suffering and give happiness? If one ponders this, it is clear that they do not" (Kiruṭṭiṇamūrtti 1968: 98). Because allopathy and homeopathy have not been successful at curing diabetes, tuberculosis, and other chronic illnesses, Kiruṭṭiṇamūrtti asks: "Have those [medical systems] understood basic, essential medical details, such as the natural classifications of the structure of the human body, the details of that structure, and the natural bases of those classifications? Without a doubt we can see they have not." He includes Ayurveda and Unani in his list of medical systems that do not clearly understand "the nature of disease, the reasons for the onset of disease, the medicines that can remove disease, the supplements that make medicine effective, and the time to give medicines. . . . Is there not a single medical system that can cure all diseases fully?" (Kiruṭṭiṇamūrtti 1968: 98).

Kiruṭṭiṇamūrtti answers his question in the affirmative, that medical practice being one that comes "from our Tamil Nadu," the medical system that is the "mother" (*tāy*) of Ayurveda and Unani, that is, "Siddha medicine," or "Tamil medicine" (Kiruṭṭiṇamūrtti 1968: 98). He claims that Siddha medicine is at least 5,000 years old, and that Siddha *vaidyas* have intuition into the human condition that practitioners of other systems lack. Tamil medical practices attend to more than the physical body of the patient, taking into account the heart (*uḷḷam*) and soul (*uyir*). Thus Siddha *vaidyas* can cure all ailments. Today's Western experts do not know how to stop disease, because they do not attend to the heart and soul (Kiruṭṭiṇamūrtti 1968: 98–100). "*Uḷḷam*" literally means that which is internal, and it more specifically refers to both heart and mind. "*Uyir*" is most simply "life," but in its more active sense, it is that which animates things, the "life breath" of things.

Because Western doctors do not consider *uḷḷam* and *uyir* important, they are inadequate in their understanding of nature. Western science sees the world as dead matter, and so it is itself lifeless, all brain and no heart. Needless to say, lifelessness is hardly a quality that one desires in any medical system that aims to master death. The particular genius of Tamil science is that it penetrates the essence of things beyond mere physicality. It is this common perception of the *depth* of Tamil tradition, its ancientness and its primacy, as well as its claim to rationality, that makes these assertions of the superiority of Siddha medicine to an immature Western science appear credible to a Tamil audience.

Siddha *vaidyas* assign a rationality to their medical knowledge that does not just parallel Ayurveda or Western science but incorporates the depth of tradition and utilizes a "sixth" sense, a "mental eye" or a "wisdom eye" that intuits processes beyond the merely physical (*Tamiḻ (Citta) Maruttuvak Kōṭpāṭu* [Principles of Tamil (Siddha) Medicine]: 5; Kastūri 1970; Velan 1963: 38). As T. V. Sambasivam Pillai, one of the most influential commentators on Siddha medicine in the twentieth century, puts it, what is required for medicine is a "holy science," a science that has "true knowledge and understanding of natural laws." These natural laws are not only physical but require intuitive modes of perception to be discerned. "The mysteries of curing and healing [are] hidden from the eyes, but open to the spiritual perception of the Wise" (T. V. Sambasivam Pillai 1993: 8). Ancient Siddha medicine is this very "perfection" of science (T. V. Sambasivam Pillai 1993: 4). The *siddhars* "were the greatest scientists both material and spiritual," and the "Siddhars' Science" is "the fountain head of all knowledge and sciences" (T. V. Sambasivam Pillai 1993: 42–43). This Tamil science is not only the mother of all science, it also is the *future* of all science, because it has already discovered what Western sciences are only now coming to understand (T. V. Sambasivam Pillai 1993: 26).

Some Tamil social reformers have advocated an approach to traditional knowledge and practices that Ramasami forcefully articulated that "Tamil Nadu will have no salvation unless she is razed to her foundation by a catastrophic deluge or storm, a flood or an earthquake, and then renewed" (Ramasami 1985: 18–19). Siddha *vaidyas*, however, are not anxious to abandon their livelihoods and begin a study of Sanskrit, Ayurveda, or biomedicine. They therefore claim the ancientness and rationality of their practices in order to ratify their knowledge as having the capability to access deeper aspects of the human body and the cosmos itself. They reject the notion that the only authority is a science of medicine or a national Sanskritic tradition that they do not possess, and instead assert that their tradition contains all the insights of science and more. Siddha medicine is not only scientific but just as importantly it is *theirs*, and it testifies to the glory of the Tamil community. As Dr. Ciṟcapai exclaims, "If siddha medicine flourishes, the Tamil land can be proud. The Tamil people will live sweetly" (Ciṟcapai 1968: 80).

CONCLUSION

In the past century, traditional medical practice in Tamil Nadu often has become part of a politics of identity that demarcates the "proper" divisions of community and knowledge as Tamil, Aryan/Sanskrit, and Western. Those practicing medicine based on texts attributed to the *siddhars* today see themselves occupying a unified medical space called "Siddha medicine" or "Tamil medicine," which is itself an essential component of a coherent Tamil tradition. Increasingly, Siddha *vaidyas* have seen the *real* divisions of knowledge and practice as lying between a Siddha medicine *system*, on the one hand, and Ayurveda,

Unani, and biomedicine, on the other.[10] Stepping back to view the effects of these changes on the *vaidya* as a historical subject, it becomes clear that shifting notions of community identity mark not only changes in the way autonomous, stable individuals view their practices, but indeed these notions have transformed the very ways that *vaidyas* view themselves. New articulations of Tamil tradition mark a transformation of the individual medical practitioner from simply *vaidya* to *Siddha vaidya* (*citta vaittiyar*), to *Tamil vaidya* (*tamiḻ vaittiyar*), and to *traditional vaidya* (*pāramparyamāṉa vaittiyar*).

When Tamil *vaidyas* argue for the development of Siddha along its own lines and close ranks in order to protect the "purity" of their knowledge, they assume a natural coherence of practices that have been splintered for as long as we know. The hope of the recovery of an "original" unity is one of the features that sets traditional medicine in modern India apart from prior conceptualizations. With the unification and systematization of Siddha medical knowledge, they claim, the full potential of Siddha practice will be realized, and Siddha medicine will (re)gain its place at the pinnacle of the medical world. The damage wrought by foreign imposition is not permanent, most contend, as the scattering of Siddha medicine has not reduced the value of each of its pieces. "The rare truths of Tamil medicine are like precious hoardings in the minds of many Siddha practitioners. Now is the time to join these as one so that they will increase" (Cuppiramaṇiyam 1940: 51).

The authority of Tamil notions of history, religion, and medicine is justified through an act of identification that links articulations of a Tamil society with reformulations of Tamil tradition. Non-Brahman Tamil leaders characterize the relationship between people, language, and knowledge as natural and organic, effectively "ethnicizing" all knowledge, even as they insist on the universal applicability of their own. The articulation of community identity and the characterization of tradition are not only historically conditioned, but they are formulated as *reflections* of each other in such a way that their conjunction appears natural. In other words, when Siddha healers situate their practice within a narrative of Tamil identity, they contribute to that narrative which in turn frames and shapes the nature of their practice. This mirroring of traditional knowledge and community identity creates the impression of an essential and eternal link between the Tamil community and particular medical practices. This is, however, a *historical* process—the constituents and character of tradition are constantly transformed by a variety of agendas, as are formulations of community identities.[11] The narratives of tradition are myths in the sense offered by Roland Barthes, transforming history into nature and the particular into the eternal (Barthes 1972: 129–41).

These characterizations of Tamil tradition share with all other ideologies the attempt to compose a particular vision of community. The qualities of the rational, the scientific, and the civilized, it seems to me, are articulated in response to depictions of Tamil traditions that have emerged out of Orientalist scholarship, colonial attitudes, Indian nationalism, and rationalist and missionary critiques.[12] These characterizations of Tamil tradition and Siddha medicine as superstitious, or as plagiarisms of the Sanskrit original, were significant enough that Tamil leaders such as Adikal and Ramasami worked to rectify a lack of respect for the Tamil people on an increasingly important world stage. They were keenly aware that science had become an important criterion through which knowledge and practice were legitimated in India and beyond, and that many educated Indians held science to have a universal legitimacy that transcends any particular culture. In this context, the promotion of a Tamil medicine that is rational, scientific, and uniquely Tamil is an attempt to invert portrayals of a superstitious Tamil society and to win for the Tamil community a more respected place in world history.

NOTES

A different version of this chapter is part of the forthcoming monograph *Recipes for Immortality: Healing, Religion, and Community in South India* (New York: Oxford University Press).

1. I use the term *Sanskrit Ayurveda* advisedly, as translations of Sanskrit ayurvedic texts are widely used, and there is much original work in vernacular languages. The term is appropriate here because Sanskrit remains the canonical language of Ayurveda, a point that is emphasized in the discourses that I will analyze in this chapter. Thanks to Dagmar Wujastyk for cautioning me on this usage.

2. "Pillai" or "Piḷḷai" is a caste marker, designating members of a *veḷḷāḷar*, land-owning caste. They have been Tamil scholars and Siddha *vaidyas* for centuries and have been particularly influential in the revival of Tamil tradition and dominate much of the contemporary literature on Siddha medicine. I transliterate "Piḷḷai" with diacritics from an original Tamil source, where spelling without diacritics indicates an English source.

3. In a relatively more recent and influential instance of this view, see Jaggi (1973: 127).

4. For a recent comprehensive history and analysis of Lemuria in its paleogeographic, occult, and Tamil incarnations, see Ramaswamy (2004).

5. This likely refers to Indologist H. H. Wilson, though Pillai does not provide a specific citation, and I have been unable to track down the specific reference. Thanks to Frederick Smith for making this connection.

6. According to T. V. Sambasivam Pillai, *baspam* (Tamil *paṟpam*, Sanskrit *bhasma*) is "oxidized white powder derived from mercury and mercuric

compounds, metals and gems," derived from a process of calcination (T. V. Sambasivam Pillai [1931, vol. 5: 247]). *Chendooram* (Tamil *centūram*, Sanskrit *sindūra*) is red arsenic, or any red chemical preparation (T. V. Sambasivam Pillai 1931, vol. 4.1: 466).

7. These writers also promote Siddha medicine vis-à-vis allopathy, which they consider true insofar as it is scientific, but still inferior to Siddha medicine in its relatively recent origin, in its foreignness, and in its absolute dependence on the empirical method. See Weiss (2003).

8. For the dating of Tamil medical manuscripts, see Venkatraman (1990: 115). For a list and an account of Siddha manuscripts, see Madhavan (1984).

9. *Amiltam* is the Sanskrit *amṛta*, Tamil *amirtam*.

10. In this way, the attempt to unify disparate practices into a single "system" resembles projects in the last 150 years to articulate a coherent religion called Hinduism, of which the most recent influential manifestation is that of the Vishva Hindu Parishad. These medical and religious attempts at unification likewise share a focus on "foreign" others who define the boundaries of tradition.

11. The modern character of this process of identification does not lie in the act of identification itself, since the linking of knowledge, practices, and vocations to particular communities has taken place in South Asia for thousands of years. What is new in this process are the contours of the articulated communities and the ways in which knowledge and practice are conceived to be both traditional and scientific.

12. These Tamil formulations of tradition do not reject everything contained in Orientalist narratives. They retain the depiction of Aryans as alien to Indian soil and of Dravidians as indigenous in arguing for their exclusive right to political control of South India.

REFERENCES

Āṉantarāmaṉ, B. 1983. Nalivuṟṟa Citta Maruttuvarkaḷ Vāḻa Vaḻimuṟaikaḷ ["Ways for Siddha doctors to survive their decline]. *Citta Maruttuva Nūl Ārāycci Nilaiyam Mupperum Viḻā Malar* [Souvenir of the Conference of the Siddha Medical Literature Research Center]. Chennai: Siddha Medical Research Center.

Barthes, Roland. 1972. *Mythologies*. New York: Hill and Wang.

Caldwell, Robert. 1998. *A Comparative Grammar of the Dravidian or South-Indian Family of Languages*. Madras: Asian Educational Services.

Ciṟcapai, Ṭākṭar. 1968. Citta Vaittiyattiṉ Ciṟappum Ataṉ Tevaiyum [The excellence of Siddha medicine and its importance]. *Iraṇṭām Ulakattamiḻ Mānāṭu Citta Maruttuva Karuttaraṅku Ciṟappu Malar*. [Second World Tamil Conference, Siddha Medicine Seminar Special Souvenir]. Chennai: 78–80.

Cuppiramaṇiyam, Eṉ. 1940. *Cittavaittiyattiṉ Muṉṉeṟṟam* [The Development of Siddha Medicine]. Taramapuram, Tamiḻ Nāṭu: Kaṉṉikāparamesvari Press.

de Camp, L. Sprague. 1970. *Lost Continents: The Atlantis Theme in History, Science, and Literature*. New York: Dover Publications.

Foucault, Michel. 1984. Nietzsche, genealogy, history. In *The Foucault Reader*, ed. Paul Rabinow, 76–100. New York: Pantheon Books.

Hausman, Gary J. 1996. *Siddhars, Alchemy, and the Abyss of Tradition: "Traditional" Tamil Medical Knowledge in "Modern" Practice*. PhD diss., University of Michigan.

Iraṇṭām Ulakattamiḻ Mānāṭu Citta Maruttuva Karuttaraṅku Ciṟappu Malar [Second World Tamil Conference, Siddha Medicine Seminar Special Souvenir]. 1968. Chennai.

Jaggi, O. P. 1973. *History of Science and Technology in India, Vol. V: Yogic and Tantric Medicine*. Delhi: Atma Ram and Sons.

Kastūri, Irā. 1970. Citta maruttuvam [Siddha medicine]. *Tiruvaḷḷuvar Īrāyiramāṇṭu Niṟaivu Viḻā Malar* [Commemorative Volume of the Celebration of Two Thousand Years of Tiruvalluvar]. Kōvai, Tamiḻ Nāṭu: Pāventar Pāratitāca- Ma-ṟam. No page numbers.

Kiruṭṭiṇamūrtti, Ilā. 1968. Citta Maruntum Iṉṟaiya Ulakum [Siddha medicine and the world today]. *Iraṇṭām Ulakattamiḻ Mānāṭu Citta Maruttuva Karuttaraṅku Ciṟappu Malar* [Second World Tamil Conference, Siddha Medicine Seminar Special Souvenir]. Chennai.

Madhavan, V. R., ed. 1984. *Siddha Medical Manuscripts in Tamil*. Madras: International Institute of Tamil Studies.

Maṟaimalaiyaṭikaḷ (Maraimalai Adikal). 1959. *Tamiḻiṉ Taṉic Ciṟappu* [The Unique Greatness of Tamil]. Ceṉṉai: Pāri Nilaiyam.

Pandian, A. J. 1935. Exhibition of Indian medicines: Opening address. *The Journal of Indian Medicine* 1:1: 32–33.

Piḷḷai, Es. Kē. Es. Kāḷimuttup. 1968. Cittar Tiṟaṅkaḷ [The powers of the Siddhars]. *Iraṇṭām Ulakattamiḻ Mānāṭu Citta Maruttuva Karuttaraṅku Ciṟappu Malar* [Second World Tamil Conference, Siddha Medicine Seminar Special Souvenir]. Chennai. 64–68.

Piḷḷai, P. Muttukkaruppa. 1968. Cittarkaḷiṉ Vayatu [The age of the Siddhars]. *Iraṇṭām Ulakattamiḻ Mānāṭu Citta Maruttuva Karuttaraṅku Ciṟappu Malar* [Second World Tamil Conference, Siddha Medicine Seminar Special Souvenir]. Chennai. 36–38.

Pillai, S. Purnalingam. 1929. *Tamil Literature*. Munnirpallam, Tinnevelly District, Tamil Nadu: The Bibliotheca.

Pillai, T. V. Sambasivam. 1931. *Tamil-English Dictionary of Medicine, Chemistry, Botany, and Allied Sciences*. 5 vols. Madras: The Research Institute of Siddhar's Science.

———. 1993. *Introduction to Siddha Medicine*. Madras: Directorate of Indian Medicine and Homeopathy.

Ramasami, E. V. (Periyār). 1972. *Irāmāyaṇap Pāttiraṅkaḷ* [Characters of the Rāmāyaṇa]. Tirucchi: Periyār Suyamariyātai Piracāra Niṟuva-a Veḷiyāṭu.

———. 1985. *The Revolutionary Sayings of Periyar*. Translated by R. Ganapati. Madras: Department of Information and Public Relations, Government of Tamil Nadu.

———. 1996. *Tamiḻar Tamiḻnāṭu Tamiḻarpaṇpāṭu* [The Tamil People, The Tamil Country, and Tamil Culture]. Cheṇṇai: Tirāviṭar Kaḻaka Veḷiyāṭu.

Ramaswamy, Sumathi. 2004. *The Lost Land of Lemuria: Fabulous Geographies, Catastrophic Histories*. Berkeley: University of California Press.

The Report of the Committee on the Indigenous Systems of Medicine. 1923. Madras: Government of Madras. Ministry of Local Self-Government.

Subramanian, S. V., and V. R. Madhavan, eds. 1983. *Heritage of the Tamils: Siddha Medicine*. Madras: International Institute of Tamil Studies.

Tamiḻ (Citta) Maruttuvak Kōṭpāṭu [Principles of Tamil (Siddha) Medicine]. No date. Chennai: Tamil Nadu Government, Department of Indian and Homeopathic Medicine.

Tarumanīti, Irāma. 1987. *Kumarikkaṇṭattu Nākarikam* [The Kumari Kandam Civilization]. Vilruppuram: Muttup Patippakam.

Thirunarayanan, T. 1993. *An Introduction to Siddha Medicine*. Tiruchendur, Tamil Nadu: Thirukumaran Publishers.

Velan, A. Shanmuga. 1963. *Siddhar's Science of Longevity and Kalpa Medicine of India*. Madras: Shakti Nilayam.

Venkatraman, R. 1990. *A History of the Tamil Siddha Cult*. Madurai, Tamil Nadu: Ennes.

Weiss, Richard. 2003. *The Reformulation of a Holy Science: Siddha Medicine and Tradition in South India* (dissertation monograph). Ann Arbor, MI: UMI.

Zvelebil, Kamil V. 1974. *Tamil Literature: A History of Indian Literature*. Vol. 10. Edited by Jan Gonda. Wiesbaden: Otto Harrassowitz.

CHAPTER 5

Ayurveda and the Making of the Urban Middle Class in North India, 1900–1945

Rachel Berger

The history of indigenous medicine in India has been predominantly concerned with debates in the interpretation of the major classical texts and with governmental regulation of practice. While these issues are integral to the study of medical history, their scope excludes the social, cultural, and political implications of the role of medicine in society and, in particular, the shifting significance of indigenous knowledge within postcolonial society. A methodology that allows for the exploration of these factors reveals that the practice and theory of Ayurveda in mid-twentieth century urban North India was shaped by the culture and preoccupations of the emerging middle class, and in turn helped the bourgeoisie cement both the practices and ideologies of their social world. At the same time, the colonial state attempted to regulate and institutionalize the practice of indigenous medicine in response to mounting demands for it to address the general health needs of the Indian population. This had the effect of recasting indigenous medicine as a vital and necessary part of North Indian society, while simultaneously establishing the practice of these systems as a respectable profession. An emerging professional identity was mediated through the Hindi public sphere, which emerged as a forum for the dissemination and discussion of ideas among a rapidly widening circle of literate, middle-class urbanites. Journals and magazines, as well as textbooks and novels, particularly from 1920 on, educated an urban public about the variety of health systems, both European and Indian. Steered by a cultural ethos that triumphed the "indigenous" over the "imposed," these authors—and consumers—resurrected the "ancient" practice of Ayurveda as the best means for curing the ills of

India. While these processes have been cast as a vital part of the development of nationalism, in this chapter I will move beyond this paradigm by suggesting that these new concepts were a vital part of social and cultural organization and were made manifest in the "project" of creating social class in the urban United Provinces (UP).

"Indigenous medicine," a term referring mostly to the ayurvedic and Unani systems of medical practice but large enough to encompass anything nonallopathic and non-Western, began to circulate toward the end of the eighteenth century. However, it only became a category of ordered information of relevance to politics in the mid-nineteenth century, as the Raj attempted to discipline all non-European systems of medicine. The first British explorers, traders, and businessmen had been interested in the "medicine of the natives," in part because of their limited access to the cures left behind in Europe.[1] It also was a subject of ethnographic interest to Orientalists and others keen to collect indigenous knowledge.[2] The first efforts of the British Raj in India to curtail the influence of indigenous practitioners over Indian public health came with the attempt to prevent the transmission of the most socially disruptive infectious diseases.[3] The state employed the notion of a threat to the "public health" to assert control over those Indian bodies who "threatened" the colonial order. The cure for these ills was the "modern," allopathic medical system and its practices, as well as its practitioners. While the limited public health measures of the latter nineteenth century were primarily restricted to the control of venereal diseases and of major epidemics, the social and cultural reach of the "body politic" of the state impinged upon the daily practices of Indian colonial subjects.[4] While the masses were free to confer with the practitioners they had always consulted, the consumption of these services, as opposed to allopathic and foreign-staffed ones, was now cast as deliberate choice.

The colonial government began to address the scientific value of remedies and treatments stemming from Indian-grown plants—and identified by native practitioners—in the late nineteenth century, through the formation of the Indigenous Drugs Committee. Relying on the expertise of doctors and scientists trained in the Western scientific schools of botany, medicine, and biology, the members of the committee came together "to consider the question of the extended use of drugs indigenous to India."[5] Over the next two decades, they produced three reports surveying and commenting on the potential of Indian drugs and updated the British Pharmacopoeia of India, neither of which had any real impact on the Indian Medical Service (IMS); the gesture, in the end, was largely an intellectual one. However, the significance of the work done by the committee had relevance long after its demise. In using "scientific" methods to reorder Indian nature, it had simultaneously held up the value of Indian botanical material while denigrating the systems that had traditionally organized this knowledge. Furthermore, the reports presented medically useful components of Indian agriculture as something that Europeans had stumbled upon, of which Indians had been unaware.

Outside the context of this committee, there was still little contact between Indian practitioners of indigenous medicine and the state in the early twentieth century. While several Hakims approached the Government of India with supposed cures for various epidemic illnesses in the years before the First World War, they were summarily dismissed as unscientific practitioners who failed to provide "reliable evidence of the efficacy of the medicine" and who were unable "to state the ingredients of which [the substance was] composed."[6] Interestingly, these Hakims only suggested cures for major epidemic diseases that the Sanitary Commission and the IMS understood as being crucial to public health, including cures for snake bites, plague, influenza, and malaria.[7] The fact that they were peddling specific, public, health-related cures for illnesses led the Raj to categorize them as attempted businessmen with some medical training, not as community-based practitioners looking to forward a particular medical system. This made it possible for the state to dismiss them as neither representative of their community nor authoritative in their knowledge. In short, they epitomized the nonprofessional, potentially exploitative quack "native" that British rationalism—guised in this instance as the benevolence of the master looking out for his subjects—was meant to impede.

These concerns with regulation, standardization, and the registration of medical practice in India were formally addressed in a series of Medical Registration Acts. From the 1910s, these acts had been developed in various provinces, and a National Act was created in 1915, entitled the Indian Medical (Bogus Degree) Bill, and drafted by C. P. Lukis, the director of the IMS. The purpose of the bill was to prevent "the grant to unqualified persons of titles implying qualifications in western medical science, and the assumption and use by such persons of such title."[8] The act defined Western medical science as "western methods of allopathic medicine, obstetrics and surgery, but [did] not include the homoeopathic or Ayurvedic or Unani systems of medicine."[9] The fine for laying claim to being a Western medical practitioner was set at Rs. 500, and it also was stated that only Indian institutions created by an act of government could grant a valid degree, thus rendering invalid the degrees of many practicing doctors. The legislation left little room for misinterpretation, and it was clear that while tolerated, indigenous medicine would not be privileged, or even considered as a part of the scientific tradition.

Despite the limits imposed by the Bogus Degree Bill, and the spirit of racial and social exclusion that was made evident in its rhetoric, its implementation grew somewhat more complicated in various regions of the subcontinent. These acts could reach only as far as the hand of government and were rather limited when dealing with the everyday lives of Indian health consumers. Furthermore, as it became evident on several occasions, most notably in Madras and Bombay in the late 1910s, indigenous practitioners who occupied positions of power in the health sector were crucial to the maintenance of the public health; their sudden illegality of position had the potential to cause major problems for local administrators.[10]

The broad reforms of Indian governance after 1919 transferred responsibility for medicine to provincial control for the first time in 1921–1923, and this was accompanied by a softening in the official attitude toward indigenous medicine. Deepak Kumar, David Arnold, and Mark Harrison have attributed the increased official patronage of indigenous medicine in the 1920s to a growing realization after the First World War that indigenous medicine and medical practitioners played a culturally and financially indispensable role in maintaining the basic health of Indians.[11] The severe strain the war had placed on the availability of medical services and supplies made it impossible to ignore established health systems, regardless of political ideology. However, this perspective has underestimated the importance of the administrative structures themselves in encouraging government to engage with practitioners. Up until 1920, the responsibility of the provinces in health care had been strictly limited to epidemics and their prevention, and even this work had been conducted under the rubric of the (national-level) IMS. The reforms introduced a new system of regional governance that brought the maintenance of basic health care under the care of provincial officials with little experience and few resources, but with much clearer channels of accountability to the local population than had previously been the case. Consequently, this new provincial responsibility represented a significant shift in the ways that health and medicine had to be approached; pragmatism had to outweigh colonial ideology, and systems already in place could not be ignored.

It is at this point that a regional focus is not only useful but necessary. Notions of qualification, standardization, and indeed professionalism itself were determined by region. While the national acts held for those medical interventions concerning government, local health care needs did not come under their jurisdiction.[12] The attempts by the government in the United Provinces to professionalize indigenous medicine illustrate how the social and cultural context shaped the practice, perception, and consumption of health services. The United

Provinces was a crucial location of discussion of the future direction of an independent India, and government policy was considered within an emerging Hindi public sphere that framed debates on the best form of health care for Indian bodies. Indigenous medicine was deemed the appropriate treatment for some bodies, but not others; moreover, the level of training of the practitioner was directly commensurate with the economic worth of the patient. The growing articulacy of supporters of indigenous medicine was reflected in a paradigmatic shift in government thinking; whereas previous stances had lumped all indigenous medicine together into a single, albeit an amorphous, category, government now attempted to untangle the multiple identities and experience of practice that characterized the different systems. At the same time this was the first attempt to consider the place of indigenous medicine in Indian society, beyond the ubiquitous comment that it was widely used by the masses; in essence, the United Provinces state government started to consider the constitution of those masses with regard to medicine.

The United Provinces government remained far behind the indigenous medical establishment, both allopathic and nonallopathic, in its understanding of these issues. From the end of the nineteenth century, Vaids and Hakims had been organizing among themselves to create some tangible efforts at uniformity. The All-India Ayurvedic Council had met annually from 1907, and smaller councils existed throughout the subcontinent.[13] For instance, Vaids and Hakims around the UP had started grassroots programs for students of Ayurveda or Unani, mainly based out of the homes of practitioners. Indian Institutions of higher learning, including Banaras Hindu University (BHU), had funded departments of Ayurveda or Unani medicine, offering some instruction in the art of "traditional" Indian medicine, alongside the practice of allopathic medicine.[14] By the early 1930s, local governments began to understand that the key to the standardization and professionalization of indigenous medicine was the creation of institutions that could produce qualified professionals of a uniform standard.

It was in the schemes to fund and aid these institutions, as well as to create a registry of acceptable institutions, that the social implications of the transformation of a traditional practice into a "new" profession began to emerge. To begin with, the notion of an "institution" was problematic; Ayurveda and Unani had been traditionally taught according to a system of apprenticeship, with a Vaid or Hakim instructing students over a long period of time, and mostly through experience. At the same time, the focus of the training would have depended on the practitioner's own expertise, and most likely on the sort of cases that confronted him. It is doubtful that elaborate guides to medical practice would have been learned in full by an apprentice.

The concept of a degree course, replete with examinations, a dictated notion of progression from subject to subject, and little hands-on experience, ran counter to the traditional process of learning. The course taught in Ayurveda and Unani Tibb conformed to the allopathic norms for medical instruction, which both local practitioners and local government felt added to the credibility of the course.[15]

The shift from "home"-based learning into the "world" of public learning was of great social and pedagogical relevance.[16] The move from one's local setting to a state-sanctioned institution almost always meant the movement from a rural to urban area, as all of the state-approved institutions were located in urban centers, even if situated outside of the major cities of the province. For instance, even schools in relatively remote cities such as Haridwar and Meerut presented a shift for students who had come from the village. This process of relocation served to eliminate the specific local illnesses and remedies that a student would have encountered when studying in a remote area in favor of providing a rounded education. In so doing, it pushed the notion that the systems being studied were universal and should not be bound by local practice. It also initiated the students into a new category of practitioner, where he or she (though there were very few women studying at the time) had more in common with his or her fellow students as official Vaids or Hakims than with those who lacked certification.

The result of this was to train a cadre of professional Vaids and Hakims capable of treating the body regardless of the illness encountered or the location at hand. The subsequent effect was the further marginalization of rural-based, untrained medical practitioners who did not conform to the system. Impacting this difference was the economic gap between the two groups. Attending an ayurvedic or Unani Tibb course was a significant financial undertaking, and only those who could afford the training could access the course, thus making the population of trained Vaids and Hakims a relatively self-selecting group. Furthermore, the income scale ensured that those with a degree certificate would make significantly more than those without it, and would have access to a more prestigious level of clientele. Those who attended institutions supported by the state were in turn granted the privilege to issue death, age, and medical certificates to those employed in government service, the trade that provided a more lucrative option than merely treating illness or vending medicines.[17] At the same time, a Vaid's or Hakim's services were still cheaper and more accessible than those of an allopathic doctor, therefore ensuring them a larger patient base. In addition, the government's decision to cut back on its costs by allowing Vaids and Hakims to issue these official certificates ensured their employment by multiple cadres of society.

Regardless of economic imperative, the choice to employ the services of a Vaid was a socially and politically charged one and reflected deeper concerns about the state of the community and one's role within it. Sanjay Joshi, in his work on the social structure of North Indian society, argues that the formation of the middle class was an often self-conscious process, fueled in part by the new opportunities for educated men and women, and predominantly occupied with the self-fashioning of social belonging through cultural production.[18] The Vaids and Hakims, newly certified by state institutions, were involved with this "project" in part because of their career status, but mostly because of their prominence in the emerging discourses of community belonging being disseminated to the Hindi-speaking public. The early decades of the twentieth century saw the massive growth of Hindi printed materials and the widespread dissemination of these works. This was fueled in part by the standardization of various Hindi dialects into a uniform language, based on *Khari Boli Hindi* (lit: upright dialect) that the Hindi used in bazaars throughout the north.[19] Within a few short decades, and despite the illiteracy of the vast majority of the population, the printed word had become an indispensable part of the performance of public life.[20] Fueled by nationalist and anticolonial sentiment and the fervor of a gradually collectivizing nation, the Hindi printed word became the forum for the dissemination and discussion of public ideals and sociocultural norms. However, the public sphere was initially engineered and later maintained by those who could participate in it directly, namely, those who could read and write; while the participation of the illiterate was made possible through the public reading of Hindi writing, their agency in determining what would be printed was not as straightforward. Ultimately, this served as another indicator of social status and conforms to Joshi's notion of public performance being central to the making of the middle class; participation in—and, in fact, control of—the public sphere was integral to this social project. At the same time, it ensured that the mores and opinions of the middle class became normative for the population of the United Provinces, despite the relatively small demographic that could participate directly.

It is in this material that we see the social and cultural implications that shaped the notion of indigenous medicine outside of the government discourse. While government insisted on holding up both Ayurveda and Unani in order to deflect accusations of communal favoritism, the former outweighed the latter overwhelmingly in public discussion. This offers insight into the reality of late colonial Indian nationalism, especially in the UP: from the 1920s on, in a context of increasing tension between communities, Hindu identity underwrote the use of Hindi as an anticolonial strategy. Hindi nationalism was only a step away from Hindu nationalism. It was in this context that Ayurveda was resurrected as the means of curing the ills of Indian "society" as well as Indian bodies. Its authority as a state-sanctioned medical system refuted the original European claim that Indian science was inherently inferior and resurrected the glory of a past era when timeless wisdom, in the form of the Suśruta- and Caraka-Saṃhitās, had been created. At the same time, it sited the nationalist discourse on a tangible object, namely, the "Indian" body, thus locating the individual's lived experience at the center of the struggle.

Medical writing made up a large part of the public sphere, and indigenous medicine was a frequent subject of debate and discussion. Hundreds of Hindi guides to *cikitsā* (medicine), *ārogya* (health), and *Āyurveda* were printed from the 1920s on, aimed at a relatively ignorant audience. The structure of the text that was most often replicated was the printing of Sanskrit *ślokas* on health and disease followed by a translation and an explanation in Hindi. The books were short, affordable, and well-demarcated, and they were broken down into useful subject headings, giving them the appearance of being user-friendly guides to common health practices. The writers varied in expertise, ranging from ayurvedic practitioners to those who attempted to maintain an "ayurvedic balance" between mind, body, and spirit in their everyday lives. Despite the strict government control over who could and could not practice, there was more flexibility in the publishing world to speak authoritatively about medicine; scientific information coupled with ideological leaning could construct authority. Common to all of these writers was a strong sense of Ayurveda and indigenous medicine as the appropriate mode of treating Indian bodies, both healthy and diseased. Their allegiance and interaction with the larger nationalist project, both in thought and in activity, varied based on the year of publication and on the author. These allegiances often made themselves felt in the tone, language, and composition of the text contained within the book, and in a few cases, in the visual imagery employed by the author and publisher.

Of all the texts published during this time, Haridas Vaid's *Cikitsā Candrodaya* seems to have been among the most detailed and most popular. Vaid published his encyclopedia, which ran into eight volumes and multiple editions, under the auspices of his own Haridas & Co. The number being published rose dramatically from a mere 1,000 copies of the 1920 version to 3,000 copies per volume in 1930. The price, however, remained at Rs. 3 per volume, no surprise, as the price per entire collection rose from Rs. 3 in 1920 to Rs. 24 in 1930, when all of the additional volumes are taken into account; Vaid took this into consideration, fixing the charge per volume at 4 *annās*. There is evidence of this being an ongoing project in the form of single, additional volumes published individually throughout the 1920s, adding on to the original 1920 edition, though it seems as if writing stopped in 1930 at the conclusion of the eighth volume.

Vaid's book differed from others of the period in both form and content, and it was undoubtedly these differentiating features that secured its popularity. Where other medical books published at this point embraced pictorial diagrams, they were normally limited to the part of the body being discussed, and they often seemed to have been drawn by hand. Vaid took a huge leap by often reproducing the entire figure of the male body, even when only one organ was being discussed, as well as inserting photographs and painted portraits of exhibited medical conditions. These depictions of illnesses and bodies bring to light the question of representation involved in a visual rendering: while the rhetoric of medical writers such as Vaid was bound up in the racial politics of nationalism, which often served to classify both disease and treatment as decisively Indian or non-Indian, the images used often depicted white men, or white body parts. While the printed and drawn diagrams were carefully demarcated as "Indian"—made visually evident by a *tīkā* mark on the forehead, a certain rendering of facial features, or the inclusion of a "Gandhi cap" on the head of the figure—there was no accounting for the discrepancy between the rhetorical and the visual.[21] This is particularly strange, as Vaid seems to think that the value of his collection came from its strong adherence to the rigors of the Indian corpus and the subcontinental environs, as well as the strong pictorial evidence he provided; the ambiguity of meaning relating to the individual pictures was left undiscussed.

Other writers of the period were more emphatic in constructing indigenous medicine as beneficial to the local body, and abhorrent to the foreign; conversely, foreign medicine, understood largely to be synonymous with the term *allopathic*, was thought to work only on the bodies of those within the region of its development. According to Shyamsundar Sharma, author of a guide to Ayurveda in 1925, "Even in England, the question of climate is often raised. Between England and France there is distance of only a few miles; but on several occasions, the doctors of France have discarded English medicines, saying that the climate of that place does not suit the patient in the country. And so have the doctors of England rejected the French medicines on the same ground."[22] This claim to an essential composition treatable only by the medicine available indigenously was a common theme among those writing medical books for popular consumption in the early twentieth century. The stock theme inspiring more than a few forewords, commentaries, book jackets, and other peripheral comments on the text boasted an understanding of the Indian body as inherently intolerant of Western medicine.

The motives behind the various points of engagement with the question of universality remain unclear or, rather, disjointed. Sharma, for instance, engages with a sociopolitical message of resistance, claiming that the allopathic response, while differentiating between European bodies, maintains that "medicine in every climate is supposed to suit an Indian."[23] He therefore hints at the racialization of medicine and at understanding it as part of an imperial agenda. He continues by making the point that "this even throws considerable light on the fact that in favouring Allopathy at the cost of indigenous medicine, commercial and mercenary motives were also prominent."[24] Others were less focused on the potential for financial exploitation contained within the colonial medical system, and instead they highlighted aspects of allopathic medicine they found problematic. For Gandhi, in one of his first books on medicine, it was the singular focus on hygiene employed by state medicine, which failed to cogently incorporate diet, lifestyle, and health into its agenda.[25] At the same time, for many of the writers the "othering" of different medical systems had more to do with domestic politics than with foreign ones; the emphasis often was on the Hindu body, the Hindu "religion," and, ultimately, the Hindu nation. Despite the binary of foreign and local employed in these texts, the Indian body in question was characterized by a very particular classed and casted identity.

Despite the variance in the text and the difference that can easily be categorized as the most significant in this instant was the inclusion of a section on women's health. Almost completely lacking in the traditional literature, every guide to health and health care in the twentieth century included at least one chapter, if not a full section, dedicated to the female body. For the most part, these sections were dominated by concerns about the reproductive system of the female, and they went into great detail on the topics of conception, gestation, delivery, and postnatal recovery. However, by the 1930s, and most prominently in Vaid's in-depth medical guide, there were discussions of extra-reproductive aspects of the female body, as well as the use of female diagrams in discussions of both the function and disease of nonreproductive parts of the body. At the same time, women began to author books and to sell them in great numbers to other women, thus increasing both the size of the audience and the amount of writing that circulated during the period.[26] Most prominent among these female authors was Yashodadevi, the daughter and wife of ayurvedic practitioners in Allahabad, who authored over forty books on women's health and the sexual life of the couple.[27] The construction of gender in her works also reveals the extent to which Yashodadevi and those who wrote similar texts were engaged in delimiting social class. In her dissemination of recipes, remedies, and health-related instructions,

Yashodadevi ignored all of these social processes associated with preparation and consumption and put forth instead an uncomplicated ideal of health nutrition that was far removed from the lived experience of cooking and eating in middle-class households. Always absent from her work were references to the labor of cooks, *dais*, domestic servants, and the myriad others who actualized the living of a middle-class life. It is in this subset of the genre of medical writing that sexuality, reproduction, and the question of population all became interlinked with notions of class, caste, and communal belonging, and came to constitute the basis for discussions of the actualization of the modern Indian nation as envisioned by its Hindu citizens.

The content and information contained within these different texts varied greatly and covered a wide range of topics from many different perspectives, ranging from the scholarly to the decidedly amateur. However, the concern of all of the authors remained similar at its center: to define Ayurveda as a visceral part of one's identity as an "Indian." This is why a discussion of bodies and their constitution provided such a fruitful ground for investigation: by linking the politics of nationalism to the everyday managing of the most basic, mundane, albeit, indispensable, routines of the individual, it made the most intimate of subjects the topic of public discussion. Furthermore, it expanded the idea of the public to incorporate women, and the parameters of acceptable debate to include sexual and reproductive functioning, thus breaking two highly entrenched taboos. At the same time, by including women as authors, consumers, and subjects of discussion, a space was secured for the medical discourse in the everyday routines of the domestic space, which worked to further ingrain it into the lives of the average, middle-class family. This had the effect of normalizing the medical information as part and parcel of everyday life, while simultaneously constructing the family that practiced healthy living techniques as the normative model in an ideal Hindu nation, represented in this instance by the microcosm of the household.

Central to this discussion is also the notion of who was left outside it. In positioning Ayurveda as the dominant medical tradition of North India, others were excluded. Most importantly, Unani medicine was rarely discussed in Hindi and was relegated instead to discussion in Urdu and discussion within the Islamic community. While Hakims still had a role to play in the Hindi public sphere, they generally did so by laying claim to the supposedly neutral notion of indigenous medicine, which was coded as Ayurveda in public discussion. Rural practices were marginalized in the same way that rural practitioners had been by the certification system; the ayurvedic system being presented had to apply to all "appropriate" bodies across a vast territory, leaving no room for regional specificity. At the same time, those living outside of the dominant communities were excluded from its reach; for instance, several Dalit writers, most notably Omprakash Valmiki in his memoir *Joothan*, have written about the difficulties in obtaining medical treatment.[28]

It was the science of Ayurveda, reincarnated in the twentieth century as a banner heading for any nonallopathic medicine practiced by Hindus, that the authors of the twentieth century used to lay claim to social and intellectual authority and political viability. These guides paid little attention to the methodological approach contained within the ayurvedic tradition, balancing medicines instead of humors, and focusing on specific instances of illness instead of taking a holistic approach to health and disease. However, by playing up the distinct "Hinduness" of Ayurveda, they could lay claim to social legitimacy for their medical claims. Similarly, they relied upon the intellectual authority of the tradition as an established school of philosophy, coupled with the social legitimacy provided by their assertion as to the specifically Hindu nature of the tradition, to claim legitimacy for the varied medical advice suddenly falling under the category of ayurvedic medicine. However, the most important and most subtle claim to legitimacy transcended the rhetoric and was instead made manifest in the form of its dissemination: the authors recorded their message and referenced the ayurvedic *shastras* in the pages of their books, if not by scholarly notation than by a mere mentioning of the traditional texts. By moving medicine out of both the technical manuals and the informal pathways of knowledge and into the printed vernacular in the public sphere, the authors of the twentieth-century guides to Ayurveda carved out a niche for their writing that evoked that of a long-gone era. At the same time, it envisioned a future where a strong Indian nation of healthy citizens, constructed in this discourse as Hindu, twice born and middle class, would live happily according to the modern interpretation of Vedic ideals.

By the late colonial period, Ayurveda had shifted significantly away from the amorphous category of indigenous medicine. Though shifts in policy had helped bring about this change, it was ultimately the public discussion of its merits, its limitations, and its value to Indian nationalism that determined its social and cultural relevance. Faced with the choice of health systems, and steered by a cultural ethos that triumphed the "indigenous" over the "imposed," these authors—and consumers—resurrected the "ancient" practice of Ayurveda as the best means for curing the ills of India. The discourse of Ayurveda in the Hindi public sphere illuminates the social networks and the consumption patterns of the emerging middle class, a key constituency of the North Indian nationalist movement. Studying the practice of Ayurveda in UP illuminates not just the social life of medicine in a colonial setting but also the class formation "project" of the Hindu middle class. Furthermore, Ayurveda was increasingly placed within a domestic context emphasizing hygiene, diet, and aspects of family well-being, thus creating a new genre of guides to middle-class life that claimed the authority of Ayurveda but mapped out the normative practices of the bourgeoisie. Finally, an exploration of this sort begins to bridge the gap between the official and social discourses of medicine and indigenous knowledge in the late colonial period.

NOTES

Many thanks to Seema Alavi, Polly O'Hanlon, Emma Reisz, and Sarah Wilkerson for comments on this work. In referencing, I have used the following abbreviations: NAI for the National Archive of India, UPSA for the Uttar Pradesh State Archive, and OIOC for the Oriental and India Office Collection.

1. See, for instance, de Figueiredo (1984); Pearson (1995).

2. The Asiatic Society of Calcutta regularly contemplated the origins of Indian medicine and their connection to the development of medicine in the West in its journal *Asiatick Researches*. See, for example, the well-known and little-read article by Sir William Jones, "On the Literature of the Hindus, from Sanskrit, Communicated by Goverdhan Caul, with a Short Commentary," *Asiatick Researches*, vol. 1 (1783–1784). Similarly, the Medical and Physical Society of Calcutta often dedicated articles about indigenous health practices in its publication, which was meant to provide information about health and medicine to doctors and surgeons around the subcontinent.

3. See, for example, Peers (1998).

4. Arnold (1993) and Harrison (1994) stress the reach of the state in their respective works on public health in India.

5. NAI Home (Medical) 15–18A (December 1895): 789–799.

6. NAI Home (Sanitary) 326 (April 1907).

7. For example, Syed Raziul Hossains prepared medicine for the cure of plagues.

NAI Home (Sanitary) 325–326 (April 1907); Mohamed Hidatayul Hasan Treatment of Malaria NAI Home (Sanitary) 187–88B (December 1909).

8. NAI Home (Medical) 174 (December 1915): 23.

9. Ibid.

10. This is particularly true in Poona. A medical dispensary that began to receive state funding many years after its inception was found to be run by a *vaid*. The state pulled its funding, and the dispensary had to close. However, the IMS officials in Poona petitioned the government to reopen the dispensary, despite the lack of allopathic involvement in its administration, claiming that the threat to the public health of the community would be in decline if this free clinic was closed. Furthermore, IMS officials argued that they were understaffed and overworked, and depended on dispensaries, even if unofficial, to play a part in the dispensation of health materials. Ultimately the Bombay Presidency Act negated the retroactive claim inherent in all of the

Medical Registration Acts throughout the subcontinent, and instead inserted a claim that no other clinics that relied on indigenous medical practitioners were to be funded by state money.

11. Kumar (1997); Arnold (1993); Harrison (1994).

12. See the chapter by Dominik Wujastyk in this book.

13. Pamphlet, All-India Ayurvedic Council, 1921.

14. See, for example, UPSA Medical, File no. 32/20, Box 7, 1920, on the Establishment of Medical Schools in the Province, and UPSA Medical File 244/1944, 1944, on the official status of BHU's faculty of Ayurveda.

15. The question of appropriate texts had been a concern of the national government from the 1910s, culminating in a survey done in 1916 of texts used in different provinces of British India by practitioners of the Ayurveda, Siddha, and Unani. NAI Home (Medical) 26-50A (June 1919), 411.

16. Partha Chatterjee (1989) has transformed Tagore's metaphor of *Ghare-Bhare* into an eloquent separation of public space and private space.

17. UPSA Medical File 165, 1923, p. 23.

18. See Joshi (2002: 2–3).

19. See Orsini (2002: 2–3).

20. See Bayly's (1996) pioneering work on the matter.

21. See Tarlo (1996). and Collingham (2001) on the importance of visual markers of racial and ethnic identification as reflected through clothing.

22. S. Sharma, *Ayurved-Mahantva* (Lucknow: 1925), 13.

23. Ibid.

24. Ibid.

25. See the introduction to M. K. Gandhi, *Arogy Sadhan* (Lucknow: 1932).

26. See Orsini (2002) and Gupta (2002) on the significance of women as authors and consumers to the development of the Hindi public sphere.

27. See Gupta (2000: 188–90) and Prakash (1999: 148–54) on Yashodadevi.

28. See Valmiki (2003: 2–43); Chauhan (2002: 10).

REFERENCES

Arnold, David. 1993. *Colonizing the Body: State Medicine and Epidemic Disease in Nineteenth-Century India.* Berkeley: University of California Press.

Bayly, C. A. 1996. *Empire and Information: Intelligence Gathering and Social Communication in India, 1780–1870.* Cambridge: Cambridge University Press.

Chatterjee, Partha. 1989. The nationalist resolution of the women's question. In *Recasting Women: Essays in Colonial History*, ed. Kumkum Sangari and Sudesh Vaid, 233–54. Delhi: Zubaan.

Collingham, Elizabeth M. 2001. *Imperial Bodies: The Physical Experience of the Raj, 1800–1947.* Cambridge: Cambridge University Press.

de Figueiredo, J. M. 1984. Ayurvedic medicine in Goa according to European sources in the sixteenth and seventeenth centuries. *Bulletin of the History of Medicine* 58:2: 225–35.

Gupta, Charu. 2002. *Sexuality, Obscenity, Community: Women, Muslims, and the Hindu Public in Colonial India.* New York: Palgrave.

Harrison, Mark. 1994. *Public Health in British India: Anglo-Indian Preventive Medicine 1859–1914*. Cambridge: Cambridge University Press.

Jones, William. 1783–1784. On the literature of the Hindus, from Sanscrit, communicated by Goverdhan Caul, with a short commentary. *Asiatick Researches*. Vol. 1.

Joshi, Sanjay. 2002. *Fractured Modernity: Making of a Middle Class in Colonial North India*. Delhi: Oxford University Press.

Kumar, D. 1997. *Science and the Raj 1857–1905*. Delhi: Oxford University Press.

Orsini, Francesca. 2002. *The Hindi Public Sphere, 1920–1940: Language and Literature in the Age of Nationalism*. Oxford: Oxford University Press.

Pearson, M. N. 1995. The thin end of the wedge: Medical relativities as a paradigm of early modern Indian-European relations. *Modern Asian Studies* 29:1: 141–70.

Peers, Douglas M. 1998. Privates off parade: Regiments and sexuality in the nineteenth century Indian empire. *International History Review* 20:4: 823–54.

Prakash, G. 1999. *Another Reason: Science and the Imagination of Modern India*. Princeton, NJ: Princeton University Press.

Tarlo, Emma. 1996. *Clothing Matters: Dress & Its Symbolism in Modern India*. Chicago: University of Chicago Press.

Valmiki, Omprakash. 2003. *Joothan*. Translated by Arun P. Mukherjee. Kolkata: Mandira Sen for SAMYA.

HINDI SOURCES CITED

Chauhan, Surajpal. 2002. *Tiraskrit (Disregarded)*. Ghaziabad: Anubhav Prakashan.

Chaube, Datt Ram Narayan. 1912. *Nutanā Cikitsā Cakravartī*. Moradabad: Nawal Kishore Press.

Sinha and Sinha. *Ayurvedīya-Koṣa: An Encyclopoedical Ayurvedic Dictionary*. Baralokpur-Ithava: Prakashak Duara Surakshit.

Gandhi, M. K. 1932. *Ārogya Sādhan*. Lucknow.

Sharma, Jagannath. 1915. *Ārogya Darpan*. Prayag: Hindihiteshi karyalaya.

Sharma, Shyamsundar. 1915. *Āyurved-Mahantva*. Lucknow: Nawal Kishore Press.

Vaid, Haridas. *Cikitsā Candrodaya*. Calcutta: Haridas and Co.

CHAPTER 6

The Ayurvedic Diaspora

A Personal Account

ROBERT E. SVOBODA

Ayurvedic traditions have long been plural all over India, but for some millennia now what most nonmedical people think of when they think of Ayurveda is the Sanskritic, professionalized, commercialized tradition that has since its inception focused on treating society's elites. However, Ayurveda, and medicine in general in India, is not now and never has been the exclusive province of physicians. Even today there are thousands of otherwise nonmedical people all over India who have somehow learned a diagnostic or treatment method and regularly use it to alleviate suffering. I have met many who follow nonprofessional traditions, including "*sādhus*" who pass on to their disciples both medical knowledge and respect for the forest, "*vanavāsīs*," for whom the forest continues to serve as home, temple, and pharmacy, and an array of local healers who treat spirit illness. The bulk of ayurvedic energy and attention has, however, been focused for more than two millennia on the professionalized tradition.

Its history has been studied, though we are still far from having arrived at a continuous and comprehensive picture. Certain phases in and aspects of the history of Ayurveda have been highlighted in historical, philological, and sociological writings, such as the early phase of ayurvedic codification; the development of ayurvedic literature; the challenges Ayurveda met with in the nineteenth century with the introduction of Western medicine to India and its support through the British colonizers; and Ayurveda's renaissance and transformation into "modern Ayurveda," which began with the cultural revivalism that swept India during the latter decades of the nineteenth century and through the entire twentieth century.

This most recent bout of re-professionalization and institutionalization, which has occurred within the confines of a social and cultural context significantly different from that of 2,000 to 3,000 years earlier, has been pursued with the best of intentions, though results have been different than anticipated. My mentor, the Aghori Vimalananda, liked to observe about the Law of Karma, "How can anyone talk about the end justifying the means, when the end IS the means!" All means employed toward whatever noble end act as causes that inevitably produce unpredicted, and often deleterious, effects. In this case, modern ayurvedic colleges and institutions developed as reactions against colonialist overlords—and a significant feature of subsequent ayurvedic polity has since been a reactionary justification of its existence via ancient customs and mores. Contemporary organized ayurvedic education began as a political act—and since that time it has never been possible to divorce politics from it. When I attended the Tilak Ayurveda Mahavidyalaya in Pune, between 1974 and 1980, different interest groups rivaled for influence on the school's education policies. These groups were the following:

1. the currently prominent political parties of the day (at that time and place the Congress, and one or another incarnation of the Socialist Party);

2. groups that supported the teaching of Ayurveda through the medium of English, and groups that insisted on the "regional language" (Marathi) alone;

3. communal groups whose ideologies were based on competition between Brahmans and Marathas (though this competition was never explicit);

4. medical groups, split into two rivaling factions—the proponents of *Śuddha Ayurveda* against those of *Miśra Ayurveda* (Pure [*śuddha*] Ayurveda) was then temporarily in the ascendancy, following the efforts of eminent *vaidyas* such as Pandit Shiv Sharma to standardize a nationwide ayurvedic syllabus in which any modern medicine would be taught solely within an ayurvedic framework. Advocates of mixed (*miśra*) Ayurveda aimed at that time to create instead a sort of giant umbrella therapeutic structure (informally termed *curopathy*) in which all effective therapies for all conditions would be gathered, regardless of their medical system of origin. Given the contemporary level of fascination with allopathy, the unspoken understanding was that allopathic remedies would have pride of place; and

5. institutional or administrative groups. For example, the school was run by a society known as the Rāṣṭrīya Śikṣan Maṇḍal, and passionate wrestling for control of this body was continual. Rumors swirled daily, most speculating on how long the then-college principal (who sat effectively in the Śuddha-English-Brahman-Congress camp) would be able to hold onto his chair against the most recent onslaught of the opposing (roughly Miśra-Marāṭhi-Marāṭha-Socialist) bloc.

The results of these machinations were as sociologically fascinating as they were academically debilitating. Of the roughly 130 students who entered the college with me in 1974, 65 eventually completed the BAMS course with me in 1980. Of these, at least 90 percent were there out of necessity rather than design, their previous examination results being a few points below the cutoff that would have permitted them to apply to allopathic colleges. These roughly 60 students openly declared their intentions to practice allopathy in their villages after graduation, no matter what their degree might say; they had entered the college with this resolve, and their six years there had for most of them merely confirmed them in it. (My friends who are currently associated with ayurvedic colleges tell me that the situation is improving, slowly, and that now only 70 percent or so of the students in the colleges would rather be elsewhere. Given conditions, this seems a positive result.)

The majority of my fellow students had had no positive personal experience of ayurvedic treatment previous to our course, and few felt they saw positive benefits from Ayurveda during the course. Most held both Ayurveda and its practitioners in some degree of self-deprecating contempt. Those who saw good results from Ayurveda generally thus became convinced of its potential efficacy; the rest mostly complained that the teachers there who were knowledgeable in Ayurveda were unwilling to part with their secrets, and so while they received book knowledge that was valuable for passing the exams, they missed out on the practical tips that would have made the book knowledge useful. In India, blood is substantially thicker than water, and any *vaidya* would tend, when considering to whom to pass on proprietary practices and preparations, to limit the list of recipients to kin alone. This hesitancy to share such secrets is a strong relic of the fact that historically Ayurveda, like other occupations in India, has been transmitted through family lineages. Indeed, these family secrets, often more symbolically valuable than practically advantageous, have served to perpetuate an ayurvedic lineage holder's "therapeutic mystique."

This charge was to some extent accurate; medicine, including allopathy, continues to be more art than science, and all good doctors will tend to find themselves besieged with patients. Experienced physicians of any "pathy" are more likely to invest the time and effort to thoroughly train selected individuals in the trade's tricks than to try to disseminate indiscriminately their hard-earned wisdom to those who may not be fit to receive it.

The question of who is fit to be taught—who is a *supatra*, a sound vessel in which knowledge can safely be poured—is one over which most serious educators anguish. The impersonal lecture system may work well for "objective" subjects such as mathematics or "pure science," in which a given problem can only have one reasonable solution. "Subjective" subjects such as medicine are, however, better taught, as was the case in India until the last half-century, via the very personalized, hands-on, mentor-pupil system.

Modern ayurvedic education arose as a reaction to the British, but only a partial reaction; the subject matter may have been indigenized, but the system itself, the organized syllabus with its lecture classes and examinations scheduled without regard for climatic conditions, was retained. Into the early 1970s a compromise was in force in ayurvedic education in which a disciple could be taught exclusively by a mentor and then licensed by the state, provided that she or he passed the exams that the students in the organized ayurvedic colleges had to pass. This arrangement ended under pressure from the professionalizers and institutionalizers who had become obsessed with educational standardization, with the result that now all students who aim to become Ayurvedists must submit themselves to the (currently five-and-a-half-year-long) BAMS degree course (and I do mean submit; how viscerally I recall the university exams, with their three hours of writing essay questions on porous paper with fountain pens during the 42-degree C. heat of mid-April, sweat dripping from my own pores, ceiling fans desultorily whirring far overhead).

Political modifications may be made by fiat, but transformations in society take their own time to develop. Human nature, and Indian nature in particular, inspires us to want to do all we can for our progeny. Particularly in a culture where one's offspring continue to be one's best hope for a relatively trouble-free old age, it is understandable that doctors, like other individuals, will prefer to teach their secrets to their children, or to the children of relatives or to other hand-picked personal students who can be expected to feel some sense of obligation to come to that teacher's aid later in life.

Well-intentioned administrators ignored human nature, however, and tried to gather together as many knowledgeable, experienced *vaidyas* as possible to teach Ayurveda to potentially well-meaning but nevertheless suspicious students. The result was that each knowledgeable, experienced *vaidya* fed the skimmed milk to the college students and kept secret the cream of their secrets, yielding a lifeless educational edifice dedicated to teaching the Science of Life.

Under such conditions few students found it possible to gain access to high-quality training in practical Ayurveda. The aptest or luckiest found gurus among the ayurvedic community or elsewhere (my mentor, though qualified in Ayurveda, did not practice it as a career); the rest had no alternative but to seek mentors elsewhere, or to do without. Given the relative plethora of allopathic physicians in Indian society, in comparison to practitioners of all other pathies, most serious students had no alternative other than to locate allopathic mentors—which only ensured that, once loosed from the ayurvedic college, they would be practicing allopathy alone. Others did without guru guidance, and some of these who stayed with Ayurveda were able to garner an admirable quantum of theoretical knowledge, but with only a fraction of the practical experience needed to put it to use.

Many of these became the next generation of ayurvedic teachers and administrators, guaranteeing that the next generation of ayurvedic students would again be provided a diet lopsided toward theory, particularly as the number of ayurvedic colleges mushroomed. For reasons too complicated to detail here, there was a time when opening an institution of higher education in Maharashtra became a favored method for earning one's fortune; the two ayurvedic colleges that existed in Pune when I arrived, for instance, have now been joined by five others, all hungry for instructors. And so, in my estimation, the current state of Ayurveda in India differs from that of three decades back, chiefly in degree, save in two important respects. First, many among those students who were serious about their studies, and who were sufficiently fortunate to find gurus, have found success in urban areas as ayurvedic consultants, inspiring a small but increasing number of students to emulate their example. Second, the road abroad opened. In the waning days of the 1970s, few students at Tilak could comprehend why I would possibly want to insert myself willingly into such a course (and there were of course days that I asked myself the same question), and many (even most) instructors saw me as a good but an eccentric student. Then one day in 1979 a plane ticket arrived for Dr. Vasant Lad from Mr. Lenny Blank, an alternative medicine entrepreneur from Santa Fe, New Mexico, and shortly thereafter Dr. Lad flew off to spread Ayurveda to the United States.

In a few short years, Dr. Lad leapfrogged from being low man on Tilak Ayurveda College's institutional totem pole to a position of international renown, from which vantage he became the object of acute jealousy directed at him by many of those whose reputations he had surpassed. Several of these set out to attempt to imitate his success, and the speed with which some of these lecturers shifted their allegiance from *miśra* to *śuddha* Ayurveda was breathtaking. One, for example, who had always taught us diligently, but solely allopathic and never any ayurvedic knowledge, suddenly began to behave as if he were pure Ayurveda's staunchest devotee.

After graduating in 1980 and completing my internship, I too found myself beginning the long, slow process of learning how to translate ancient Indian wisdom into a modern postindustrial, non-Indian idiom, watching the transformation of Ayurveda as it spread from its homeland to other terrain. Initial makeovers occurred simply by extension into new countries with different cultures and customs, educational and clinical and norms, languages, medical practices, and medicinal substances. Rarely did conditions in these new lands facilitate traditional ayurvedic practice, except perhaps in "India-town" ghettoes, as in Toronto, which gave shelter to two or three *vaidyas* whose influence is effectively limited to Gerrard Street.

When Ayurveda has been able to break away from such bridgeheads, it has tended to carry its preexisting *"doshas"* along (as I had assumed it would). Some of the rough edges of contemporary Ayurveda have been rubbed off as it has tumbled in the drum of the world, but others have become sharper, in particular, its politics. Ayurveda is thus far insufficiently important in terms of numbers or sums to attract the serious attention of established politicians or political parties (in contrast, for example, to homeopathy, which has Charles, Prince of Wales, as an aficionado; or the serious political support that the well-funded lobbyists for the supplement industry in the United States have been able to generate in Congress). Though it would clearly benefit Ayurveda to have its devotees speak with one voice on such matters, the questions of whether and/or how to integrate Ayurveda into the medical establishments of other countries, and of what advocacy groups will best serve Ayurveda's interests in this regard, produce forceful debate among those who band together to try to generate influence in those countries.

In the United States, three ayurvedic associations currently exist, and efforts over several years to unite them into one body have thus far signally failed. The transmission of Chinese medicine to the West has had a similar history in that (1) its various proponents have often been unable to unite, and (2) some of its therapeutic methods, such as acupuncture, have become more popular than others, leading to fragmented therapies taken out of their epistemological context and exploited by unqualified practitioners. Very basic acupuncture technique is easy and quick to learn, as one need not know any theory in order to push needles into acupuncture points.

However, Chinese medicine has had a better reception in the West than Ayurveda, due to its overseas community. For one thing, it seems the Overseas Chinese are better organized and more unified than are non-resident Indians (NRI); in most medium to large cities in the United States there is but one large Han Chinese organization, and a veritable plethora of Indian ones, organized along communal or linguistic lines: the Maharashtrians in one, the Gujaratis in another, the Kannadigas with their own organization, the Hindu Punjabis meeting separately from the Muslim Punjabis, and so on.

Secondly, even within such Indian organizations abroad ("abroad," since Ayurveda is incarnating in the East, South, and North, as well as in the West), there is far less sympathy for Ayurveda than there is appreciation for Chinese medicine within Chinese organizations abroad. Most NRIs are well educated, and a substantial proportion of educated Indians are products of a system that tends to disparage Ayurveda as being unscientific, if for no other reason than because it is ancient and has lost its position of dominance in its homeland. Any appreciation for the Indianness of such things Indian (particularly when comparisons are being made with other cultures) usually competes within the appreciator with sometimes acute embarrassment over how obsolete these fields of endeavor seem. Add to this mix the fact that what support Ayurveda gets from the Indian government is more symbolic than practical, and that within India it is rare to be able to get the proponents of one style of Ayurveda to say much good about any other style (the mutual disdain that North Indians and South Indians share in most regards is particularly pronounced within the ayurvedic realm), and the overall result is that the image projected from Ayurveda's native country to the rest of the world is often one more of shame than of pride.

In any case, there continues to be a dearth of well-trained ayurvedic physicians in countries other than India. The United Kingdom, where some estimates have it that upward of 200 college-educated *vaidyas* live, probably hosts the most, though perhaps as few as twenty of them actually practice Ayurveda. I would guess that not more than two or three dozen BAMS *vaidyas*, many of them nonpracticing and uninvolved in Ayurveda education, currently live in or regularly visit the United States. Many of the best of India's ayurvedic physicians have no interest in leaving India, seeing little to be gained by pulling up stakes, abandoning a thriving practice, and deserting loved ones to seek fame and fortune in foreign realms. Others would love to come but cannot get visas; some do come but find the food, economy, lifestyle, or some other factor intolerable and succumb to homesickness. Yet fewer are the non-Indians who have traveled to India and returned home bearing Promethean ayurvedic wisdom. A few non-Indian ayurvedic graduates are physicians qualified in their own countries in other systems of medicine (particularly allopathy) who have taken shorter ayurvedic diploma courses. Though few, these are substantially more than the number of degree-possessing ayurvedic physicians who are actually from outside India or the Indian diaspora, who I believe can continue to be counted on one hand. I was the first, after which it took at least a decade for the second. One is Japanese, another (I am told) a Spaniard, and recently a Swede completed a BAMS degree in Varanasi. I have heard rumors that one or two others are currently in the pipeline.

There is little that I can add to Claudia Welch's summary in this book of the reasons that admission to Indian Ayurveda colleges is nearly impossible for foreigners to obtain. As for me, I am certain that the Tilak Ayurveda Mahavidyalaya would never have admitted me had it not been for the personal letter I carried from Pandit Shiv Sharma directing them to admit me. I was fortunate to appear at Tilak during that one year in which they provided for an English-medium batch; the next year fifty of the roughly 150 entering students tried to join the six of us (one Sindhi, one Malayali, one Gujarati, one Tamil, one Maharashtrian, and me), at which the Marathi partisans among the powers-that-were shut down further movement in that direction. Yet more fortune came my way in the person of Dr. Vasant Lad, whom the college assigned to look after me, both because his English was adequate and because he could not refuse. Despite being thus put upon, Dr. Lad and his family accepted this task with genuine enthusiasm, for which they have my undying gratitude. Dr. Lad was not the first *vaidya* to go abroad, but he has certainly (despite his own often intense homesickness) become Ayurveda's most prominent face there (Dr. Deepak Chopra being disqualified from this competition by his allopathic credentials). Dr. Lad's kind, patient ways with his patients and his ability to relate well to foreigners certainly helped him gain acceptance, as did his sound theoretical knowledge of Ayurveda and his extensive clinical experience, gained during his many years as medical officer in the college's teaching hospital. He was a great favorite among us students at Tilak by virtue of being one of the few instructors who was eternally ready to answer questions and offer assistance with any problem or mystery.

Dr. Lad's success and his many good qualities derive fundamentally from his sincere, dedicated spiritual practice, guided first by his guru Hambir Baba, who directed him to study Ayurveda, and then by my own mentor, Vimalananda, who helped direct his path after Hambir Baba's demise. For the thirty years that I have known him, in dearth and affluence alike, Dr. Lad has continued to treat Ayurveda more as a spiritual calling than as a money-making enterprise. In this he follows the advice of the *Caraka Saṃhitā*:

> He who practices medicine out of compassion for all creatures rather than for gain (*artha*) or for gratification of the senses (*kāma*) surpasses all. Those who for the sake of making a living merchandise medicine, bargain for a heap of dust letting go a heap of gold. No benefactor, moral or material, compares to the physician who by severing the noose of death in the form of fierce diseases brings back to life those being dragged towards death's abode, because there is no other gift greater than the gift of life. He who practices medicine while holding compassion for creatures as the highest religion is a man who has fulfilled his mission. He obtains supreme happiness. (*Cikitsāsthāna* 1.58–62)

We have of course no real idea of how far *vaidyas* of that era followed this advice, but that it made it into Caraka's text is significant. In Sanskrit, a student is a *vidyārthī*, "someone whose *artha* (here: purpose or aim) is *vidyā* (knowledge)," not *artha* (here: wealth), *kāma* (sensual pleasure), or even *mokṣa* (liberation). Clearly, even then students were tempted to chase *artha* or *kāma* rather than the *dharma* of studying the *vidyā* alone, a temptation that has only worsened as money has become a bigger part of Ayurveda's environment. To all the previously enumerated problems from which moden Ayurveda suffers, we may now add the commercialization of Ayurveda in an unprecedented culture of consumerism, enticing Ayurvedists to indulge the modern consumer, affluent or otherwise, in Ayurveda as a commodity, encouraging their delusion that knowledge and health can be bought.

Ayurveda may have thus far resisted complete commercialization in its homeland, but it will be far more difficult for it to escape that fate in the West. Many in the West, perhaps particularly in America, eye any potential course of study from the perspective of how quick and easy it will be to exploit the knowledge thereby gained for profit. Yoga has already been extensively subjected to this process; Ayurveda's turn has now arrived. Open any "New Age" publication and you will find a plethora of advertisements for ayurvedic practitioners, counselors, bodyworkers, and detoxification specialists. New "ayurvedic" supplements appear daily, and therapeutic institutions of every kind are rushing to add panchakarma treatments to their product lines. The majority of these resources are ayurvedic in name alone.

A few months ago when I looked casually into one of the several ayurvedic journals that have appeared in the West, I spied an erratum: apparently the periodical had previously published a transliteration of two well-known Sanskrit mantras from the "*Devinagari*" [*sic*], and one eagle-eyed reader had identified mistakes in the transliteration. The amended transliterations were duly republished as correct—though they still contained mistakes. A few pages later the magazine offered an article that equated *kāya-kalpa* with hot oil spa treatments. While I believe that the spa environment may eventually provide a decent context in which to introduce both Ayurveda's techniques and its spirit, I doubt that the path to follow toward this end is the drastic devaluation of its tradition. The traditional ayurvedic prescription for *kāya-kalpa* or extreme rejuvenative treatment involves an enforced and extended retreat from the world, away from one's normal haunts, in a dark, quiet hut, during which the patient is subjected, after proper preparation, to cathartic purification, after which the disorganized organism is reintegrated and reorganized into (ideally) a superior state of function and being. Specifically, the ayurvedic texts state, one's skin, hair, nails, and teeth fall out and then regrow. Whether or not such a process ever succeeded in full (for a testimonial see *Maharaj*, the account of the life of Tapasviji Maharaj, most recently published by the Dawn Horse Press) is immaterial; the clear implication is that transformative rejuvenation requires ample time, calm, and personal effort.

The average spa regimen is by no means so ambitious, but the long European tradition of retreat from polluted, overcrowded cities into more salubrious climes to "take the cure" is sufficiently similar to the ayurvedic approach to rejuvenation that a useful dialogue with nature may yet arise, at the point where the asymptotes of spa and Ayurveda intersect. Long a staple of the Western scene, the spa culture has now gone global, and spas of all levels of luxury all around the world are today enthusiastically integrating ayurvedic treatments into their armamentaria of services. But before this process can go further forward, Ayurveda will itself have to undergo substantial cathartic purification and reintegration.

Today, as tradition is being devalued to facilitate business by such means as the creation of journals to "serve the ayurvedic community," one is forced to ask whether the combination of a few trained ayurvedic practitioners with a cohort of soi-disant "Ayurvedists" constitutes a viable "ayurvedic community" or rather a substantial downgrading of Ayurveda's self-vision. The upgrading of self-esteem within the "ayurvedic community" has provoked some groups to devote their energies to establishing licensing and regulation procedures in key states (licensing of health care professionals in the United States is done at the state and not the federal level). The very concerns that drove Ayurveda's first efforts at professionalization thousands of years ago in India are thus resurfacing as dreams of legitimation abroad.

So it is alarming that the American ayurvedic community's concern for status and earnings often outweighs its concern for the *vidyā* itself. To be sure, I am sympathetic to the apprehension that some people feel regarding the tenuousness of Ayurveda's current hold outside of India, and I can respect their efforts to regularize the profession via registration and licensing procedures. But no state will license a profession that contains but a few competent members, and I am unable to see what Ayurveda will gain by padding practitioner rolls in order to "grandfather in" ill-trained and/or incompetent therapists. Speedy regulation can only be accomplished by a substantial dilution of standards. To those who argue that this is a reasonable price to pay to permit students to put quickly into practice what they have quickly learned, I answer that standards once diluted take much time to stiffen, and that by the time Ayurveda's presence matures, its simplified image will have solidified. This process is already ongoing; those mainstream periodicals that have taken any interest in Ayurveda are already equating it to evaluation of constitution (*prakṛti*) and applications of hot oil. Even a recent introduction to Ayurveda published by the in-house journal of Bastyr University (Seattle's naturopathic university, which mandates that all of its incoming students take an ayurvedic overview course) was illustrated with a photo of a massage and a *prakṛti* chart.

This process may to some degree be inevitable in a sound-bite society like ours, for ayurvedic theory is difficult to simplify without making it sound risible to the Western ear, and most ayurvedic categories do not translate easily into English. One example of the conceptual oversimplification of Ayurveda is the facile notion that the three humors, *vāta*, *pitta*, and *kapha*, are the "essence" of Ayurveda, as if Ayurveda can be so easily essentialized. Like any complex organism or epistemological system, Ayurveda studied in depth resists essentialization.

Ayurveda thus seems well along the path toward commodification, toward its fifteen minutes of fame: Specialists outside of the "ayurvedic community" see prospects for profits in certain segments of the ayurvedic world; the multibillion-dollar dietary supplement industry, for example, is always looking for new herbs and formulas to be commodified. Spas are taking to ayurvedic oil treatments, and yoga studios offer "Yoga for your dosha type." The upcoming conference of NAMA (the National Ayurvedic Medical Association, of whose advisory board I am a member) addresses an open invitation to practitioners and teachers of yoga and bodywork, to spa specialists, to health care professionals, and to the general public. These are no doubt Ayurveda's natural constituencies in the West, as Ayurveda is only likely to develop within a commercial framework; and commercial activity provides one avenue for the NAMA and other ayurvedic organizations to communicate meaningfully with the general public. Difficulty arises, however, when fidelity to the subject being studied collides with the drive to simplify and commodify.

Many of those who sincerely wish Ayurveda well happen also to be integrated into our current consumerist consensus reality, our society of the spectacle, participating in the conceptualization of an "ayurvedic community" that can quickly, easily, and (relatively) painlessly fit into the consensus that the spectacle codifies. Having resolved that becoming "ayurvedic" is a simple matter of self-selection, a conceptualized "ayurvedic community" quickly develops, after which suppositions promptly run riot (e.g., that membership in this "community" equips one to learn mantras off a printed magazine page or undertake *kāya-kalpa* at a weekend massage spa). Once conceptualized, the "ayurvedic community" proceeds (via its internal logic) to educate and professionalize within the confines of its conceptual bubble. This pathology seems to characterize much of what passes for Ayurveda, both within India and beyond its borders; the speed of life increases, and the propagation of illusion also speeds up.

CHAPTER 7

An Overview of the Education and Practice of Global Ayurveda

CLAUDIA WELCH

When we look at Ayurveda's place in the modern world, it is impossible to depict it as having a single flavor. As the microcosm reflects the macrocosm, Ayurveda is currently reflecting a polarized world. If we consider the present state of ayurvedic education and the possibilities Ayurveda offers as a profession, then we find a great deal of uncertainty, whether it is in India or in the West. Two main educational paths are available for the modern Indian student of Ayurveda, the institutional and the traditional. The former is associated with the BAMS (Bachelor of Ayurvedic Medicine and Surgery) degree, which can then lead to higher degrees. The latter is associated with lineage, where a student may serve or even live with a teacher, gaining his trust and wisdom over many years. This has a rich history in India, from Arjuna learning from his charioteer Krishna in the *Bhagavad Gītā* to the *gurukula* system of education, in which knowledge of a particular field is passed from the guru to the disciple. This was the near-universal system of ayurvedic education in India until the establishment of ayurvedic colleges in the early twentieth century. The first ayurvedic college was the Keraliya Ayurveda Samajam in 1902, established in Shoranur, Kerala (http://www.samajam.org). This was followed soon by the Arya Vaidya Sala, established in the same year in Kotakkal, Kerala, by P. S. Varier (http://www.aryavaidyasala.com). Since that time, institutional degrees have assumed the greatest importance, as they have in other areas of education.

This is not to say, however, that learning through lineage is lost; indeed, it survives in a few places in India, including among the *aṣṭavaidya* physicians in Kerala, where a student is trained in a family lineage in addition to receiving the BAMS degree. However, very few students of Ayurveda in India currently participate in both tracks, while nearly all undertake their ayurvedic educations only in the five- or six-year BAMS course in the government of private Ayurveda colleges. For at least the last thirty or forty years, a significant percentage of the students in the Ayurveda colleges have been students who were unable to secure admission to the allopathic medical schools. Generally, the government programs are more competitive and well regarded than the private colleges, into which admission is usually easier to obtain and which are usually extraordinarily expensive and, therefore, prohibitive, for all but wealthy students to attend. The private colleges often demand large "capitation fees" as a condition of admission. In addition, their level of instruction is sometimes questionable, and their degrees are often not recognized in states outside of that in which the school is situated (and sometimes not even there).

One of the main areas of contestation has been the purity of ayurvedic instruction. Whether in government or private institutions, there has been, and continues to be, a polarization between instructors and physicians who wish to teach and practice "pure" Ayurveda versus those who wish to teach it together with allopathic principles, as Robert Svoboda has discussed in this book. The curriculum, as it stands now, offers enough allopathic medical education that if a BAMS graduate so chose, he or she could legally approach the practice of medicine from solely an allopathic perspective and upon graduation dispense allopathic pharmaceutical drugs. This is very attractive to students, many of whom were turned down for admission into allopathic medical colleges. In this way they achieve at least some of the prestige, wealth, and clientele that would ordinarily be the property of allopathic physicians, especially in urban areas. This also is attractive to many of the faculty at the Ayurveda colleges, for these same reasons and because it confers a measure of prestige on their institutions.

This is borne out by my own experience. While trying to gain admission into a BAMS program in India in the period 1992–1993, I visited a number of private and government colleges. I was told by many students, in all of these colleges, that they would rather have attended a college for allopathic medicine, but the competition for seats was so prohibitive that they settled for admission into an ayurvedic medical program. These students were planning to treat with allopathic drugs and principles—not ayurvedic principles—when they graduated. Often the students expressed a nearly embarrassed or apologetic sentiment regarding Ayurveda as compared to allopathic medicine.

This attitude also is at least partially responsible for the fact that BAMS students routinely submit papers that emulate a "Western" approach to medicine. Among the topics for these papers, which follow the research of the faculty at these institutions, are experiments in which the active ingredients of herbs are isolated, after which they are tested on control groups. They also test these substances on mice (this happens, for example, at the government ayurvedic college in Lucknow).

Change is beginning to occur, however, in part due to the increased interest in Ayurveda in the West. While Indian students increasingly admire Western science and lifestyles, many in the West have awakened to the riches of Indian knowledge and lifestyles. Much of these parallel phenomena are the products of the idealization and romanticization of the other, the desire to escape from the boundaries of one's own respective culture. Nevertheless, it remains the fact that such idealization is, in some instances at least, being used consciously and purposefully to influence the current ayurvedic students in India. For example, in January 2006, an international conference was organized in Mahabalipuram, a famous temple city south of Chennai. Its stated goal was to "educate the Indian Ayurveda community about global trends wherein the move from reductionism to holism is on the rise and thus motivate Ayurveda students to aspire to study and apply Ayurveda in its authentic totality." It was not an accident that most of the invited speakers—both Indian and foreign—were practitioners in Western countries. Whether this conference is able to establish a trend in ayurvedic education (which has always experienced a shortage of seminar-based educational opportunities) or more substantively succeeds in altering the perspective of students of Ayurveda within India remains to be seen, but it does mark a formal, clear representation of the influence of Western practitioners on Indian ones. At the moment, however, this is expressed more in terms of morale than in evidence of bringing to students the "authentic totality" of Ayurveda (however this may be construed).

EDUCATIONAL POSSIBILITIES FOR STUDENTS OF AYURVEDA OUTSIDE OF INDIA

Although the influence of the West on India in terms of the study of Ayurveda is just now beginning to emerge, the influence of India on the West is equally unmistakable. India is the home of Ayurveda and has therefore not only introduced Ayurveda to the West but also has influenced the manner in which it is introduced.

As is the case within India, outside of India as well there are two educational paths for the modern student of Ayurveda. Students who seek an education in Ayurveda in the West also are offered routes that are predominantly institutionalized or predominantly traditional, as described earlier, though with important differences from the way these appear in India. Whereas within India the formal route is associated with a BAMS degree, this is not at present an option outside of India. Even dedicated non-Indians experience great difficulties when seeking admission to Indian ayurvedic colleges. Though language may constitute a problem, this is not to be counted as one of the most insuperable when seeking admission. As mentioned above, one problem is that degrees from ayurvedic medical colleges are not usually recognized outside of the Indian states in which they are granted. This is particularly true of the private Ayurveda colleges. Another problem is the issue of "reservations," the Indian system of affirmative action. Whether or not administrators of the government schools profess to want foreign students at their institution or not, the problem of "reserved seats" often intercedes, especially at government schools.

At most of the colleges, a significant number of "seats" are reserved for certain communities, castes (e.g.,"OBCs," or "other backward castes," a designation that carries weight in the politics of Indian education), descendants of "freedom fighters," and so on. A few seats may occasionally be reserved for students from outside of the state. However, these almost invariably go to students from Indian states that do not have their own Ayurveda college, or to students from Sri Lanka or Nepal with histories of ayurvedic practice. Because getting into college at all is an extremely competitive prospect in India, it is the rule that all these seats are filled. If a foreigner would like to apply for one of these seats, then he or she could end up waiting, sometimes for years, and in the end admission will still be turned down, and by then one's visa will have expired, with little chance for renewal.

This was my experience, as well as the experience of many other non-Indians. In short, the politics of education in India makes it extremely unlikely that even a vacant "seat" could be relinquished. One possible solution would be to lobby the government to create seats in various institutions for (non-Nepali or Sri Lankan) foreigners. But this can hardly be done by the applicant himself or herself. This would entail institutional and governmental cooperation involving a number of ministries in New Delhi.

That said, other formal options are available. Though the traditional route of a *gurukula* apprenticeship is not readily available to non-Indian students, many of the ayurvedic physicians who guide non-Indians at institutions in the West have managed to impart a lineage-based flavor to their teaching. This has received a very positive reception by the students, as it conveys not only knowledge of Ayurveda but a sense of intimacy with the cultural and scientific traditions in which Ayurveda is embedded. Thus whether this student is studying in a seminar format or in a longer program, he or she can choose between the more formal, standardized approach and a more lineage-oriented approach.

STANDARDIZED AND LINEAGE-BASED AYURVEDIC OPTIONS IN THE WEST

A few institutions in the United States, including the Kripalu School of Ayurveda in Massachusetts and the American University of Complementary Medicine in California, offer curricula taught by highly experienced and/or educated teachers from varied backgrounds, many of whom are Indians who have earned the BAMS degree. These institutions offer in-depth education on ayurvedic theory and as much clinical experience as is possible in a country where there is no recognized licensing and regulation for the practice of Ayurveda. One benefit of this approach is an exposure to different valid viewpoints, resulting in a tolerance to multiple approaches within the study and practice of Ayurveda.

In addition to efforts to standardize ayurvedic education in the United States, a product of the development of curricula at instutions such as those mentioned, in which courses are designed to be taught by a number of faculty members from different lineages, some institutions carry the distinct imprint of specific ayurvedic lineages. These institutions will generally have a charismatic founder whose name is linked inextricably to the institution, as is the case with Dr. Vasant Lad of the Ayurvedic Institute in Albuquerque, David Frawley, founder and sole instructor at the American Institute of Vedic Studies in Santa Fe, New Mexico, and Dr. Marc Halpern, founder of and primary instructor at the California College of Ayurveda.

Other institutions reach more deeply into lineage-based authority. In such cases, the primary instructor or founder may be a respected author and leader within the ayurvedic community who also has taken on the role of spiritual guru to at least some of the students. This is the case with Lad at the Ayurvedic Institute. In my position as an instructor at this institute, I have not infrequently heard students there declare that Lad is their guru, regardless of whether or not he has accepted that role. So too with the Wise Earth Monastery in North Carolina, founded by Sri Swamini Mayatitananda (formerly Maya Tiwari), whose Web site (as noted in the Introduction to this book) describes her as the "spiritual head of Wise Earth School of Ayurveda" and as a "pre-eminent spiritual Mother who emanates silence and wisdom" who "belongs to India's prestigious Vedic lineage—Veda Vyasa."

To some extent at least, this reflects the sort of person who is interested in adopting Ayurveda as part of his or her active practice in America. This presents a complex set of comparisons to Ayurveda, present and past, in India. I cannot enter too deeply into this in this chapter, but it should be noted that in lineage-based Ayurveda in India, which was the dominant system for millennia until roughly the

1930s, a physician or *vaidya* who had (1) mastered the primary texts of his respective tradition (e.g., *Aṣṭāṅgahṛdaya-Saṃhitā* in Kerala, or *Caraka-Saṃhitā* in North India), (2) mastered the equally authoritative and more recent Sanskrit and vernacular medical literature, (3) had a command of the pharmacopoeia, (4) was recognized as a good doctor and healer, (5) had at one time devoted himself to his guru, and (6) was a practitioner of various spiritual arts and was recognized not just as a medical expert and teacher by his students but as their guru as well. It is this combination of attributes that made such a *vaidya* a lineage holder in the local medical tradition. It is for this reason that it sometimes appears that Ayurveda is not easily separable from its religious or spiritual contexts. And it is this context that is attractive to many Western ayurvedic aspirants.

While a single instructor is not sufficient to meet the needs of an institution, these lineage-flavored institutions often hire only, or predominantly, graduates of their own home institution to teach their courses. No matter how charismatic the leader, however, lineage-flavored programs in the West differ from those in India in another major way. While the *gurukula* system in India encouraged knowledge to be passed to only a small number of deserving pupils who would then receive significant attention from the guru, modern institutions, even those that hire predominantly their own graduates (which remains the norm in India, even if it has moved away from the *gurukula* system), graduate large numbers of students, while the main instructor, with no pretensions to spiritual authority, may not even remember the names of the students by the following year.

Another difference is the student's loyalty to one lineage. While a mentor in India would take the student through the basics of Ayurveda through to clinical proficiency, in the United States these programs are a few years at the most and can only take the student through the theory and a minimum of clinical work. Thus the student of Ayurveda has few options to turn to for a serious level of ayurvedic fluency if the accessible venues are insufficient. If they are fortunate, they are able to establish both a working and a spiritual connection with a mentor willing to guide the student's education beyond the routine course offerings. If not, the student may wander from one instructor or institution to another trying to complete and mature her or his education. For example, the student may study at the California College of Ayurveda with Dr. Halpern, then attend the Ayurvedic Institute under the graces of Dr. Lad, and then study for a month in India with Dr. Sunil Joshi of the Vinayak Ayurvedic Center, also in Albuquerque, without ever developing the bond necessary to comprehend the heart of Ayurveda from any of them, to truly internalize an ayurvedic way of thinking and being.

This practice of wandering from one instructor to another as often as not fosters distrust of those instructors, who, usually more than the students, are sensitive to the dynamics of the teacher-student, guru-disciple relationship, with its often unarticulated but always implicit sense of reciprocal loyalty. In such cases, then, it is unlikely that any teacher will impart her or his lineage-based secrets. This quest for knowledge and meaning in Ayurveda, coupled with a quest for spiritual enlightenment, usually takes the form of a quest for healing or medical secrets that makes sense to the ayurvedic aspirant's spiritual or religious vision. Often these teachers never impart such secrets; indeed, they might not have secrets to impart. This can be frustrating to the teachers as well as the students. I mention this because quite often I have seen an interest in Ayurveda deeply embedded within personal spiritual quests. This vision of Ayurveda as an aspect of a spiritual system is one of the defining features of Ayurveda in America, though by no means do all students share this perspective.

Let us look for a moment at these "secrets" that are sought by such students. First, it is nearly tautological to state that if a student is looking for secrets (and this is not infrequent), then the student does not know what he or she is looking for. Such secrets, unbeknownst to the seekers, are not esoteric mysteries, nuggets of privileged knowledge, or spiritual experience; rather, they are mental and emotional patterns that are part of the constitution of the teacher and that enable the teacher to live and practice medicine in a certain way. And it is possible that this can only be imparted if there is a long-term connection and intimacy. Historically, ayurvedic lineages are defined as much by such heritages of intimacy as they are by the intimacies of textual knowledge.

Whatever the limitations, there also may be benefits to such lineage-based education in the West, whether it is expressly spiritual, as in the case of the Wise Earth Monastery, or whether the institution simply has a charismatic leader, as in the case of the Ayurvedic Institute. These benefits include a sense of belonging to a community of practitioners with a shared sense of affirmation that they have an acceptable grasp of Ayurveda. This is particularly salient in the West, where larger national communities do not have educational standards through which to prove their proficiency in Ayurveda. Another result often found in this type of program—and this is a negative one—is that its graduates tend to feel competitive with graduates of other lineage-based programs, with an attendant disrespect of the practices of other lineages. Needless to add, this is not a healthy sign for the future of Ayurveda in the West.

PROFESSIONAL CLIMATE AND POSSIBILITIES FOR AYURVEDA IN THE WEST

Currently no recognized standards of ayurvedic education exist in the United States, nor is there recognized licensing for practicing Ayurveda that either significantly protects or determines the practitioner's scope of practice or that serves to educate the public about the qualifications or education of the practitioner. This means that the public is unable to distinguish between an ayurvedic practitioner with twelve hours of education from one with 4,000 hours and, perhaps more seriously, that practitioners themselves may remain unaware of the proficiency and depth possible in the field. This problem is exacerbated by the fact that many students of Ayurveda in America already have healing practices of their own, such as massage, Reiki, chiropractic, and so on. Studying a little (or a lot) of Ayurveda enables them to add that to their portfolio. However, the client (or patient) often does not know the degree to which Ayurveda enters into their actual practice or how well trained they are. For example, a massage therapist who incorporates a few principles learned in a weekend seminar may have no idea that Ayurveda is a comprehensive medical system, or that there are entire hospitals in India that are dedicated to treating only with ayurvedic principles and medicines. And the client knows even less. Thus the very term *Ayurveda* in public awareness has become diminished in many areas of discourse and practice to that of a minor appendage of other healing systems.

When Ayurveda is practiced in a context that exceeds the practitioner's skill level, questions of safety arise that potentially threaten the reputation of Ayurveda. These concerns however, are not generally foremost in the minds of modern practitioners, who may simply be trying to figure out how to make a living using and/or applying ayurvedic principles to the best of their abilities.

Whatever the educational background of the Western ayurvedic student might be, a number of different options exist for employing it as a viable practice. Because Ayurveda is not a licensed modality of health care, a practitioner has the option of practicing it under another health-related license as far as the scope of the dominant practice will allow. For example, massage therapists can determine for themselves the client's probable psycho-physical constitution (*prakṛti*) and its leading modifications (*vikṛti*) and determine appropriate massage oils and techniques. But they may not diagnose conditions, prescribe herbs, or perform other services that lay outside of the scope of their practice of massage therapy. Another example is of Doctors of Oriental Medicine (OMD), which is to say those with degrees in Traditional Chinese Medicine (TCM), who may legally practice most ayurvedic therapies under their scope of practice laws. Naturopaths, medical doctors, doctors of chiropractic, and other licensed health care practitioners also may practice in this way.

Students of Ayurveda also may incorporate ayurvedic principles into health-related fields, such as yoga therapy and health spa services, fields that are currently flourishing and expanding in America. Indeed, any "New Age" magazine rack is likely to feature at least one article relating Ayurveda to yoga or to spa services.

Incorporating Ayurveda into spa settings is uniquely challenging because the ayurvedic treatments that are most appealing to spas also are used as a precursor to panchakarma treatments. These are, as such, to be monitored and administered with certain precautions that are not necessarily understood or adhered to in the context of a spa setting. However, is it not possible to expand on those challenges here?

Suffice it to say that most ayurvedic practitioners of any level or knowledge and skill who are able to make a living using Ayurveda do so in one of the aforementioned ways. At present, Ayurveda must be an adjunct practice, as no full five- or six-year courses of study are available (or even possible) in the West, licensing is practically nonexistent, and the full pharmacopoeia is neither available nor approved for use by drug-regulating agencies in the West. Thus for the moment at least, what we have in the West is an altered form of Ayurveda.

CONCLUSION

Whether inside or outside of India, the dissemination of Ayurveda may occur through either a more institutionalized approach or through one that attempts to retain a certain regional and textual lineage. This picture reflects two approaches to the study of Ayurveda: one emphasizes the spiritual nature of the medicine, along with the empirical side, and the other emphasizes only the empirical science of Ayurveda.

It is of great importance to recognize that both approaches are present in the classical texts. In the first chapters of the *Bṛhat-trayī*—the "great three" classical ayurvedic texts, the *Caraka-Saṃhitā*, the *Suśruta-Saṃhitā*, and the *Aṣṭāṅgahṛdaya-Saṃhitā*—the story is told of enlightened *rishis* gathering in the Himalayas to learn and disseminate Ayurveda from the Gods to the masses. Ayurveda is then embedded in a context in which its origins and dissemination are valorized as divine and divinely transmitted. And, indeed, it has been presented in this context throughout much of its history, including in the modern medical colleges. Thus many ayurvedic practitioners in India and in the West approach it from this standpoint, even if they teach and study it as an empirical or a scientific system. In the attenuated shape that Ayurveda has been forced to assume in the West, for the reasons discussed earlier, it is easy (and not at all wrong) to study it with these perspectives in the ascendant.

Nevertheless, the overwhelming bulk of material in the classical texts addresses the more empirical aspects of Ayurveda, including complex recipes for medicines, detailed descriptions of treatments, delineation of disorders, full accounts of a variety of diagnostic procedures, and in the case of *Suśruta* even surgery (which is still practiced effectively in a few places in India). And, it is important to note, it is common to find ayurvedic practitioners who emphasize this empirical medicine and who may minimize or ignore entirely the spiritual aspects of the texts. This is visible in high-volume practices in India and in parts of South India, where Christian and Muslim practitioners of Ayurveda who may not easily relate to the Sanskritic contexts of Ayurveda may be found in relatively large numbers (most often trained in the colleges established by the Arya Vaidya Sala).

It is, then, a modern-day challenge of the study, dissemination, and practice of Ayurveda to find a balance between and synthesis of these two perspectives.

CHAPTER 8

Ayurvedic Pharmacopoeia Databases in the Context of the Revitalization of Traditional Medicine

UNNIKRISHNAN PAYYAPPALLIMANA

Traditional medicine in South Asia includes the three "codified" systems—Ayurveda, Siddha, and Unani—Tibetan medicine, and countless "noncodified" oral traditions. Codified systems are grounded in a theory of physiological functioning, disease etiology, and clinical practice. They have formal traditions of training and possess a vast array of written documents recording the *materia medica*, specialized subjects related to medicine and surgery, clinical procedures, and medical ethics. The noncodified or folk traditions, such as those represented by bonesetters, birth attendants, pediatric specialists, veterinary healers, poison healers, and local specialists in specific diseases, such as jaundice, eye diseases, gastrointestinal diseases, and so on, have been transmitted as oral traditions for generations through a person-to-person process. Another feature of folk traditions is that they are ethnic community and ecosystem specific, and thus they embody tremendous geocultural diversity. Folk medicine also includes what is popularly known as grandmothers' remedies, the household knowledge of primary health care, dietary remedies, seasonal health regimens and health customs, rituals, and so on.

Though local health practices have evolved alongside the codified knowledge systems, they also have closely interacted with them in a relationship of reciprocal influence. Ayurvedic texts are replete with examples attesting to this relationship. For example, *Suśruta* (Sū 38.10) states: "One can know about the drugs from cowherds, ascetics, hunters, forest dwellers, and those who subsist on roots and tubers."[1] One can thus say that local health practices are living expressions of the theories and concepts mentioned in the codified texts. However, since this relationship is complex, a detailed study of it would be required to reveal its exact nature.

HISTORICAL CONTEXT

Folk medicine and the classical systems of medicines have evolved differently in India. In the post-Independence period, Ayurveda and other codified systems of medicine, most notably Siddha and Unani, were professionalized through the establishment of university programs and medical and research councils. Because of its very nature, however, folk medicine was excluded from these policies until 2002. Except for a few stray, unsuccessful attempts to integrate traditional birth attendants (TBAs) into the national health program, folk practitioners were completely neglected in the past. The nationalistic and pluralistic ideology of the Independence movement contributed to guaranteeing a respectable place for Ayurveda and other codified medical systems in modern India. However, even after more than fifty years of government support, Ayurveda remains in a rather unhealthy condition (Shankar 2004). Let us examine some of the recent history that has led to this sorry state of affairs.

During the Independence movement, a debate that had its roots in the "Swadeshi" movement arose over strategies for revitalizing Ayurveda. Two distinct ideological positions were developed: (1) Ayurveda must remain classical or pure (*śuddha*), and (2) it should be integrated with other, more dominant medical systems. Those who were overwhelmed by the advancement of modern science and possessed a pragmatic and liberal view held the position that the classical tradition needed to be enriched by modern technology and methods. Conversely, the opposing group advocated a purist view. However, no systematic study was ever conducted on the influence of modern concepts and methods on the epistemology of traditional medicine in order to objectively assess its value. Nevertheless, the result was an alteration in the nature of a number of fundamental aspects of Ayurveda, including education, research, and clinical practice (Shankar 2004). The issue is still not settled, hence this ideological confusion persists today in Ayurveda and other traditional medical systems.

Until the late nineteenth century the education of Ayurveda was purely through *guru-śiṣya paramparā*, an experiential learning where the student (*śiṣya*) stays with the teacher. But this began to change around the period of Indian Independence, with the establishment of ayurvedic university programs. At present, there are more than 300 Ayurveda colleges in India for graduate and postgraduate courses with syllabi designed along the lines of those of allopathic medical education. In addition, all states in India have medicine councils that grant registration to graduates, and only those who are licensed by these councils are allowed to practice. Even though this institutionalization was designed to improve the quality of medical education, in fact the quality of learning deteriorated after the introduction of fixed syllabi and formal courses designed by individuals outside of the institution (Shankar and Manohar 1995). For example, pulse examination (*nāḍī parīkṣā*), a method of diagnosis that can only be acquired within the setting of a slow and careful experiential learning process, is widely practiced today by traditional physicians. Yet in the university system, many such fascinating methods and practices are not being taught at all, or they are taught in an incomplete and very defective manner in a week or two. Many ayurvedic graduates tolerate this, however, because they regard their ayurvedic education as an entry to a private allopathic practice.

In the area of research, after Indian Independence, the Indian Council of Medical Research (ICMR) assumed responsibility for the pharmacological and clinical evaluation of Indian Systems of Medicine (ISM) drugs. After the formation of the Central Council for Research in Ayurveda and Siddha (CCRAS) in 1978 (see http://www.ccras.org/index.htm), this responsibility was turned over to them. Today most ayurvedic research programs are based on modern medical methods and parameters. Even after thirty years of research in ISM, these bodies have not released any comprehensive publication that can advise Indian medical professionals on how and what aspects of ISM can be integrated with mainstream Indian medical practice. In the area of research, for want of a proper intercultural research methodology, Ayurveda is losing its identity in a struggle to prove itself to modern science. The shortage of peer-reviewed publications on Ayurveda that meet international standards is another lacuna in the area of research.

With respect to economic resources, ISM still suffers from government neglect. During the Seventh, Eighth, and Ninth National Plan periods (1987–1992, 1992–1997, 1997–2002, respectively), ISM (including homeopathy, naturopathy and yoga) received around 3 percent of the national health budget. State allocations varied, with only the government of Kerala allocating 13 percent of its medical budget for ISM and Bengal allocating less than 0.5 percent. ISM health delivery services in rural and urban areas are not linked to the national primary health care services. India has approximately 23,000 ayurvedic, Unani, and Siddha dispensaries funded by state governments in various parts of the country. They are effective and popular in some states, including Kerala and Tamil Nadu, while in other states their impact is negligible. They function without any orientation to national health goals, and there has been no review in postindependent India of how to make the ISM health services sector more effective (Shankar 2004).

On the whole, as described earlier, development in the field of Ayurveda and other traditional medical systems is facing an epistemological crisis, along with social and political disregard. The poor quality of education, research, and clinical practice, lack of appropriate political and social support, loss of self esteem among practitioners, marginalization by mainstream knowledge systems, issues related to intellectual property rights, lack of serious efforts to generate fundamental and collaborative research, and large-scale depletion of the natural resources are some of the major issues confronted by traditional medicine in India today.

In this context of crisis, a nongovernmental organization, the Foundation for Revitalization of Local Health Traditions (FRLHT), was founded in 1993 (see http://www.frlht-india.org/). The FRLHT has two broad objectives: the revitalization of the Indian medical heritage and the conservation of natural resources used by traditional medical systems. Over the last ten years, the FRLHT has established an effective medicinal plant conservation program through public-private partnership in many states in India. It also has developed a number of comprehensive multidisciplinary databases of medicinal plants of India and related traditional knowledge. Partnering with government organizations in each of its projects, the FRLHT also has been able to play a key role in advocacy for traditional medicine. It has been involved in training, extension activities, and development of products to serve various interests groups of the traditional medical community (i.e., practitioners, professors, and students) as well as scientists, public health workers, and the general public. Among the extension activities are the documentation of local knowledge and the promotion of effective practices for primary health care in the form of home herbal gardens. In addition, there are ex situ and in situ conservation initiatives for medicinal plants. Among the products the FRLHT is developing are CD-ROM databases, books, field test kits, and medicinal formulations. The following section describes the ayurvedic databases, one of the FRLHT's successful projects.

AYURVEDIC PHARMACOPOEIA DATABASES

It is estimated that traditional medicine in all of its manifestations in India uses approximately 7,500 medicinal plants.[2] Out of this number,

Ayurveda uses approximately 1,750, of which around 880 are traded in various marketplaces. According to one study, nearly 300 plants used in traditional medicine are considered rare, endangered, or threatened.[3] The reasons for this are overexploitation and unsustainable harvests.

In 1993, at its inception, the FRLHT launched a conservation project in three southern states of India, which was to be handled both in situ and ex situ. Part of this project was the preparation of a comprehensive checklist of medicinal plants and related background information. For this, a database project was initiated. This project included various topics, including distribution mapping, trade, threat status, propagation, traditional medical information, and other relevant information. Under the traditional medicine databases, Ayurveda, Siddha, and Unani databases were built. A number of challenges were faced in the process of developing these databases, some of which remain unsolved. One of these was nomenclature correlation, primarily problems linking Sanskrit plant names to botanical equivalents. Another major challenge was simply identifying a substantial number of plants used in Ayurveda and named in the classical literature. The following pages highlight some of the experiences and the insights gained during the process of trying to break through these problems.

The objective of the traditional medicine database is to identify and locate the medicinal plants described and employed in the codified medical traditions. In the case of Ayurveda, the first effort was to build a state-of-the-art database correlating Sanskrit names with botanical names mentioned in the nonclassical secondary literature. The textual sources for this database included twenty-one books belonging to the last 100 years of works by Ayurvedists, botanists, and pharmacognosists that correlate Sanskrit names with botanical names. This work culminated in a correlation of more than 20,000 Sanskrit names with 1,750 species belonging to 830 genera. The following (see Table 8.1) are the selected ayurvedic sources (see References at the end of this chapter for full cites).

Subsequently, many more secondary textual sources were included from different medical systems (Siddha, Unani, Tibetan, and folk). At present, this nomenclature correlation database has more than 550 textual sources and a listing of more than 150,000 names from 35 languages correlated to 7,673 botanical names. This is one of the most comprehensive databases of medicinal plants in India.

The building up of the Ayurveda database enabled the staff of the FRLHT to understand a number of nomenclature correlation-related issues. Ayurveda follows a polynomial system of nomenclature in which a plant is described with multiple names. Each of these names pertains to a specific character or feature of the plant. By grouping the names together in the manner found in the versified Sanskrit glossaries

Table 8.1. Ayurvedic Sources

No.	Name of the Work	Author	Year
1	*Pharmacognosy of Ayurvedic Drugs*, Vols. 1, 2, 3, 10	K. N. Iyer, A. N. Namboodiri, and M. Kolammal	1951 1957 1979
2	*La-Hārita Saṃhitā*	Alix Raisom	1974
3	*Aṣṭāṅgahṛdaya-koṣa*	Anonymous	1936
4	*Ayurvedic Pharmacopoeia of India*, Vol. 1	Ministry of Health and Family Welfare	1989–
5	*Ayurvedic Formulary of India*, Part 1	Ministry of Health and Family Planning	1978
6	*A Dictionary of Economic Products of India*	George Watt	1889
7	*Indian Medicinal Plants*, 4 vols.	Kirtikar and Basu	1935
8	*Handbook of Medicinal Plants*	P. N. V. Kurup	1968
9	*A Catalogue of Indian Synonyms*	Moodeen Sheriff	1988
10	*Single Drug Remedies*	N. S. Mooss	1976
11	*Gaṇas of Vāhaṭa*	N. S. Mooss	1980
12	*Indian Pharmaceutical Codex*, Vol. 1	B. Mukherji	1953
13	*Indian Materia Medica* 2 vols	K. M. Nadkarni	1954
14	*Indian Medicinal Plants*, Vols. 1–5	S. Raghunath Iyer	1993–1996
15	*Dravyaguṇavijñāna*, Vols. 2 and 5	P. V. Sharma	1994
16	*Ayurvedic Drugs and Their Plant Sources*	Sivarajan and I. Balachandran	1994
17	*Glossary of Vegetable Drugs in Bṛhattrayī*	Thakur Balwant Singh and Chunekar	1972
18	*Nighaṇṭu Ādarśa*, Vols. 1 and 2	Vaidya Bapalal	1968
19	*Some Controversial Drugs of India*	Vaidya Bapalal	1982
20	*Studies on Medicinal Plants in Dhanvantarīya Nighaṇṭu*, Vol. 1	Vaidya D. K. Kamat	1972
21	*Materia Medica*	Whitelaw Ainslie	1984

or lexicons (*nighaṇṭu*), the plant and its uses can usually be determined. For example, *Guḍūcī*, which is correlated to *Tinospora cordifolia*, is assigned approximately seventy names in the classical literature, including *amṛta* (nectar of immortality), *somavalli* (soma vine), *somalatikā* (climber with nectarlike properties), *cakralakṣaṇa* (having a wheellike appearance in cross section), *maṇḍalī* (circular), *kuṇḍali* (entangled), *nāgakumārī* (like a young snake), *tāntrika* (spreading nature), *chinnarūha, chinnodbhava, chinnāṅgi* (grows when cut and put in soil), *śyāma* (with a bluish-black color), *rasāyaṇī* (rejuvenative), *vayastha* (age regulating), *jīvantī* (life promoting), and *jvarāri* (pacifying fever) (Manohar 1994).

Another nettlesome problem is that different plants often share the same name (Meulenbeld 1974: 424, 509). For example, *kṛṣṇa* is a name for *pippali* (*Piper longum*) as well as *arjuna* (*Terminalia arjuna*). Because the texts do not address this issue, it is sometimes difficult to determine the plant to which a text is referring. In other words, many of the correlations that we and others have made between Sanskrit and botanical names are guesswork, as it is impossible to substantiate references in the absence of either physical specimens or more detailed descriptions, which unfortunately is not done in a majority of these materia medica.

This problem is further highlighted by the authors of such materia medica who hail from different regions of India. Naturally they tend to correlate their local plant to the Sanskrit name, but this will often turn out to be a different plant than the one that goes by that name elsewhere. For example, for the plant *śankhapuspi*, a Keralan author gives *Clitoria ternatea*, whereas a North Indian author correlates it to *Convolvulus microphyllus* (Kareem 1997). Indeed, it is estimated that nearly 50 percent of the plants currently used have multiple botanical sources. Two examples of multiple numbers of botanical species correlated to the same name follow (see Table 8.2).

Another problem was peculiarities in the transliteration of Sanskrit names. Various authors spelled or transliterated the Sanskrit names

Table 8.2. Examples of Multiple Correlations of Botanical Names

śaṅkhapuṣpi	*pāśānabheda*
1. *Clitoria ternatea*	1. *Aerva persica*
2. *Evolvulus alsinoides*	2. *Aerva lanata*
3. *Convolvulus microphyllus*	3. *Ammania baccifera*
4. *Canscora decussata*	4. *Bergenia ciliata*
5. *Canscora diffusa*	5. *Bergenia stracheyi*
6. *Lavendula bipinnata*	6. *Bridelia montana*
7. *Cannabis sativa*	7. *Bridelia retusa*
8. *Xanthium stumarium*	8. *Didymocarpus pedicellata*
	9. *Homonoia riparia*
	10. *Kalanchoe pinnata*
	11. *Nothosaerva brachiata*
	12. *Ocimum basilicum*
	13. *Plectranthus amboinicus*
	14. *Rotula aquatica*

differently. For example, the local names for the botanical name *Acalypha indica L.* are, variously,

> *ariṣṭamañjari* (VB), *arittamanjarie* (KM), *arittamunjariye* (KB), *arittamunjari* (IP), *arittamunjayrie* (GW, WH), *haritamañjari* (VA), *manshinka* (WH), *muktavarcca* (VB).

At times, even such slight variations indicate a completely different entity. Thus one of the challenges was to standardize the transliteration. This was possible only by checking the description of the plant in the relevant classical text, by checking the etymology (*nirukta*) of the name, or through other detailed textual study.

In general, an in-depth understanding of ayurvedic plant nomenclature was lacking among these authors. Thus we understood that a detailed study of classical texts with their chronological linkages was necessary to address issues related to nomenclature correlation and multiple identity. This challenge led us to the building of a database comprised of primary literature source material.

NOMENCLATURE CORRELATION DATABASE BASED ON PRIMARY SOURCES

The effort to develop a nomenclature database based on primary sources—the classical texts of Ayurveda—required the study of twenty classical texts covering a chronological period of two millennia. The texts chosen are those that represent the major milestones in *dravyaguṇa* (pharmacology) and are in contemporary use, regardless of whether they are generally known (such as the *Suśruta-* or *Caraka-Saṃhitās*) or are specific to different geographical locations (see Table 8.3). Thus various text types were consulted, including *saṃhitās* (foundational treatises), *saṃgrahas* (compendia), and *nighaṇṭus* (lexicons). The purpose of this broad selection was a database project that would aspire to comprehensiveness, that is, to bring together the maximum number of variations in plant names and uses.

STRUCTURE OF THE CLASSICAL NOMENCLATURE (*NĀMAJÑĀNA*) DATABASE

Though this database consists primarily of plant identifications, it also covers animals, minerals, and metals from select texts. The following fields are in the database:

Table 8.3. Reference Books

S No.	Text Name	Chronology	Author	Region	Plant Ref. No.
1	*Caraka-Saṃhitā*	500 BCE–400 CE	Agniveśa Caraka Dṛḍhabla	Himalaya, Kashmir	12,850
2	*Suśruta-Saṃhitā*	500 BCE–500 CE	Suśruta Nāgārjuna	Kāśī Sindhudeśa	9,650
3	*Astāngasaṃgraha*	500 CE	Vāgbhaṭa	Sindhudeśa	20,500
4	*Aṣṭāṅgahṛdayam*	600 CE	Vāgbhaṭa	Sindhudeśa	9,900
5	*Aṣṭāṅga Nighaṇṭu*	800 CE	Vāgbhaṭa		2,100
6	*Paryayaratnamālā*	900 CE	Mādhava	Śilahṛda (?)	1,900
7	*Dhanvantari Nighaṇṭu*	200–1000 CE	Unknown	Unknown	3,250
8	*Cakradatta*	1075 CE	Cakrapāṇidatta	Vaṅgadeśa	12,300
9	*Dravyaguṇasaṃgraha*	1075 CE	Cakrapāṇidatta	Vaṅgadeśa	320
10	*Mādhavadravyaguṇa*	1250 CE	Mādhava	Unknown	750
11	*Śārṅgadhara-Saṃhitā*	1300 CE	Śārṅgadhara	Devagiri	4,200
12	*Nighaṇṭu Śesa*	1200 CE	Hemacandra	Unknown	2,950
13	*Siddhamantra*	1210–1247 CE	Keśava	Unknown	950
14	*Hṛdayadīpaka Nighaṇṭu*	1260–1271 CE	Bopadeva	Unknown	820
15	*Madanapāla Nighaṇṭu*	1374 CE	Madanapāla	Kāsṭhanagara	3,000
16	*Bhāvaprakāśa*	1550 CE	Bhāvamiśra	Kāśī, Kanyākubja	11,200
17	*Bhāvaprakāśa Nighantu*	1550 CE	Bhāvamiśra	Kāśī, Kanyākubja	2,600
18	*Rāja Nighantu*	1700 CE	Naraharipaṇḍita	Kaśmīra	7,300
19	*Śāligrāma Nighaṇṭu*	1896 CE	Śāligrāmavaiśya	Murādābād	4,200
20	*Siddhabheṣajamaṇimālā*	1896 CE	Kṛṣṇarāmabhaṭṭa	Jayapura	620

Source: FRLHT databases

- Sanskrit name
- Plant/animal/mineral/metal
- Gender
- Whether plant, plant part, product, group, relation with time, space
- Chapter
- Section (*sthāna*)
- Verse

The database field "Sanskrit name" pertains to resource names, which are classified into plant, animal/mineral and metal. The gender of the Sanskrit name is important, as some names in the feminine gender indicate vines, while the masculine counterpart indicates trees. For example, *amṛtā* (*Tinospora cordifolia*) is feminine, while *amṛta* (*Terminalia chebula*) is masculine. To differentiate this, "gender" is taken as a separate field. The plant parts, products, and groups are differentiated by tags. The same is the case for temporality and space relations. With respect to the former, for example, an unripe (*āma*) banana (*kaḍali phalam*) must be formally distinguished from a ripe (*pakva*) one; and with respect to the latter, for example, water from different locations is distinguished in the texts, for example, *sahyaja* (water from Western ghats).

At present, this consists of approximately 23,000 Sanskrit names drawn from 122,000 references in twenty texts. Tentative botanical correlations have been created using information derived from earlier databases and interface facilities that enhance the search capacities for synonyms and basionyms found in individual texts.

The database is now very helpful in analyzing and searching a variety of data for research purposes. For example, an analysis of *nighaṇṭus* composed between the eighth and nineteenth centuries reveals that around 70 percent of the materials used in Ayurveda is derived from plants, 20 percent from animals, and 10 percent from minerals during this period (Unnikrishnan 1997).

One of the challenges in building this classical, text-based database was the selection of texts. The main problem was the difficulty in defining a classical text. Can the many ayurvedic texts in regional languages, such as Malayalam or Marathi or Hindi, which are in common use in their language domains, be considered classical? These also may be in Sanskrit, but only in local use, or in a mixture of Sanskrit and a regional language. For example the Kerala tradition uses the *Cikitsāmañjari*, the *Sahasrayogam*, the *Yogāmṛtam*, the *Vaidyamanoramā*, the *Ārogyarakṣakalpadrūmam*, and others that were composed in Malayalam and are thus not used elsewhere in India. As a first criterion, we selected only Sanskrit texts that have not incorporated modern views or botanical correlations. Another criterion was that the text must be in the mainstream of ayurvedic thought and used or known in different parts of the country. This effort also attempted to address major chronological milestones in the development of Ayurveda and different geographical locations in order to demonstrate how Ayurveda and its pharmacopoeia might be different in various places in India.

Ascertaining the chronology of these classical texts was often difficult, as there are differences of opinion, though now Meulenbeld's chronology presented in his *History of Indian Medical Literature* must take precedence. Another issue is the dearth of critical editions. Various editions of these texts often show differences in verses or variations in *śloka* (verse) numbers. For the purpose of standardization, foundational verse texts (*mūlagranthas*) with or without Sanskrit commentaries, published in widely accepted editions, were selected. We are aware, of course, that more often than not these texts cannot be considered critical editions.

Another issue that often presented itself was irregular Sanskrit grammar. As mentioned earlier, even the slightest variation in the word, its gender, or a suffix or prefix (*pratyaya*) indicated a change in the identity of the plant. For example, *pippalī* and *pippala* are different, as are *mṛṇāla, mṛṇālī,* and *amṛṇāla, veṇu* and *veṇī; madhuka* and *madhūka, pataṅga* and *pattaṅga, padma* and *padmā, ariṣṭa* and *ariṣṭaka, nyagrodha* and *nyagrodhī, parpaṭa* and *parpaṭakī, palāśa* and *palāśī, sarala* and *saralā,* and *śāla* and *śāli,* to name just some.

Often the same plant name appears in slightly variant forms. For example, *yaṣṭi, yaṣṭika, yastīka, yastikāhvika, yaṣṭimadhūka, yaṣṭīmadhūka, madhūka, madhuyaṣṭika, madhuyasti,* and so on. All of these appear to be variants of the more commonly designated *yaṣṭimadhu,* but all must be considered separately before determining this.

A difference in names in various time periods was another problem. For example, *kokilāksa* is the name Suśruta uses for Caraka's *ikṣuraka* (see Ḍalhaṇa on Suśruta cikitsāsthāna 26.33), while *bhūmyāmalakī* and *tāmalakī* and *cākṣuṣya* and *kulatthikā* are said by *nighaṇṭu* authors to be identical. Yet another issue was collecting commentators' views on a plant in case of doubt. In a number of instances, differences of opinion among commentators with scant descriptions complicated the issue.

While compiling the references, contextual differences had to be considered. For example, in one context *kuṣṭha* means a skin disease, whereas elsewhere it is a plant name. Similarly, the term *tikta* means "bitter," but it is elsewhere identical to the plant names *kaṭukā* and *kirātatikta,* thus these references had to be carefully screened.

Similarly, we found a number of synonyms used in the same text in different contexts. Since the effort of this database was to prepare a complete list of plant names from each of these texts, it was necessary to group the variants and synonyms of each plant and link them to a primary name. This we did by grouping the references. This was, however, difficult without complete descriptions and commentators' views on each plant.

Another difficulty in grouping was that of classification of the parts used. At times the part has a different name altogether and is considered a separate entity. For example, *mocarasa*, the exudate of *śālmalī* (*Bombax* sp.), is mentioned as a different entity, as are *kuṭaja* (*Holarrhena pubescens*) and *indrayava*, the seed of this plant. Similarly, there are differences in plant names at different stages of maturity, for example, *ārdraka* (fresh ginger) and *śuṇṭhī* (dry ginger). Such references had to be identified and grouped separately. As mentioned earlier, the same names are used in the classical texts for different plants. For example, *uṣṇa* is a name used for *pippalī* and *marīca*, *kṛṣṇa* for *pippalī* and *arjuna*. Similarly, *citra* is used for *urubūka*, *eraṇḍa* and *dantī*, *tikta* for *kaṭurohinī* and *kākatiktā*, and *amṛta* for *guḍūcī* and *harītakī*. In these cases, each reference had to be searched for common names and synonyms.

The texts allow us to extract a few broad general principles for understanding the nomenclature. These principles, which we may regard as the units that contribute to definitions, are *jātiliṅga* (reproductive characteristics), *ākṛti* (physical characteristics), *varṇa* (color), *vīrya* (potency), *rasa* (taste), *prabhāva* (specific action), and so on. For example, *guḍūcī* (Tinospora cordifolia) is called *kuṇḍalī* or *maṇḍalī* due to its circular shape (*ākṛti*), or *kīrāṭatikta* (*Andrographis paniculata*) is called *tikta*, literally "bitter" because of its taste (*rasa*).

The texts also state that synonyms should be determined according to the meaning, context, tradition (*sampradāya*, *paramparā*), and reasoning (*tarka*). The term *tikta*, just noted, is also an example of this. Similarly, the term *kuṣṭha* is both a plant name and a disease name. Thus each contextual reference becomes important.

The references selected for this work did not represent the regional non-Sanskrit literature, such as the *Sahasrayogam*, *Cikitsāmañjarī*, and *Ārogyarakṣakalpadrūma*, all in Malayalam, in which much additional information is available. Thus this database is not yet a comprehensive inventory, because some plants that are in common use in Ayurveda do not appear in it. For example, *saptacakra* (*Salacia oblonga*) is described in the *Sahasrayogam*, but it does not appear in the database, as regional literatures are not included. Around 200 materials that are unique in their usage in Keralite medical tradition are documented in old issues of *Dhanvantari*, a journal published from Arya

Vaidya Sala, Kottakkal, a few decades ago. But many of these entries may not have been entered in this database.

The lack of proper software for Sanskrit also has proved somewhat problematic. The GIST software, produced by the Center for Development of Advanced Computing (CDAC) in Pune, has proved useful, though database style and programming have changed considerably since the inception of the project. The lack of good software for database operations in Sanskrit remains an unsolved issue, even today. As of this writing, the software for multilanguage databases compatible with Sanskrit remains inadequate. Fonts are available, but not complete software that can perform all of the necessary database operations.

Even after completion of this database, the major issue of critical nomenclature correlation remains unsolved. We learned that the issue of nomenclature correlation could only be advanced by a combination of approaches, including specialized studies of classical literature, documentation of the knowledge of ayurvedic and Unani physicians (*vaidyas* and *hakims*), and pharmacognostic and pharmacological/clinical studies.

For such an in-depth study, a mere reference database is not sufficient. All of the contextual details in each reference are necessary. Thus detailed individual text databases have been prepared. These include databases on the *bṛhattrayī*, the three great foundational compendia of Ayurveda, the *Caraka-Saṃhitā*, the *Suśruta-Saṃhitā*, and the *Aṣṭāṅgahṛdaya-Saṃhitā*, and databases of *nighaṇṭus*, specifically the *Dhanvantari Nighaṇṭu*, the *Madanapāla Nighaṇṭu*, the *Bhāvaprakāśa Nighaṇṭu*, and the *Rāja Nighaṇṭu*.

The database is bilingual, in Sanskrit and English, and the references are grouped by *nāma* (name), *rūpa* (form/identity), *guṇakarma* (quality and action), *varga, yoga,* and *gaṇa* (all indicating classification or formulation), *kalpana* (pharmaceutical preparation), and *prayoga* (clinical application). Sections also include the views of major commentators, including Cakrapāṇidatta (on Caraka) and Ḍalhaṇa (on Suśruta). Nomenclature is further classified into *svarūpabodhaka* (revealing form), *guṇabodhaka* (revealing quality), *karmabodhaka* (action), *rudhi* (traditional usage), *deśyokti* (habitat), and *itarahvaya* (names prevalent in other regions or due to other factors). For example, *kuṇḍalī, maṇḍalī,* and *cakralaksaṇa* are *svarūpabodhaka*; *tikta, āmlika,* and *kaṭuka* are *guṇabodhaka*; and *jvararī, bhedanī,* and *meharī* are *karmabodhaka*. A glossary is then prepared for the Sanskrit terms. Because similar problems exist for nomenclature correlation in disease names, and because we have not attempted a detailed study in this area for the database, we resorted to secondary sources for the preparation of this glossary.

After building the individual text databases, we used the following methodology to group the synonyms and locate the unique plants in each text:

- Collection of plant references
- Collection of commentators' views on these references
- Fixing of tentative basionym—based on commentaries and frequently used names
- Marking of grammatical variants linked to basionyms
- Marking of synonyms based on suggestions of commentators
- Marking of gender variations, if any
- Marking of plant names that pertain to groups, for example, *triphala, daśamūla*
- Marking of plant names as basionyms, if the plant name correlated by the commentator is not found marked under synonym or variant name
- Comparing of botanical correlations recorded by subject experts.
- Fixing status of identification by flagging them as noncontroversial, controversial, or unidentified, based on these studies

This analysis has now culminated in the following data for the *Caraka-Saṃhitā*: Of the 12,870 references to plants recorded in Caraka, 620 are calculated to be unique plant names, determined after grouping synonyms. Out of this number, 508 are identified and correlated to 630 botanical species. There are approximately 500 synonyms, 817 variants, and 56 group names in Caraka (Venugopal 2001). Of these, 305 plant names are noncontroversial, 203 are controversial, and 112 are unidentified. Furthermore, Caraka records approximately 1,630 formulations, the contents of which may be broken down. All of this adds up to a unique inventory of plants in the *Caraka-Saṃhitā*. Finally, based on the conservation databases at the foundation, we have ascertained that 56 plants identified in Caraka are presently under threat.

The database project is continuing along these lines. Similar work is now being carried out on other texts, and it is expected that after a few more years we will arrive at a better picture of the plants of Ayurveda.

Apart from this, as part of this project, similar work is being done on the Siddha and Unani systems of medicine. A number of other databases also are being developed on traditional quality standards, malaria, plants grown at home for primary health care, clinically important plants of Ayurveda, and rapid assessment of local health practices. These are linked to the master nomenclature correlation database (secondary sources of Ayurveda, Siddha, Unani, and folk medicine). Another master nomenclature database is based on nonclassical secondary sources published during the last 100 years. This database links the local language names to botanical names. The languages represented are the eighteen national languages and Sanskrit. Each botanical name has a standard identification number that is linked to any database developed at the FRLHT. Besides contributing to the study of nomenclature correlation, these databases also support efforts at conservation, education, research, clinical practice, pharmaceutical development, determination of intellectual property rights, and local health traditions assessment programs for primary health care.

CONCLUSION

During the process of developing these databases, the FRLHT has learned that nomenclature correlation of Sanskrit names of ayurvedic classical literature to botanical names is a complex task. A long history of casual and noncritical methodologies in correlation is the primary reason for the abundance of controversial, multiple, and confusing botanical identities. Only a systematic approach that considers equally the classical texts and commentaries, the regional literature, and the experience of living traditions, combined with pharmacognostic and pharmacological works, can shed proper light on Indian medical botany and serve as a springboard for solving problems of conservation and development.

NOTES

1. *gopālās tapasā vyādhā ye cānye vanacārinaḥ/ mūlāhārāś ca ye tebhyo bheṣajā vyaktir iṣyate//*. See also *Caraka* Sū 1.120-21: *auṣadhir nāmarūpābhyāṃ jānante hy ajapāvane/ avipaścaiva gopaś ca ye cānye vanavāsinaḥ//.*
2. See Saradamma (1990). This is one of a number of related studies.
3. Shankar (1998).

REFERENCES

Ainslie, Whitelaw. 1984 [1826]. *Materia Medica; or, Some Account of Those Articles Which Are Employed by the Hindoos, and Other Eastern Nations, in Their Medicine, Arts, and Agriculture . . . , etc.* Delhi: International Book Distributors.

Aiyer, K. N., A. N. Nambodiri, and M. Kolammal. 1957. *Pharmacognosy of Ayurvedic Drugs*. Vol. 3. Trivandrum: Pharmacognosy Department.

Anonymous. 1951. *Pharmacognosy of Ayurvedic Drugs*. Vols. 1 and 2. Trivandrum: Pharmacognosy Department.

Anonymous. 1978. *Ayurvedic Formulary of India, Part I*. New Delhi: Ministry of Health and Family Welfare.

Anonymous. 2001. *The Ayurvedic Pharmacopoeia of India. Part I, Vol. 1*. New Delhi: Ministry of Health and Family Welfare, Department of Health, Government of India.

Bāpālāl, Vaidya G. 1968. *Nighaṇṭu Ādarśa (Pūrvārdha)*. Vidyābhavan Āyurveda Granthamālā 54. Varanasi: Chowkhamba Vidyābhavan.

——. 1982. *Some Controversial Drugs in Indian Medicine*. Jaikrishnadas Ayurveda Series No. 33. Varanasi: Chaukhamba Oreintalia.

——. 1985. *Nighaṇṭu Ādarśa (Uttarārdha)*. Vidyābhavan Vidyābhavan Āyurveda Granthamālā 54. Varanasi: Caukhambā Bhāratī Ākādemī.

Kamat, Vaidya D. K. 1972. *Studies on Medicinal Plants in Dhanvantarīya Nighaṇṭu*. Poona: D. K. Kamat and S. D. Mahajan.

Kareem, A. 1997. *Plants in Ayurveda*. Bangalore: Foundation for Revitalization of Local Health Traditions.

Kirtikar, K. R., and B. D. Basu. 1935. *Indian Medicinal Plants*. 8 vols. 2nd ed. (with 1033 plates). Allahabad: Lalit Mohan Basu. Revised, enlarged, and mostly rewritten by E. Blatter, J. F. Caius, and K. S. Mhaskar. Dehradun: International Book Distributors/Delhi: Periodical Expert book Agency, 1981.

Kolammal, M. 1979. *Pharmacognosy of Ayurvedic Drugs*. Vol. 10. Trivandrum: Pharmacognosy Department.

Kurup, P. N. V., et al. 1968. *Handbook of Medicinal Plants* (revised and enlarged). New Delhi: Central Council for Research in Ayurveda and Siddhas.

Manohar, Ram. 1994. *Nomenclature and Taxonomy of Vṛkshāyurveda*. Coimbatore: Lok Swasthya Parampara Samvardhan Samithi.

Meulenbeld, G. J. 1974. *The Mādhavanidāna and Its Chief Commentaries, Chapters 1–10, Introduction, Translation, and Notes*. Leiden: E. J. Brill.

———. 1999–2002. *A History of Indian Medical Literature*. 3 vols. Groningen: Egbert Forsten.

Mioodeen Sheriff. 1978 [1869]. *A Catalogue of Indian Synonyms of the Medicinal Plants, Products, Inorganic Substances, Etc., Proposed To Be Included in the Pharmacopoeia of India*. Delhi: Periodical Experts Book Agency/Dehradun: International Book Distributors.

Mooss, N. S. 1976. *Single Drug Remedies*. Kottayam: Vaidyasarathy Press.

——. 1980. *Gaṇas of Vāhaṭa*. Kottayam: Vaidyasarathy Press.

Mukerji, B. 1953. *Indian Pharmaceutical Codex*. Vol. 1. New Delhi: Council of Scientific and Industrial Research.

Nadkarni, A. K. 1954. *Dr. K. M. Nadkarni's Indian Materia Medica, with Ayurvedic, Unani-Tibbi, Siddha, Allopathic, Homeopathic, Naturopathic, and Home Remedies*. Vols. 1 and 2. Bombay: Popular Book Depot.

Raghunath Iyer, S. 1993–1996. *Indian Medicinal Plants*. Vols. 1–5. Madras: Orient Longman.

Raisom, Alix. 1974. *Le Hārītasaṃhitā, texte médical sanskrit, avec un index de nomenclature āyurvédique*. Pondichéry: Publications de l'Institut Français d'Indologie No. 52.

Saradamma, L. 1990. *All India Coordinated Research Project on Ethnobiology, Final Technical Report—Phase-1 (1987–1990)*. Trivandrum: Regional Research Institute. Unpublished.

Shankar, D. 1998. *India's Medical Heritage: New Awakening*. Bangalore: Foundation for Revitalization of Local Health Traditions.

———. 2004. *Contemporary History in Challenging the Indian Medical Heritage*. Edited by D. Shankar and P. M. Unnikrishnan. Ahamedabad: Center for Environment Education.

Shankar, D., and Ram Manohar. 1995. Ayurvedic medicine today—Ayurveda at the Crossroads. In *Oriental Medicine—An Illustrated Guide to the Asian Arts of Healing*, edited J. V. Alphen and A. Aris, 99–105. London: Serindia Publications.

Sharma, P. V., 1994. *Dravyaguṇa Vijñāna*. Vols. 2 and 5. Varanasi: Chowkhambha Bharati Academy.

Singh, Thakur Balwant, and K. C. Chunekar. 1972. *Glossary of Vegetable Drugs in Brihattrayi*. Varanasi: Chowkhamba Sanskrit Series Office.

Sivarajan, V. V., and Indira Balachandran. 1994. *Ayurvedic Drugs and Their Plant Sources*. New Delhi: Oxford and IBH.

Unnikrishnan, P. M. 1997. An insight into Ayurveda's understanding of medicinal plants. *Amruth* (August supplement): vol. 1, issue 10, 1–20.

Vaidya, K. M. 1936. *Aṣṭāṅga Hṛdaya Koṣa, with the Hṛdaya Prakāsham (with a Critical and Explanatory Commentary)*. Vols. 1–4. Trichur: Mangalodayam Press.

Venugopal, S. N. 2001. Medicinal plants of Caraka Samhita—A close-up. *Amruth* 5:3: 5–14.

Watt, George. 1889. *A Dictionary of the Economic Products of India*. Vols. 1–6. Calcutta: Gordhan and Co.

CHAPTER 9

The Woes of *Ojas* in the Modern World

G. JAN MEULENBELD

Scire velim quare totiens mihi, Naevole, tristis
occurras, fronte obducta ceu Marsya victus

Tell me, Naevolus—why, whenever we meet, do you wear
a gloomy scowl, like Marsyas when he had lost the contest?

—Juvenal, *Satura* 9.1–2
Trans. N. Rudd: The Woes of a Gigolo

To Henk Schoonhoven, my unrivaled teacher of Latin

What is *ojas*? Is it relevant to the world in which we live? These are the questions I wish to address and to call attention to.[1] What is intended with the title "Woes of *ojas*"? Is the genitive of the subjective or objective type? Is *ojas* in trouble, or is the one observing its conditions of life worried? Is the state of *ojas* at stake or the mental position of the examiner? Is the history of *ojas* a tale of woe, or is its suffering due to present circumstances?

These and similar questions will crop up as I discuss the status and functions of *ojas* in classical ayurvedic theory, its origin in Vedic religion, the sweeping alterations to which it has been subject in contemporary Ayurveda, and my attitude toward these radical innovations.

Ojas is an old notion, yet wanting to survive, searching for means to succeed, seeking employment, even a promising post that may go hand in hand with rich rewards. Will it attain this aim? The outcome hangs in the balance. The sky is full of dark clouds.

This situation reminded me of similar vicissitudes in the life of a character called Naevolus, a professional gigolo who is growing old in ancient imperial Rome. He is in dire straits and fosters the hope not to fall victim to poverty and misery, which would make him dependent on the liberality of more fortunate ones who could pay him for his services.

In this emotional state he is depicted by Roman poet Juvenal, imagined as his patron, a wealthy man, walking through the streets of the city. This rich person runs into Naevolus and addresses him with these words:

> *Scire velim quare totiens mihi, Naevole, tristis*
> *occurras, fronte obducta ceu Marsya victus.*
> Tell me, Naevolus—why, whenever we meet, do you wear
> a gloomy scowl, like Marsyas when he had lost the contest?

What is the reason for my comparing *ojas* to a gigolo? My answer is that *ojas* has developed into a jack-of-all-trades, a factotum.

First I would like to introduce Juvenal, one of my favorites among Latin poets. He lived in the second half of the first and the first quarter of the second century of the Common Era under poor circumstances. Sixteen satires of his hand, composed in hexameters, have been preserved. These poems denounce the meanness and folly of Roman society of his times. He was a man who experienced the world as being out of joint. Bitterly, but accurately, his compositions describe the perpetrators and victims of the vices prevalent all around him.

The quoted ninth satire has, not surprisingly, been qualified as Juvenal's literary masterpiece and as a repulsive dialogue in which a catamite expounds the troubles of his vocation. It belongs to the pieces omitted from anthologies of Latin poetry for students. I feel no such need for shielding anyone from Roman frankness, though even famous commentators on Juvenal had not the mettle to extend their explications to this and other examples of Juvenal's candor and vitriolic sarcasm.

Ojas represents an archaic idea, concretizing and visualizing an abstract vital force as a material substance, a *dravya*, a fluid with a fixed number of qualities (*guṇas*).[2] Will it remain alive and flourish in a culture that rejects reification of abstract concepts?

It is for similar reasons that Naevolus, getting on in years, exclaims in desperation in the poem:

> *Quid agam bruma spirante? Quid, oro,*
> *quid dicam scapulis puerorum aquilone Decembri*
> *et pedibus? Durate atque expectate cicadas?*
> So what shall I do when the blizzards blow, I ask you

what shall I say to my lads in December, when their feet
and shoulders
are chilled by the cold north wind? Hold on, and wait for
the cicadas?

Ojas, endowed with a human voice, could have uttered the same complaints.

Originally *ojas* belongs to the worldview of the Vedic seers. The term *ójas* is found 166 times in the *Ṛgveda*, 53 times in the *Atharvaveda* (Dumézil 1969: 82, 86–87). The terms *ojmán, ójasvant*, and compounds with *ójas* as the second member also are known from the mentioned *saṃhitā*s. The boundaries between abstract ideas and concrete substances are blurred in these texts.

Two famous scholars, Jan Gonda and Georges Dumézil, have written on the term *ojas* and its meanings. Gonda evolved the view that *ojas* is a "Daseinsmacht," a power substance, that provides deities, humans, things, and natural phenomena with something beyond understandable common experience and that rather vaguely can be designated as a kind of vital energy.[3]

Dumézil arrived at the contrasting conclusion that *ojas* is a purely physical force, directed at the outside world. Accordingly, he argues that the term is distinctive of what in his theory is the second order, that of the warriors, the *kṣatriya*s. Though he refrains from going into the details of Gonda's earlier published monograph, his perspective is almost diametrically opposed to the latter's, as Ana Salema observes in her thesis, where she sides with Gonda. In my own opinion, Salema is right in her appraisal. Gonda is more comprehensive and many-hued in his monograph, being not blinkered by a fixed view, as Dumézil is, who was obsessed by his theory of the three orders in old Indo-European communities.[4] This notwithstanding, it must be conceded that Dumézil had a keen and discriminating eye for details making *ojas* an element of a masculine universe.

The Vedic *saṃhitā*s do not evenly distribute *ojas* over the deities. The largest share is allotted to Indra (94 times in a total of 116 in the *Ṛgveda*) (Dumézil 1969: 82). The Maruts, Indra's attendants, also receive a fair portion (16 times). Different contexts are much less frequent, to Dumézil's satisfaction, who considered Indra the preeminent representative of the second order.

The notions intimately joined to *ojas* in *Ṛgveda* and *Atharvaveda* are not without consequence, belonging as they do to a coherent set of ideas. Gonda (1952) collected a great deal of this material. Three concepts stand out and have to be kept in mind, being crucial to future interpretations of *ojas*. These concepts are designated by the terms *bala*, *sahas*, and *tejas*. All three remain conjoined to *ojas* in later texts.

The medical classics handle *ojas* in a way both similar and dissimilar to the Vedic ideas about it. Unfortunately, documentation on the intermediate stages is virtually absent. Speculations only can fill up this gap in the "fossil record." It may, however, turn out that there simply are no missing links, since Vedic and ayurvedic thought can be supposed to be two different structures, originating from a common ancestor that can no longer be traced. In that case we would be faced with a situation familiar to palaeontologists; the latter tend more and more to give up their search for continuous sequences of evolving organisms in the conviction that new species originate by branching (Gould 2002: 776–81).

In Ayurveda *ojas* is no longer a force inherent in divine beings who can bestow it on human beings, nor a power possessed by outstanding holy men and sages, as in post-Vedic texts examined by Gonda.

It has been transformed into a fluid substance, a constituent of all human beings, both male and female. This component is essential for the preservation of life and health. In spite of this, its position within the theoretical framework of Ayurveda is ill-defined from the beginning and has remained so. It was and is a problematic substance.

Prior to dealing with other aspects, it seems best to turn first to the thorny and vexed question of whether or not there is one single type of *ojas*. This topic is much talked of in the commentaries and the secondary literature. To avoid longwindedness, I restrict myself to the *Caraka-Saṃhitā* and the *Suśruta-Saṃhitā*, together with their commentaries.

The issue finds its origin in some verses of Chapter 17 of the *Sūtrasthāna* of the *Caraka-Saṃhitā* (17.73–75 and an additional verse), where *ojas* is characterized as follows:

> When *ojas* has diminished, one is afraid, weak, and constantly worried, the organs of sense do not function normally, one's complexion is not healthy, nor are the mental faculties, dryness and slimming prevail.
>
> The *ojas*, which resides in the heart in a (human) body, is considered to be pure and of a reddish and yellowish colour: its loss leads to death.
>
> *Ojas* is the first (constituent) to arise in the body of bodily beings; it has the color of melted butter, the taste of honey, and the smell of fried paddy.
>
> In the same way as honey is collected from fruits and flowers by bees, *ojas* is collected in human beings by the *guṇa*s through their actions.[5]

First the symptoms of diminution (*kṣaya*) of *ojas* are listed. The second verse deals with the properties of *ojas* and adds that death ensues when it is annihilated (*nāśa*). The third stanza enumerates properties again, totally disagreeing this time with what precedes. The fourth verse, probably interpolated, contains a simile—*ojas* and the way it arises in the body are compared to the collection of honey by bees.

This short sequence of verses strikes the eye as being odd. The two characterizations of *ojas* are not in conformity with each other. The added stanza changes the tone and waxes poetic.

This presented the commentators with a set of difficulties. Their first concern was to find out whether one or two varieties of *ojas* were meant, one so essential to the going on of life that the loss of one drop was equivalent to death (Cakrapāṇidatta ad Ca.Sā.30.7) and another one that, when subject to decrease, ends in disease.

In my view, one may legitimately ask if it is unavoidable to create this conundrum, for it may well be that a diminished amount of *ojas* entails the onset of disease, and that death is the outcome of total loss. This line of reasoning is indeed adopted by the nineteenth-century commentator Gaṅgādhara and a few more recent authors.

Caraka's commentator Cakrapāṇidatta, however, posits the existence of two kinds of *ojas*. It is an amazing spectacle to watch how slavishly a majority of Ayurvedists bow to his authority. He bases his case on the distinction between *nāśa* and *kṣaya*, but the strongest prop comes from some unspecified treatise he quotes. This unknown text declares that eight drops (*bindu*) of *ojas*, the support of *prāṇa* or the *prāṇas*,[6] are present in the heart. Following this tack, Cakrapāṇidatta adds that this is the *aṣṭabinduka* (i.e., consisting of eight drops) or *para ojas*. The other type is the one mentioned as measuring half an *añjali* in the *Caraka-Saṃhitā*. I shall return to the latter.

It is remarkable that most ayurvedic scholars embrace Cakrapāṇidatta's doctrinal pronouncement, despite the fact that neither the *Caraka-Saṃhitā* nor the *Suśruta-Saṃhitā* ever refers to a quantity of eight drops of *ojas*. Even Gaṅgādhara, who confutes Cakrapāṇidatta's division into two types of *ojas*, does not dismiss the eight drops. However, he argues that eight drops amount to half an *añjali*,[7] the standard amount of the second kind of *ojas*.

To further support his interpretation, Cakrapāṇidatta refers to a passage of the *Caraka-Saṃhitā* (Sū.30.7) in which *para ojas* is mentioned as being situated in the heart.

The meaning of *para ojas* in this context needs to be discussed. As the *Caraka-Saṃhitā* nowhere makes explicit mention of two kinds of *ojas*, it is implausible that it does so here only. Although most Ayurvedists agree with Cakrapāṇidatta, I prefer the assumption that the adjective *para* is chosen to highlight *ojas* as a superior and an excellent bodily constituent.

Another piece of evidence employed by Cakrapāṇidatta to corroborate the distinction of two kinds of *ojas* is the occurrence of the expression *ślaiśmikaujas* in the *Caraka-Saṃhitā* (Śā.7.15).[8] It is found once only in a prose passage specifying the quantities of a number of bodily constituents in an average human being, measured in *añjalis*. The amount of *ojas* is settled at half an *añjali*, precisely the same quantity as that of brain tissue (*mastiṣka*) and semen (*śukra*).

Again, I do not see a cogent reason to discern a particular variety of *ojas*, as Cakrapāṇidatta is wont to do. What is intended may simply be that *ojas* has properties in common with *śleśman* or *kapha* (the third *doṣa*, often rendered as "phlegm"), as the preceding items, brain tissue and semen, have. Actually, Cakrapāṇidatta comments in this sense, remarking that both elements are *samānaguṇa*, that is, they have the same or similar qualities.[9] Support of this interpretation is provided by the *Suśruta-Saṃhitā*, which characterizes *ojas* as having the nature of water (*somātmaka*) and as being cold (*śīta*), qualities suitable to *śleṣman*.

Ojas, though having no intrinsic affinity for the *doṣas* whatsoever, is associated with *śleśman* on a second occasion in the *Caraka-Saṃhitā* (Sū.17.117). A noteworthy and puzzling verse puts *śleśman* in its normal state (*prākṛta*) on par with *bala* (physical force) and *ojas*. This stanza gives proof that some unspecified kind of kinship is supposed to exist between *śleśman* and *ojas*.

What to make of this?[10] My preference goes to regarding *ojas* as possessing qualities in common with *śleśman*, maybe not with the latter as a *doṣa*,[11] but as a *mala*.[12] One ayurvedic authority, the late C. Dwarkanath, wrote a lengthy exposition on *ojas* in one of his books (*Introduction to Kāyachikitsā*). He underscores an intimate affinity of *śleśman*, *ojas*, and one of their effects, namely, stability and integrity. This issue requires more study and has to be left for another occasion.

Provisionally, the conclusion is that the *Caraka-Saṃhitā* recognizes one single, homogeneous kind of *ojas*.

The picture we get from the *Suśruta-Saṃhitā* is in various respects at variance with the *Caraka-Saṃhitā*. There are no clues in it that give reasons to differentiate two kinds of *ojas*. *Ojas* is one single, undivided substance, so closely yoked to *bala* as to make the two terms interchangeable. *Ojas* is pictured as the essence of all the *dhātus*, the series of seven types of tissue. It is the source of unhampered functioning of all the organs of sense (*indriya*). Bodily strength (*bala*) also finds its ground in *ojas*. The heart is its seat, thence it is transported through vessels and carried throughout the body.

Three disorders of *ojas* are acknowledged, which constitute three degrees of depletion: *visraṃsa*, *vyāpad*, and *kṣaya*. The last of these three may result in death. This series, mounting in severity, is unknown to the *Caraka-Saṃhitā*. Suśruta's *kṣaya* resembles Caraka's *nāśa* without being identical.

Ojas is highlighted as the quintessence of the *dhātus*.[13] Interestingly, it is called their *para tejas*. The term *tejas* is not found in the context of *ojas* in the *Caraka-Saṃhitā*, where it is designated as an essence (*sāra*) or the *sneha* (literally, a fatty substance) collected from the whole body (Sū.30.8–12ab). Ḍalhaṇa, the commentator on the *Suśruta-Saṃhitā*, remarks that *tejas* should be taken metaphorically: *ojas* is the essential part (*sneha*) of all the *dhātus*, as ghee is the essential part of milk. Even though the *Suśruta-Saṃhitā* literally pronounces *ojas* and *bala* to be one and the same, Ḍalhaṇa emphasizes that, actually (*paramārthatas*), this is not true at all. *Ojas*, being a substance (*dravya*), possesses properties (*guṇa*), whereas *bala*, as a power, a potential activity, such as the ability of carrying burdens, is devoid of them. In summary, the *Suśruta-Saṃhitā* depicts *ojas* as one single substance, the essence of all the bodily elements and the fountainhead of physical force.

Some of the details found in the *Suśruta-Saṃhitā* deserve closer inspection. To be noted first is that, unexpectedly, Suśruta's text displays more affinity for the Vedic data than the *Caraka-Saṃhitā*. *Ojas* is affiliated with *bala* and *tejas* in Vedic texts.

Tejas[14] is an ambiguous term in ayurvedic literature. In a large number of instances it is synonymous with or closely related to *pitta* (e.g., Su.Sā.15.23). It also may designate an inherent force, for the *doṣas* are endowed with an *ātmatejas* (Su.Sā.15.36; Ḍalhaṇa: = *śakti*), which means that each *doṣa* possesses its own type of *tejas*. In general, *tejas* is a kind of fiery energy, denoting brilliance, brightness, glare. This explains its kinship to *agni*, the digestive and, in general, transforming fire, and to *pitta*, not to *ojas*, which is watery and cold. The interconnectedness of terms from the sphere of *ojas* should be taken into consideration consistently and accepted as consequential in interpreting particular passages. The term *sahas* also belongs to this category. P. V. Sharma published a short article on the relationships of *ojas*, *bala*, and *sahas*, which is a little gem, written in Hindi. There, Sharma points out that these three terms, not found consecutively in ayurvedic texts, do occur in a series, even repeatedly, in the *Bhāgavatapurāṇa*, as three forms of *bala*. The commentator Śrīdharasvāmin gives in his *Bhāvārthadīpikā* (ad 25.26; edition used not indicated) the following three equivalents: *indriyaśakti*, *manaśakti*, and *dehaśakti* (power of the sense organs, the mind, and the body). Sharma does not refer to *Ṛgveda* 5.57.6, where *sahas*, *ojas*, and *bala* are said to reside in the arms of the Maruts (see Gonda 1957: 19).

He argues, in the same vein as Ḍalhaṇa, that *ojas* and *bala* are not identical. In his opinion, *ojas* is an inner (*ābhyantara*) *bala* with *prāṇadhāraṇa*, support of the life forces, as its function; it is the cause of *vyādhikṣamatva*, a term that still needs to be discussed. *Bala* sensu stricto is directed to the outside world (*bāhyabala*) and is the source of the actions of the various parts of the body.

Sahas plays a minor role in ayurvedic texts. The word is more common in Vedic literature and often joined to *ojas* and *bala*. P.V. Sharma considers *sahas* the limit of *bala*. It is connected to endurance and stamina. *Sahas* ought to be kept in reserve for extreme circumstances, and physical exercise should not exceed the half of one's *bala*. Action on the level of *sahas* is called *sāhasa*, or *ayathābala*;[15] its abuse causes diseases, such as *uraḥkṣata*, *śoṣa* and *rājayakṣman*.[16]

As pointed out in the foregoing, *ojas* also is connected to *śleśman* or *kapha*. Caraka's *ślaiśmikaujas* may have contributed to this, as well as Cakrapāṇi's comments on the term, claiming that *ojas* and *śleśman* have the same or similar properties, and that *ojas* is the essence (*sāra*) of *śleśman*. Caraka's verse about the identity of *ojas*, *bala*, and *prākṛtaśleśman* also may have provided further grounds for this development.

The status of *ojas* among the other constituents of the body is inquired into by the commentators.

Cakrapāṇidatta expatiates on the subject (ad Ca.Sū.30.7). He rejects that *ojas* is the same as *rasa*,[17] despite Caraka's declaration (Ni.4.7) that the *rasa* called *ojas* is one of the corruptible constituents (*dūṣya*) in *prameha*,[18] and another claim of Caraka's (Ci.8.41) saying that a small amount only of the ingested food is converted into *ojas*. Cakrapāṇidatta regards *ojas* as the essence of all the *dhātus*. He adds that some consider *ojas* a secondary *dhātu* (*upadhātu*). A *dhātu*, however, supports the body (*dehadhāraka*) and nourishes it (*poṣaṇa*), whereas *ojas*, as any *upadhātu*, is only *dehadhāraka*. Hence, it is unjustified to call *ojas* the eighth *dhātu*. Others again bring to the fore that *ojas* is a particular kind of *śukra* (semen). Cakrapāṇidatta does not agree with that idea. Finally, he gives his consent to the view that *ojas* consists of the collection of the essences of all the *dhātus* (*sarvadhātusārasamudāya*), is not distinct from them, and is neither a *dhātu* nor an *upadhātu*. The nature of an essence is not elucidated and remains mysterious.

Cakrapāṇidatta maintains the same stance elsewhere (ad Su.Sū.15.19): *Ojas* is an assemblage or mixture of the *prasāda* parts of the bodily elements (*[dhātu]prasādamelakarūpa* and *saptadhātuka*).[19]

In the context of contemporary views on *ojas* one cannot possibly refrain from considering the term *vyādhikṣamatva*, resistance against a disease or disease in general. This notion is found in the *Caraka-Saṃhitā* (Sū.28.7), in an elaborate exposition on the problem that proneness to disease and its effects varies from person to person, and that the degree of resistance depends on a multiplicity of factors.

Cakrapāṇidatta distinguishes two types of resistance in his comments on the passage: resistance against the force (*bala*) of a present disease entity (*vyādhibalavirodhikṣamatā*) and resistance against the etiological factors of a disease (*vyādhyutpādavibandhakatva*). This resembles another dichotomy: Drugs can be effective against a disease entity itself (*vyādhipratyanīka*) or against the cause of a disease, consisting of a *doṣa* (*doṣapratyanīka*).

Vyādhikṣamatva is a term with a wide range in the *Caraka-Saṃhitā*, comprising all of the elements that bear upon the rise of a disorder, its symptoms, and its course. An immediate relationship with *ojas* cannot be detected.

Nevertheless it has become a widespread habit in contemporary ayurvedic circles to conjoin the terms intimately and even specifically. The two, frequently along with *bala*, are now considered to designate immunity. The history of this evolution is still to be traced.

Before diving deeper into current assumptions and convictions, a glance at the diverse interpretations of *ojas*, ancient and recent ones, may illustrate that my comparing *ojas* to a gigolo is not unfounded. History teaches that the concept is at the disposal of anyone wishing to fill up a gap perceived or imagined in ayurvedic theory, particularly after the penetration of Western medicine.

The coupling of *ojas* to *bala*, *tejas*, and *kapha*, the essence of the *dhātus*, and to *vyādhikṣamatva* has already been examined. Ḍalhaṇa (ad Su.Sū.15.19) adds *rasa*, *ūṣman*[20] and *jīvaśoṇita*,[21] terms that I shall not discuss, as equivalents of *ojas*.

New inventions and interpretations of ayurvedic technical terms thought up or concocted by Ayurvedists after they had become more conversant with advances in the life sciences nicely reflect the course of development in these disciplines. Some articles of Indian authors provide us with a motley list of such mostly unfounded renderings. Regrettably, the sources of these inventions are rarely disclosed.

One of the authors supplying such an inventory, Prabhañjan Ācārya, connects *ojas* to albumine, glycogen (oddly called *drākṣāśarkarā*, which is glucose), vitamins (*jīvanīyadravya*), pituitrine (a hormone from the pineal gland, but, unintelligibly, referred to as *pīyūṣagranthisāra*), the internal secretions of testicles and ovaries, and the prostatic secretion (*aṣṭhīlāsāra*).

An article by Aśvinī Kumār Śarmā and Kanak Prasād furnishes an even longer list of twelve possible meanings of *ojas*: *śukrasāra* (the essence of semen), *śukramala* (the impurity derived from semen), *śukropadhātu* (the *upadhātu* of semen), *śukrasnehabhāga* (the fatty part of semen), *śukrajanaka* (that which generates semen), *rasa* (lymph or plasma), testosterone, *śleśman* (phlegm), *rasayoga*, *rakta* (blood), the *para tejas* of the seven *dhātus* = *bala*, *pīyūṣagranthisrāva*.[22]

The equalization with semen, sexual hormones, and similar chemical substances is the most stunning because of the absence of correlations between *ojas* and virility or fertility in general since Vedic times. Śarmā's and Prasād's claim can therefore easily be rebutted.

More of these identifications will probably be detected in combing the literature.

An outstanding example is properdin, proposed as a serious definition of *ojas* by Dwarkanath (1959) in his *Introduction to Kāyachikitsā*. He describes this nowadays forgotten substance as a lipoprotein, present in the blood, with antibacterial and antiviral properties. A lengthy and detailed exposition is devoted to this subject.

All of this tinkering, taken together, composes a variegated scene, bearing witness to the fuzziness of *ojas*, making it multi-serviceable. Its assistance can be called for when Ayurveda is impotent in performing a particular function, and when a hiatus is observed compared to Western medicine. *Ojas* is multifaceted and multipurpose in character and a kind of passe-partout.

This smells of Juvenal's poem. The protagonist of his poem reminds his patron of debts toward him. Albeit wealthy, this patron, unable or unwilling to have intercourse with his wife, has two legal children thanks to Naevolus and ought to shower more liberal gifts on him. I quote, omitting outspoken and lewd passages, his words:

> *Instabile ac dirimi coeptum est iam paene solutum*
> *coniugium in multis domibus servavit adulter.*
> *Quo te circumagas? Quae prima aut ultima ponas?*
> *nullum ergo meritum est, ingrate et perfide, nullum,*
> *quod tibi filiolus vel filia nascitur ex me?*
> A tottering crumbling marriage just on the verge of collapse
> has, in the case of many a house, been saved by a lover.
> Why prevaricate? How can you frame a respectable answer?
> Does it count for nothing, nothing at all, you ungrateful
>   swindler,
> that, thanks to me, you possess a little son and daughter?

Ayurvedists of our age resort to Western medicine for the rescue of *ojas*, and, as to be expected, this request is granted with a vengeance.

The medical events of our times demonstrate that ayurvedic practice cannot equal the successes of modern medicine in fighting infectious diseases. The search for antibacterial and antiviral compounds from Indian medicinal plants is therefore (and has been for many years already) one of the preferred areas in pharmacological literature.

The difficulties encountered by contemporary scientists in discovering and designing efficient antiviral drugs have prompted ayurvedic pharmacologists to search for medicinal plants containing such substances. As a result, a wealth of articles has been poured out on vegetable substances acting on viruses and, especially, on those influencing the immune system. Publications on immunomodulatory drugs from Indian medicinal (ayurvedic) plants are almost countless. The intensity of these efforts is comprehensible. Discovering an efficacious drug deriving from one of these plants would boost Ayurveda tremendously.

In this situation ayurvedic scholars see themselves faced with the task of how to integrate knowledge about immunity in their theory. Those familiar with the resourcefulness of advocates of Ayurveda will not look on in wonderment observing the ease in solving this apparent crux.

The assistance of *ojas* is invoked. Its kinship to *bala* facilitates a partnership. The feature that *ojas* is transported in vessels and carried throughout the body as an essence of all of its components is a concomitant advantage.

Thus it has come about that a large number of Ayurvedists nowadays assert that the ancient *ojas* is involved in immunity or, more accurately, constitutes the basis for a well-functioning immune system (*rasasāra*). As a rule, the differences between humoral and cellular immunity are, for the sake of convenience, overlooked.

It also has become habitual to couple *ojas* directly with *vyādhikṣamatva* and its varieties, the latter being the effect of the former. A textual ground for this tight bond is not discoverable, and the marriage is in my eyes illegal. These high expectations, stemming from a preset and channeled perception, derail the ability to read the texts literally and to remain within the bounds of their teaching. In the wake of these developments, a whole new vocabulary has come into vogue.

Aśvinī Kumār Śarmā, for example, employs the following terms:

> *Vyādhibalavirodhikṣamatā* = acquired and artificial immunity
> *Vyādhyutpādapratibandhakakṣamatā* = natural or congenital immunity

In many articles this author recommends, for strengthening the immune system, drugs useful for *rasāyaṇa* purposes, as well as drugs that promote strength (*balya*) and body mass (*bṛṃhaṇa*), and, in particular, those that increase *ojas* (*ojovardhaka*).[23]

Immunity and its disorders have come into prominence since the spread of the human immune deficiency virus (HIV) and its attendant, AIDS. Ayurveda does not stay out of the battle, and its literature abounds in articles on the subject. In this case, too, a special vocabulary has sprung up.

An Indian author, Ayodhyā Prasād Acal, coined the term *mānavapratirakṣānāśakaviṣāṇu*[24] for the virus and *pratirakṣākṣamatālakṣaṇasamūha*[25] for the AIDS syndrome.

The most common term for AIDS is nowadays *ojakṣaya*, a word found in a large number of articles and books. The majority of the authors give first an account of HIV infections and AIDS in conformity with scientific knowledge at the time of writing, followed by proposals for ayurvedic treatment. The high number of drugs recommended is striking. Gyanendra Pandey's monograph on the subject enumerates no less than 122 useful plants and 155 formulations. This abundance evinces an actual poverty and means that a specific and more or less satisfactory way of treatment has not been discovered so far. Reports about the results of ayurvedic therapy are rare. A burgeoning literature is devoted to experimental studies with plants and their constituents.[26] One of the articles records two case reports, and another refers to a treatment proclaimed successful by hearsay.

In sum, while *ojas* plays only a minor and vaguely defined role in classical ayurvedic theory and therapy, it is given special attention and emphasis in the contemporary ayurvedic scene. The rise of immunology in Western medical science has challenged the ayurvedic world, which has responded not only with envy but in a competitive spirit, hoping for rich rewards thanks to its enticing *ojas*.

Juvenal's character exclaims, toward the end of the poem:

O parvi nostrique Lares, quos ture minuto
aut farre et tenui soleo exorare corona,
quando ego figam aliquid, quo sit mihi tuta senectus
a tegete et baculo? Viginti milia faenus
pigneribus positis, argenti vascula puri,
sed quae Fabricius censor notet, et duo fortes
de grege Moesorum, qui me cervive locata
securum iubeant clamoso insistere circo.
O little household gods of mine, whose aid I am wont
to secure with meal, or grains of incense and a simple garland,
when shall I net a sum that will save me, when I am old,
from the beggar's mat and crutch? An income of twenty thousand
from a well-secured principal, some plain silver (a few little pieces,
which censor Fabricius, however, would ban), a couple of brawny
Moesian[27] porters to take me upon their shoulders, and let me
Ride[28] serenely above the crowd at the noisy racetrack.

The question presents itself whether rivalry with Western medicine in the area of immunology and its applications makes any sense. Is it beneficial or detrimental to Ayurveda and its position in the world at large?

My answer is that it harms Ayurveda to overshoot its mark. Coming back specifically to *ojas*, I incline to the opinion that Ayurvedists should weigh the pros and cons of retaining the concept or dropping it. If retained, I see no chances that any interpretation can stand the test of acceptability. Discarding it would have no tragic or fatal consequences as far as I can discern and would be no reason for dismay.

Pursuing this line of reflection, I propose to deliberate on the conditions for a theory to be still called ayurvedic. What are the minimal requirements, its conditions sine qua non? This is a legitimate inquiry in my eyes. Stephen Jay Gould (2002), the famous palaeontologist, has applied it masterfully in his last book *The Structure of Evolutionary Theory*. He developed an image for the basic assumptions of his science, a tree with three main branches, not one of which can be chopped off without destroying the basic structure of Darwinian thought; the secondary and tertiary branches, however, may be cut away, giving scope for new growths.

Evolutionary theory, however, is not the most suitable object of comparison, being a scientific structure based on verifiable facts. A more congruent model is psychoanalytic theory which, as its ayurvedic counterpart, is not of a scientific nature because it is neither falsifiable nor verifiable. In psychoanalytic theory, a consensus about its minimal requirements has, unfortunately, not been attained.

The case of Ayurveda may be less complicated. It may turn out to be built on a three-pillared (*tristhūṇa*) foundation, for example the *doṣa-dhātu-mala* system,[29] though I am afraid I would make demands on a fourth one, *agni*,[30] despite the awareness that Ayurveda dislikes even numbers.[31]

The basic framework could remain intact, while the secondary and tertiary branches[32] could be removed, giving new growths the chance to develop, flower, and bear fruit. This image is more attractive to me, because it bears resemblance to Johann Wolfgang von Goethe's ingenious scheme of letting the whole plant kingdom sprout from three simple formative principles.[33]

Last, but not least, I cherish the idea that theories are models, helpful for practice, and that the results of actual practice are the things that matter most. That is why it is useful to return to comparing Ayurveda to psychoanalysis, which, notwithstanding its precarious theoretical status, can boast of practical successes, as my own experience has taught me. The same holds true for Ayurveda. Practical results will be the standards for its merits and demerits.

NOTES

Marsyas was a satyr and an expert musician; he challenged the god Apollo to a contest in playing the *aulos*. Apollo, having defeated him, took advantage of an agreement that the winner should do as he liked with the loser and flayed him alive.

1. The notion of *ojas* constitutes a significant common element in Vedic and ayurvedic thought, which would justify a much more comprehensive study than the one presented in this chapter.

2. See *Caraka-Saṃhitā, Sūtrasthāna* 17.74–75; *Suśruta-Saṃhitā, Sūtrasthāna* 15.21; *Aṣṭāṅgahṛdaya-Saṃhitā, Sūtrasthāna* 11.38; *Aṣṭāṅga-Saṃgraha, Sūtrasthāna* 19.29cd.

3. The related adjective *ugra* points to anything that has a share in it. Its comparative, *ojīyas*, and superlative, *ojiṣṭha*, also are worth studying.

4. The three orders represent authority, defense, and fertility.

5. The translation of the last verse is tentative because of the uncertain meanings of *guṇa* and *karman* (action). The *guṇas* are usually the properties of the ingested food; this sense may be applicable here, because *ojas* is described as the first bodily constituent to arise. The meaning of *karman* (*svakarmabhyaḥ* in the text) is hard to determine; in medical theory, strictly taken, a *guṇa* has no *karman*, since this is applicable to a substance (*dravya*) only.

6. The *prāṇa* and the group of *prāṇas* are vital forces.

7. An *añjali* is the quantity of fluid that can be held in the open hands placed side by side and slightly hollowed.

8. The text has *tāvad eva ślaiṣmikasyaujasa iti; tāvad eva* refers to half an *añjali*, the same quantity as that of the preceding items *mastiṣka* (brain tissue) and *śukra* (semen). Indian translator Kaviratna reads *ojas* and translates: of the *ojas* the measure is the same (as above). He remarks in a footnote that some manuscripts have *śleṣman ojas*, which is evidently incorrect, because *ojas* is not regarded as any kind of phlegm. Commentator Gaṅgādhara accepts the reading *śleṣman ojas*; his comments are rather enigmatic when compared to earlier statements ad Ca.Sū.17.73–75. He says: *Śleṣman ojas* is a particular type of *śleṣman* called *ojodhātu*; the *ojas* present in a quantity of eight drops (*bindu*) is not subject to decrease or increase, for death results from its *nāśa*; a *bindu* is the same as a *karṣa*, and eight of them amount to half an *añjali*. A parallel passage from the Saṃgītaratnākara (1.2.116cd–118) is interesting, which gives the same quantity as the *Caraka-Saṃhitā* but reads *śleṣmasāra* instead of *ślaiṣmikaujas*. In the *Kāśyapa-Saṃhitā* (p. 78), the quantity of *ojas* is the same as that of kapha.

9. Cakrapāṇidatta states that not the *aṣṭabinduka ojas* is intended, but the second type, transported through the whole body and having the same properties as purified *śleṣman*.

10. Kaviratna remarks that normal phlegm is called bodily strength; it is the phlegm that is also called the *ojas* in the system. K. R. Sharma and Bhagwan Dash translate: "The *kapha* in its natural state promotes strength in the form of ojas." P. V. Sharma renders: "*Kapha*, in normal state, is (responsible for) strength; in other words, the normal *kapha* is said as *ojas*."

11. The *doṣas* are the three fundamental morbific entities of Indian medical theory.

12. The *malas* are impurities, excretory products, to be removed from the body.

13. The *dhātus* are the seven bodily elements, or main types of tissue.

14. See, on *tejas*, Gonda (1957) and Vogel (1930).

15. The *Caraka-Saṃhitā* employs the term *ayathābala* in Ci.8.13.

16. Literally an injury to the chest, desiccation, and wasting.

17. *Rasa* usually designates the first (the nutrient fluid) of the series of seven bodily constituents called *dhātu*.

18. *Prameha* comprises a series of urinary disorders, among which is what is diagnosed as diabetes mellitus today.

19. Each bodily element is separated into a pure (*prasāda*) part and waste matter during metabolism.

20. Literally heat; the term is employed for both the digestive fire and *pitta*.

21. See, on this term, Das (2003: 119–20, 133–34, 481, 532).

22. See also Singh, Gaur, and Shukla (1977).

23. Plants regarded as *ojovardhaka* are: *aśvagandhā*, *balā*, *nāgabalā*, *śatāvarī*, and *vidārigandhā* (Devāṅgan and Kulśreṣṭh 1991).

24. Literally human immunity destroying virus.

25. Literally immunodeficiency syndrome.

26. S. K. Agarwalla (1992) claims that six plants have demonstrated to possess anti-HIV activities in in vitro studies: *Andrographis paniculata* (*Burm*.f.) *Wall. ex Nees*, *Centella asiatica* (*Linn.*) *Urban* = *Hydrocotyle asiatica Linn.*, *Glycyrrhiza glabra Linn.*, *Hypericum perforatum Linn.*, *Hyssopus officinalis Linn.*, and *Momordica charantia Linn.* Mungantiwar and Phadke (2004) mention as plants that have shown anti-HIV activity: *Cichorium intybus Linn.*, *Glycyrrhiza glabra Linn.*, *Grifola frondosa*, *Punica granatum Linn.*, *Curcuma longa Linn.*, and *Aloe vera Linn.* See also Ahn et al. (2002); Valsaraj et al. (1997); Premanathan et al. (2000).

27. The Moesians were a Thracian tribe living on the lower Danube and renowned for their bodily strength.

28. In a palanquin.

29. The pillars of medical theory are these three groups of bodily constituents and their interactions. The triad is a prominent element of the Aṣṭāṅgahṛdaya-Saṃhitā.

30. The transforming fire(s). See: Meulenbeld, *Some Neglected Aspects of Ayurveda, or the Illusion of a Consistent Theory* (forthcoming).

31. The *doṣas* are three in number, there are five *mahābhūtas*, seven bodily elements, two sets of three tastes, and five procedures constituting *pañcakarman*; opposite examples also can be adduced, for example, the two sets of ten *guṇas*.

32. A secondary branch of the primary branch of the *dhātus* would be *ojas*, with its two varieties as tertiary branches.

33. Original publication J. W. von Goethe, *Versuch die Metamorphose der Pflanzen zu erklären*, Gotha, 1790. See Gould (2002: 281–91). These three principles consist of the archetypal leaf, progressive refinement of sap up the stem, and three expansion-contraction cycles of vegetation, blossoming, and bearing fruit (ibid., 288).

TEXTS AND TRANSLATIONS

Carakasaṃhitā, with the commentary of Cakrapāṇidatta. Edited by Vaidya Jādavji Trikamji Āchrya. Bombay: Nirṇaya Sāgar Press, 1941.

Carakasaṃhitā, with the commentaries of Cakrapāṇidatta and Gaṅgādhara. Vol. 1. Edited by Narendranāth Sengupta and Balāicandra Sengupta. Calcutta: Dhanvantari Steam Machine Press, 1927.

Caraka Saṃhitā. 2d rev. ed. Vols. 1–5. Translated by A. Chandra Kaviratna and P. Sharma. Delhi: Indian Medical Science Series No. 41, Sri Satguru Publications, 1996–1997.

Caraka-Saṃhitā. Agniveśa's treatise refined and annotated by Caraka and redacted by Dṛḍhabala (text with English translation). Edited and translated by Prof. Priyavrat Sharma. Vol. 1 (Sūtrasthāna to Indriyasthāna). Varanasi/Delhi: Jaikrishnadas Ayurveda Series 36, Chaukhambha Orientalia, 1981.

Agniveśa's *Caraka Saṃhitā*. Text with English translation and critical exposition based on Cakrapāṇi Datta's Ayurveda Dīpikā). Edited and translated by Dr. Ram Karan Sharma and Vaidya Bhagwan Dash. Vol. 1—Sūtrasthāna. Varanasi: The Chowkhamba Sanskrit Studies Vol. XCIV, Chowkhamba Sanskrit Series Office, 1976.

Juvenal. *The Satires*. Translated by Niall Rudd, with an Introduction and Notes by William Barr. Oxford: Clarendon Press, 1991.

Juvenalis *Saturae. Ediderunt P. de Labriolle et Fr. Villeneuve*. Paris: Les Belles Lettres, 1963.

Kāśyapa *Samhitā* (or *Vṛddhajivakīya Tantra*) by Vṛddha Jīvaka, revised by Vātsya, with Sanskrit Introduction by Nepal Rajaguru Pandit Hemarāja Śarmā, with the Vidyotinī Hindi commentary and Hindi translation of Sanskrit Introduction by Āyurvedālankār Śrī Satyapāla Bhiṣagāchārya. Banāras: The Kashi Sanskrit Series 154, Caukhambā-Saṃskṛt-Sīrij, 1953.

Saṃgītaratnākara. Śārṅgadeva, with two commentaries (Kalānidhi of Kallinātha and Sudhākara of Siṃhabhūpāla). Edited by Pandit S. Subrahmanya Sastri. Vol. 1. Madras: The Adyar Library Series No. 30, the Adyar Library, 1943.

Suśrutasaṃhitā. Edited by Vaidya Jādavji Trikamji Āchārya and Nārāyāṇ Rām Āchārya. Bombay: Nirṇaya Sāgar Press, 1938.

REFERENCES

Acal, Ayodhyā Prasād. 1996. *Eḍs—Svarūp, nidān evaṃ upacār*. *Sachitra Ayurved* 48:9: 847–51.

Agarwalla, S. K. 1992. A multiapproach comprehensive therapy model for HIV infection and AIDS. *Sachitra Ayurved* 44:11: 741–45.

Agravāl, K. M. 2002. *Madhumeha, ojobal evaṃ rasāyan prayog*. *Sachitra Ayurved* 54:8: 577–84.

Ahn, Mi-Jeong, Chul Young Kim, Ji Suk Lee, Tae Gyun Kim, Seung Hee Kim, Chong-Kyo Lee, Bo-Bin Lee, Cha-Gyun Shin, Hoon Huh, and Jinwoong Kim. 2002. Inhibition of HIV-1 integrase by galloyl glucose from *Terminalia chebula* and flavonol glycoside gallates from *Euphorbia pekinensis, Planta Medica* 68: 454–57.

AIDS rog cikits. 1990. Āyurved Vikās, Viśeṣāṅk.

Aṃśumān, P. S. 1991a. *Eḍs aur āyurved. Sudhānidhi* 11.
———. 1991b. *Eḍs par ek vicār āyurvedik paripreksya me. Svāsthya* 10.
———. 1991c. *Eḍs paricaya. Sudhānidhi* 11.
———. 1994a. *Eḍs evaṃ manaḥkāyik vikṛtiyāṃ kuch sandarbha. Svāsthya* 5.
———. 1994b. *Eḍs kī āyurvedīya cikitsā parikalpanā. Sachitra Ayurved* 9.
———. 1994c. *Eḍs meṃ rasāyan kalp kī upādeyatā. Āyurved Mahāsammelan Patrikā* 12.
———. 1998. *Eḍs (AIDS): Āyurvedīya cikitsā: Kuch rogī. Sachitra Ayurved* 51:3: 200–204.
———. 2000. *Oj visraṃs—Ek vicār. Sachitra Ayurved* 53:6: 413–16.
Candra, Sureś. 2003. *Eḍs evaṃ ojkṣaya meṃ tulanātmak prastuti. Sachitra Ayurved* 56:3: 186–88.
Das, Rahul Peter. 2003. *The Origin of the Life of a Human Being—Conception and the Female according to Ancient Indian Medical and Sexological Literature, Indian Medical Tradition.* Vol. 6. Delhi: Motilal Banarsidass Publishers Pvt. (See index verborum: *ojas*; see in particular 530–535.)
Devāṅgan, Pradīp, and Dīpak Kulśreṣṭh. 1991. AIDS—*Ādhunik evaṃ āyurvedīya dṛṣṭikoṇ. Sachitra Ayurved* 43:10: 659–60.
Dumézil, Georges. 1969. *Idées Romaines*. Paris: Gallimard.
Dwarkanath, C. 1959. *Introduction to Kāyachikitsā*. Bombay: Popular Book Depot.
Editorial. 1986. AIDS (acquired immune deficiency syndrome)—(Ayurvedic view). *Ancient Science of Life* 5:3: 137–38.
Filliozat, J. 1964. *The Classical Doctrine of Indian Medicine*. Delhi: Munshiram Manoharlal [pp. 27, 166–68, 187: *ojas*].
Gangadharan, G. G. and R. Ram Manohar. 1994. Concept of immunology in Ayurveda. *Ancient Science of Life* 14:1–2: 2–9.
Gonda, J. 1952. Ancient-Indian *ojas*, Latin **augos*, and the Indo-European nouns in *-es/-os*. Utrecht: N.V.A. Oosthoek's Uitgevers Mij.
———. 1957. *Some Observations on the Relations between "Gods" and "Powers" in the Veda apropos of the Phrase Sūnuḥ Sahasa*. Gravenhage: Mouton and Co.
Gould, Stephen Jay 2002. *The Structure of Evolutionary Theory*. Cambridge, MA, London: The Belknap Press of Harvard University Press.
Gupta, L. P., S. P. Sen, and D. S. Gaur. 1967. Study of *para-ojas* in relation to a cardiotonic principle lodged in the heart. *Journal of Research in Indian Medicine* 2:1: 97–104.
Hattori, Toshio, Shojiro Ikematsu, Atsushi Koito, Shuzo Matsushita, Yosuke Maeda, Masao Hada, Michio Fujimaki, and Kiyoshi Takatsuki. 1989. Preliminary evidence for inhibitory effect of glycyrrhizin on HIV replication in patients with AIDS. *Antiviral Research* 11: 255–61.
Hoffman, A. J. 1998. New protocol for the treatment of cancer and AIDS utilizing *Aloe vera barbadensis*. *Ayurveda Education Series* 67: 44–51.
Hussain, S. M. 2003. Role of Unani medicine in management of AIDS. *Sachitra Ayurved* 56:4: 308–309.
Ito, Masahiko, Akihiko Sato, Kazuhiro Hirabayashi, Fuminori Tanabe, Shiro Shigeta, Masanori Baba, Erik De Clercq, Hideki Nakashima, and Naoki Yamamoto. 1988. Mechanism of inhibitory effect of glycyrrhizin on replication of human immunodeficiency virus (HIV). *Antiviral Research* 10: 289–98.

Jha, Ram Deo. 1988. Ayurvedic medicine for AIDS cure. *The Times of India*, November 29.

Krishnamurthy, J. R. 1993. Drugs for the treatment of AIDS in the Siddha system of medicine.

Kulkarni, P. H. 1998. Role of diet in the treatment of cancer and AIDS. *Ayurveda Education Series* 67: 23–30.

Lin, Yuh-Meei, Herbert Anderson, Michael T. Flavin, Yeah-Huei S. Pai, Eugenia Mata-Greenwood, Thitima Pengsuparp, John M. Pezzuto, Raymond F. Schinazi, Stephen H. Hughes, and Fa-Ching Chen. 1997. In vitro anti-HIV activity of biflavonoids isolated from *Rhus succedanea* and *Garcinia multiflora*, *Journal of Natural Products* 60:9: 884–88.

McKee, Tawnya C., Heidi R. Bokesch, Jinping L. McCormick, Mohammed A. Rashid, Dirk Spielvogel, Kirk R. Gustafson, Maria M. Alavanja, John H. Cardellina, and Michael R. Boyd. 1997. Isolation and characterization of new anti-HIV and cytotoxic leads from plants, marine, and microbial organisms. *Journal of Natural Products* 60:5: 431–38.

Mishra, Lakshmi Chandra, ed. 2004. *Scientific Basis for Ayurvedic Therapies*. Boca Raton, London, New York, Washington, DC: CRC Press.

Mohapatra, S. C. 1994. Prevention of AIDS in Indian context. *Medicine Update* (The Association of Physicians of India—UP Chapter).

Mungantiwar, Ashish A., and Aashish S. Phadke 2004. Immunomodulation: Therapeutic strategy through Ayurveda. In *Scientific Basis for Ayurvedic Therapies*, ed. Lakshmi Chandra Mishra, 63–81, in particular 76–77.

Narayana Swamy, V. 1987. *Ojas*—Ayurvedic concept of energy in human body. *Āryavaidyan* 1:1: 21–25.

Panda, Srikanta Kumar, Banwari Lal Gaur, and Om Prakash Upadhyaya. 2000. Role of *rasāyana* as an immunomodulator for the management of AIDS. *Sachitra Ayurved* 53:1: 52–53.

Pandey, G. 1990. *AIDS-pratikār meṃ upayogī auṣadhi yojanā. Āyurved Vikās*. (AIDS special issue): 137–48.

Pandey, Gyanendra. 2003. *Anti AIDS (Ojaksaya) Drugs of Ayurveda*. Delhi: Indian Medical Science Series No. 152, Sri Satguru Publications.

Pāṇḍey, Jñānendra. 1991. *Eḍs rog meṃ karkaṭak kī sambhāvit upayogitā*, *Sachitra Ayurved* 44:1: 15–17.

Pathak, Nagardas M. 1957–1958. A plea against the classification of *oja* as *para* and *apara*. *Journal of the Oriental Institute* (Baroda) 7: 86–89.

Patil, M. A. 1998. *Sapta-dhatu-gata jwar* and HIV infections/AIDS—A correlation. *Update Ayurveda* 2: 3.

Prabhañjan Ācārya. 2000. *Āyurved meṃ oj kā mahatva*. *Sachitra Ayurved* 53:5: 365–66.

Pradeep Kumar, V., R. Kuttan, and G. Kuttan. 1991. Effect of *rasayana* on cellular immunity in mice. *Amala Research Bulletin* 15: 77–82.

Premanathan, M. et al. 2000. A survey of some Indian medicinal plants for anti-human immunodeficiency virus (HIV) activity. *Indian Journal of Medical Research* 112: 73.

Pulse, Tl., and E. Uhlig. 1990. A significant improvement in a clinical pilot study utilizing nutritional supplements, essential fatty acids, and stabilized aloe vera juice in 29 serpositive ARC and AIDS patients. *J. Adv. Med.* 3: 209.

Raj Kumar, and Lok Nath Sharma. 2000. AIDS—An Ayurvedic outlook. *Sachitra Ayurved* 52:8: 815–16.

Salema, Ana. 1999. *Essai d'anthropologie du corps: Savoirs, pratiques et expériences—Enquête sur la psychagogie ayurvédique,* thèse, Université Paris IV, Sorbonne.

Sankunni, Lily. 1982. Physiological and pathological study of *ojas. Vagbhata* 1:2: 34–35, 56.

Śarmā, Anil Kumār, and Añjalī Śarmā. 1992. *Aupasargik oj-kṣaya (Eḍs)—ek āyurvedik dṛṣṭikoṇ. Sachitra Ayurved* 44:11: 733–36.

Śarmā, Aśvinī Kumār. 2003. *Vyādhi kṣamatā* (immunity). *Sachitra Āyurved* 56:5: 339–44.

Śarmā, Aśvinī Kumār, and Kanak Prasād. 2000. *Eḍs rog kā ojkṣaya ke paripreksya meṃ naidānik adhyayan evaṃ rasāyan prayog—ek vicār. Sachitra Ayurved* 52:9: 857–63.

Śarmā, Hariprapanna. 1926–1927. *Rasayogasāgaraḥ.* Vol. 1. Bombay.

Śarmā, Priyavrat. 1998. *Ojas, sahas aur bal. Sachitra Ayurved* 51:6: 407.

Śaṅkar, Tārā. 1996. *Eḍs yā phiraṅg rog. Sachitra Ayurved* 48:10: 905.

Saraswathy, A. 1994. Traditional medicine in the management of AIDS. *Ancient Science of Life* 14:1–2: 91–98.

Singh, I. P. 1966. *The study of* ojas *in relation to body resistance and effect of ojovardhak drug.* Thesis, Banaras Hindu University.

Singh, K. 1990. Concept of *ojas* and the effect of *rasayanas* in the management of cancer. *Proceedings of the Ayurveda Seminar on Cancer, Thrissur* (March 10, 1990): 15–18.

Singh, L. P., D. S. Gaur, and H. C. Shukla. 1977. The concept of *ojas* in Ayurveda. *Sachitra Ayurved* 29:8: 576–83.

Sukla, C. P. 1995. *Eḍs arthāt ojakṣaya (āyurvedīya dṛṣṭi se). Sachitra Ayurved* 48:5: 527–31.

Tewari, L. C., R. G. Agarwal, G. Pandey, and M. R. Uniyal. 1991. Screening of some important herbal drugs for potent therapeutic agents recommended for cure of AIDS in Ayurveda. *Sachitra Ayurved* 44:6: 428–33.

Thirumulpad, K. Raghavan. 1994. AIDS—An Ayurvedic view. *Ancient Science of Life* 13: 3–4: 245–47.

Uniyāl, Māyārām. 2000. *Śukrakṣayajanya oj kṣaya evaṃ aupasargik vyādhi Eḍs kā āyurvedik vivecan. Sachitra Ayurved* 52:12: 1100–1104.

Valsaraj, Raghavan, Palpu Pushpangadan, Ulla Wagner Smitt, Anne Adsersen, Soren Brogger Christensen, Archibald Sittie, Ulf Nyman, Claus Nielsen, and Carl Erik Olsen. 1997. New anti-HIV-1, antimalarial, and antifungal compounds from *Terminalia bellerica. Journal of Natural Products* 60:7: 739–42.

Vogel, J. Ph. 1930. *Het Sanskrit woord tejas (= gloed, vuur) in de betekenis van magische kracht.* Amsterdam: Mededeelibgen der Koninklijke Akademie van Wetenschappen, Afdeeling Letterkunde, Deel 70, Series B, No. 4.

Yadav, C. L. 2000. A concept of AIDS and *rasayana*—based on Ayurvedic *samhitas. Sachitra Ayurved* 53:2: 145–48.

Yadava, R. K., K. J. Dave, and S. K. Dave. 2001. Role of *achara rasayana* and *sadvrta* in the prevention of AIDS. *Ancient Science of Life* 20:3: 62–64.

CHAPTER 10

Ayurveda and Sexuality

Sex Therapy and the "Paradox of Virility"

JOSEPH S. ALTER

INTRODUCTION

In the study of South Asia, sex is regarded as a central problem in understanding mythology (O'Flaherty 1973, 1980, 1987; White 1996), social psychology (Carstairs 1958; Kakar 1990; Roland 1988), religion (Babb 1983; Parry 1985; Wadley 1975), nationalism (Alter 1994, 2000; Nandy 1980, 1983; Caplan 1987), gerontology (Cohen 1998), and the cultural construction of identity, broadly defined (Edwards 1983; Lynch 1990; Marglin 1985; Nanda 1990). Most recently, Hugh Urban (2003) has provided a critical analysis of sex and sexuality in the imagination of scholars and the public at large who have sought to understand or practice Tantra.

Building on the idea that sex and sexuality are not natural categories (Foucault 1990; Fausto-Sterling 2000; Laqueur 1990), my concern is less with how sex can be used to make sense of a domain of experience—in this case, medicine—than it is with the classification of sex as a particular kind of experience. Although pleasure and procreation would seem to define the terms of this experience, there is no reason to understand sex in this limited way. Even the *Kāma Sūtra*—an iconic and fetishized text if ever there was one in the global discourse of sexuality—builds on, but cannot be reduced to, the principles of pleasure and procreation. Moreover, as Zysk (2002) makes clear, the broader discourse on love and sex in medieval India is one that is public, open, and meticulously detailed. It is not a discourse about what cannot easily be spoken about. Lest we forget, sex is a physiological act, and the physiology of sex has a direct bearing on experiences that relate to individual health as against more inherently plural configurations that produce pleasure and/or children. In particular, it has a bearing on what I am calling the paradox of virility, which is a particular manifestation of the much more general—and perhaps paradigmatic—tension between being chaste and being a libertine, the extreme articulations of the question: to have or not to have sex. It is important to note, that whereas in the context of European history this question is framed by what Foucault has called "the slow formation, in antiquity, of a hermeneutics of the self," and the essential problem of how the self as a "subject of desire" is formulated (1990: 6), in the context of South Asian history, the problem of sex is, in large part, a problem of physiology, where "the hermeneutics of the self" is intimately linked to an understanding of semen as a substance, as distinct from a symbol of power.

Based on research conducted on physical fitness and yoga (Alter 1992, 1994, 1995, 1997, 2000), it has become increasingly clear that concepts of embodied, masculine health in India are linked to the production, retention, and internalized flow of semen. The physiology of sex is also central to the theory and practice of Ayurveda and other South Asian medical systems (Gonda 1952; Kakar 1990; Marriott 1990; White 1996; see also Daniel and Pugh 1984; Filliozat 1964; Jolly 1977; Zimmer 1948; Zimmermann 1987). The last two of the eight branches of ayurvedic medicine—*rasāyaṇa* and *vājīkaraṇa*, elixirs and aphrodisiacs, respectively—are explicitly concerned with the production, retention, and ejaculation of semen.

One of the ironies reflected in Ayurveda and its associated disciplines, both in terms of contemporary practice and historical development, is the contradictory concern with increasing masculine sexual virility, on the one hand, and, on the other, advocacy for celibacy and self-control as a means by which to promote an ideal of embodied power. In contemporary India vocal groups assertively advocate absolute asexuality and self-control in terms of a theory of contained vital body fluids, and yet there is as large a group of men—constituted by the clientele of virility clinics and sex therapists—that subscribes to therapeutic regimens for the development of sexual potency wherein those same bodily fluids are produced and accumulated precisely so that they can be spent, and spent both more often and with greater effect (see Srivastava 2004). Since both celibacy and sexual potency seem to be based on a single theory of embodied vital power, this situation may be referred to as "the paradox of virility."

Given that the importance and rationale for celibacy is widely understood in the context of history, iconic mythology, and contemporary practice (see Alter 1994, 1996; Carstairs 1958; Kakar 1990; Obeyesekere 1976; O'Flaherty 1973), my purpose here is to understand how and why virility clinics—which are anathema to those who advocate celibacy—have become increasingly popular in contemporary India. They have become popular, at least in part, because a colonial and postcolonial legacy of self-ascribed "cultural feminization"—including the advocacy for celibacy and asexuality—has provoked a virile, masculine response to the so-called "self-image of effeteness" (Rosselli 1980; see also Nandy 1983; Chatterjee 1993: 68–72; White 1996: 335–52). In this context, a modern cultural ideal of virility—enhanced, to be sure, by global modernity and increasingly public articulations of sensuality and eroticism (see Gupta 2001)—is rationalized in terms of an ayurvedic theory of good health, embodied power, and potent masculinity. This very modern discourse of sexuality—as quite distinct from discourses about the physiology of sex—disconnects *vājīkaraṇa* therapy from *rasāyaṇa*, and then fuses them together and confuses them with one another, producing a paradox of virility in the context of what might be called a crisis of masculinity, first in the colonial and then the postcolonial period.

Quite obviously, sexuality is now a transnational concept and experiential frame of reference. Without trying to sort out the various tangents of flow and trace the specific lines of historical transformation, it is clear that ideas that relate to sex in South Asia have been influenced by the history of sexuality in many other parts of the world, most directly Europe. And, as Hugh Urban (2003) has pointed out, ideas about sex, power, and eroticism flow in a multitude of directions. In light of this, it is important to note that the paradigmatic concern of Ayurveda with semen is one that is at least incipiently sexual, and therefore directly relevant to a discourse of sexuality that has emerged in colonial and postcolonial India. One might say that the structural and functional importance of semen to health in the *Caraka-Saṃhitā* and other medical texts anticipates the problematic idea that one's whole self is linked to one's sexuality. But the way in which semen is linked to the whole self is in its relation to the whole body rather than in terms of the specific and problematically delimited conditions under which it is made to flow out of the body.

SEX, SEXUAL FLUIDS, AND AYURVEDIC MEDICAL THEORY

As is the case in the *Ratiśāstra* literature (Zysk 2002: 11), sex in the classical ayurvedic texts is about reproduction. More fundamentally, however, it is an issue that is relevant to health in general and to digestion, and the suppression—or, rather, nonsuppression—of natural urges. It is about the embodiment of immortality in particular. The essential logic of immortality—that is, the cyclic process of creation and recreation—is manifest in procreation. And it is for this reason, rather than the more intuitive one, that a discussion of sex must begin with conception and the mixing of sexual fluids.

REPRODUCTION

A complete analysis of reproduction and what the ayurvedic literature says about pregnancy, gestation, and fetal development is beyond the scope of this chapter and has, in any case, been thoroughly analyzed by Rahul Peter Das (2003), Julia Leslie (1994) and, most recently, Martha Selby (2005). However, it is very important to note—even though it should come as no surprise—that in the context of this discussion sex is about the mingling and transmutation of substance. In relation to reproduction, the act of sex is described in terms of friction. Friction produces heat. Heat in conjunction with wind dislodges both semen and ovum, and these come together in the uterus. Although friction is the force that causes flow and mingling, as we will see with regard to the singular male body, in which semen is located, the process is one of forceful, mechanical extraction based on the action of squeezing (*Caraka-Saṃhitā, Cikitsāsthāna* 2:46–49). In any case, the mingling of ovum and semen produces what Ramachandra Rao (1987: 88) refers to as an elemental "material mass." In terms of duality, this mass is a combination of lunar and solar properties—manifest, respectively, in semen and ovum—a very common cosmic theme that is integral to tantric as well as yogic theories of physiology and physiological transubstantiation. Significantly, however, this mass is lifeless and inanimate. It contains all of the five elemental properties of matter, earth, water, fire, air, and ether, but these alone and nothing else. As such, the mass can be said to manifest a perfect, pre-creation, *prakṛtic* state of balance. As Rao (ibid.) puts it, the five elements are in a state where they are "mutually beneficial, mutually supporting, and mutually fusing."

With the advent of the "inscrutable soul," which is incorporated into the mass after the fluids have combined—after, since the motive force of karmic fate is not manifest in the friction of sex and its entailments—the mass is enlivened and set on a course that will end in death. The first stage of this process—which enables the mass to grow into a fetus and everything that follows—is the transmutation of the elemental mass into an entity with the subtle form of the three *guṇas*. Conception, therefore, is microcosmic creation, with the first stage being, most significantly, the reproduction of unmanifest reality and elemental being apart from time. That is, it is the reproduction of pre-creation. In this sense, life begins very soon after conception, but the first stage of conception is the reproduction of *avyakta* ("the unmanifest"), "when the three constituent *guṇas* are in a state of perfect balance [known as] *sāmyāvasthā*" (Rao 1987: 161). "The foetus will be in the form of a gelatinous substance (*kalala*) in the first month of gestation. It is an amorphous (unstructured) mass of all the material ingredients (substances and properties) mixed indistinguishably (*avyakta-vigraha*) (*Caraka, Śārīrasthāna* 4)" (Rao 1987: 89).

Throughout the nine to ten months of gestation the fetus develops, and a newly born child can be said to manifest a condition of near perfection. It has taken on the form of a human being but has only just begun the process of growth and development. Significantly, growth and development ensue from the destabilization of *sāmyāvasthā* perfection and is comparable to the *Sāṃkhya* notion of evolution known as *vṛttyantara-pariṇāma*. The key point to note here is the almost direct correspondence between sex and reproduction, on the one hand, and the cosmic logic of creation, which entails the mixing or union of *puruṣa* and *prakṛti*. However, one must not think of this correspondence in terms of either gender duality or sex roles as such, wherein *puruṣa* is paradigmatically male and *prakṛti* paradigmatically female. Both male and female sexual fluids combine to produce a mass that is *prakṛtic* in nature. If one must think in terms of gender duality, it is the inscrutable soul that is masculine. Sex and sexual fluids are feminine.

THE NONSUPPRESSION OF NATURAL URGES

It is a common tendency to think of sex, in both medical and nonmedical terms, as a unique entity. From a masculine perspective, the ejaculation of semen and everything that leads up to it is thought of in terms of pleasure and/or reproduction. The idea of sex most certainly produces an urge for it. But this urge is not often conceptualized as an urge that is analogous to belching, sneezing, or farting. Freudian interpretations notwithstanding, ejaculation is not the kind of urge associated with hunger and the satisfaction of that urge. What is unique about Ayurveda, therefore, is the way in which the urge for sex—and more specifically the urge to discharge semen, since we are here speaking of somewhat unconscious, involuntary urges—is classified along with a broad range of other urges: farting, defecating, urinating, sneezing, being thirsty, being hungry, being sleepy, coughing, huffing and puffing, yawning, crying, vomiting, and belching (*Caraka, Sūtrasthāna* 7:6–19). In fact, it is impossible to find the appropriate phrasing in English, since "being aroused erotically" is an emotional state, whereas what is at issue for Caraka is simply and directly the flow of semen out of the body, as is the case with regard to other substances such as tears, feces, urine, and different manifestations of air.

Needless to say, in declaring that urges should be satisfied, the ayurvedic literature does not advocate libertinism or uninhibited self-indulgence of the sort that was embodied, famously, by the Greek cynics. As directly linked to the flow of semen out of the body, Caraka, Suśruta, and Vāgbhaṭa advocate moderation in all things, including sex. In this context, certain mental impulses—as different from, but related to, bodily urges—need to be suppressed, even though it is acknowledged that they are natural. Thus one must restrain feelings of avarice, jealousy, hatred, envy, and anger (*Aṣṭāṅgahṛdaya-Saṃhitā, Śārīrasthāna* 1.4, 24), along with lust, it is presumed, although the latter is not mentioned as such.

Regardless, there is a degree of ambiguity manifest in the ayurvedic discussion of natural urges, daily routine, health, and hygiene. The intake of food and water can be calibrated, as can the precise length of time, and on which side and where, to sleep. Similarly, exercise can be regulated in terms of measures of exertion. And, of course, when you gotta go, you gotta go. But what does it mean to have sex in moderation? Once a day, once a week, once a month, only in the winter, and not in the summer? It is unclear, or else articulated differently in various texts and differently, both directly and by implication, at various points in the same text. In any case, classifying ejaculation—as distinct, one must assume, from the feeling of an orgasm—as a natural urge that is linked to health in general clearly means that the key health issue here is not the exchange of bodily fluids but the production, retention, and flow of vital fluids as such. My sense is that the ambiguity concerning the question of how much sex is too much—and how little too little—is directly linked to the ambiguous problem of good health. What is good health, since by definition the very action of the *guṇas* means that the body is always in a state of disequilibrium? The goal is to achieve balance. But, given the "inscrutability of the soul" (as Rao puts it), what degree of balance is possible, since perfect balance was a momentary, embryonic phase and is a transcendental state—the change in tense defining the time we live in? What can realistically be achieved and maintained on a daily, weekly, monthly, or annual basis as the body ages? These are questions that link the paradox of virility to questions of health and physical fitness.

DIGESTION AND THE PRODUCTION OF SEMEN: THE WELL-COOKED BODY

Whether or not it is considered a form of exercise, in fact—as the *Caraka-Saṃhitā* provocatively suggests (Rao 1987: 49)—celibacy is considered a pillar of health. Semen is the condensed essence of a metabolic, biochemical process wherein blood, muscle, fat, bone, and marrow are "distilled" down through a series of stages to produce energy. In almost all instances in which celibacy is advocated as the key to health, semen is thought to express itself in the body as a whole, rather than as a discrete fluid unto itself. It produces generalized vitality rather than particularized virility. Thus the physically strong, healthy, masculine body is said to "shine" and "glow" with an aura of power that encompasses physiology, character, and intellect.

Both celibacy and sexual potency are keyed not just to semen but also to a substance known as *ojas*, for which there is no English equivalent (cf. Meulenbeld in this book; Wujastyk 1998: 29–30). *Ojas* could be translated as "energy," if the abstract potential of energy could be imagined as having material form unto itself. *Ojas* is thought to be the distillate of all of the body's constituent substances (*dhātu*), but in particular the distillate of semen (White 1984). Most authors indicate that it is regarded as a minute, extremely subtle substance that pervades the whole body but emanates from the heart. *Ojas* is, in essence, the most basic force of life. A loss of *ojas* shortens life and brings on death.

There are a number of interesting and significant points about the relationship between semen and *ojas*. As in the case of all *dhātus*, *ojas* is "cooked" or metabolized; it is the "cooked" or digested "subtle aspect" of gross semen. The chain of transformation from *rasa* through blood, flesh, fat, bone, marrow, and semen ends with *ojas*, which only supports (*dhāraṇā*) the body but does not nourish (*poṣaṇa*) it, as is the case with the other seven (Rao 1987: 219). Unlike all other *dhātus*, it has no concrete aspect, leading some commentators to classify it as a meta-*dhātu*. However, there is a significantly broad range of perspectives reflected in the primary literature, some redactors calling it a *dhātu*, others referring to it as a meta-*dhātu* (*upadhātu*), and still others regarding it as a special kind of substance that, like honey made from the nectar of many flowers, derives from the essence of each *dhātu* and all *dhātus* collectively. It is not different in kind from the *dhātu*, but it has a different function. Regardless, *ojas* is very much a material substance that flows throughout the body. It is said to measure eight drops in volume and be located—although not contained—in the heart. From the heart it emanates outward to "support the body and provide the necessary force or energy for all functions, bodily and mental" (Rao 1987: 219). Its location in the heart is correlated, very significantly, to the heart also being the seat of consciousness—the place in which one has an inscrutable soul.

Two different views are reflected in the literature concerning the relationship between *ojas* and conception. One view holds that *ojas* is the very essence of the embryo (*sāram ādau garbhasya*), although it is unclear whether this is before or after the advent of the soul (*Caraka*

Sū.30.8, cited in Rao 1987: 218). Another view is that it develops in the eighth month, most likely following the structural logic of *dhātu* transubstantiation mapped onto the stages of gestation and pregnancy. In any case, it is easy to understand the logic of theorizing vitality as an incipient, embryonic force that derives from the mixing of semen, ovum, and consciousness.

RASĀYAṆA, REBIRTH, AND IMMORTALITY

Ayurvedic literature contains many references to the value of conserving semen, but a study and analysis of some of the core texts (Alter 1999) shows that the medical literature is focused on two other, very different concerns regarding semen—virility and immortality. The term *Ayurveda* itself is translated by Wujastyk as "the knowledge or science of longevity" (1998: 3), clearly indicating that the key problem in this system of medicine is not illness but the problem of life itself as bounded by time. Balance and flow are functions of time.

The branch of Ayurveda known as *rasāyaṇa* details a therapy wherein a person drinks an elixir that causes his body to become immortal. Suśruta describes one of the most detailed procedures that involves drinking *soma*. The initial effect of *soma* is dramatically and purposefully violent and destructive, if not of the body as such most certainly to the way in which the body is linked to time. But as more elixir is drunk, the body of the aging patient is reconstituted in eternal youthfulness and perfect beauty. Although less radical and not as physiologically precise or therapeutically complex, what seems to be the most dramatic *rasāyaṇa* therapy in Caraka's text is described as follows. After drinking "in full quantity" the juice of any one of a number of herbs, including *soma*, the king of herbs that grows and blooms in concert with the waxing and waning of the moon

> . . . [a person] should sleep naked in the covered tub made of wet *palāṣa* wood and anointed with ghee. (After a while) he disappears and reappears in six months. Then he should be maintained on goat's milk. In six months he becomes similar to the gods in age, complexion, voice, face, strength, and luster; all knowledge appears intuitively, he attains divine vision and audition, movement up to a thousand *yojanas* (8,000 miles) and an unafflicted lifespan of a thousand years. (*Cikitsāsthāna* 1.4.7. Sharma 1992: 29–30)

An analysis of this branch of medicine within the broader paradigmatic structure of Ayurveda indicates that immortality is the embodiment of a theoretical ideal—perfect balance between all constituent substances, and absolute purity—that is logically impossible given the nature of time and the corresponding mortal process of aging. As scholars have argued, *rasāyaṇa* is an organic formulation of inorganic Siddha alchemy wherein base metals are transubstantiated into gold (Babb 1983; White 1996). In theory, it also is linked, through Sāṃkhya philosophy, to the metaphysics of yoga and the immortality of embodied, transcendental consciousness (Eliade 1969).

Rasāyaṇa does not directly involve sex as an act, but it is all about sexual fluids and the relationship of those fluids to the aging body. The first stage of the most elaborate process is known as *kuṭapraveṣa,* "in which the patient is sequestered within the triply enclosed (*trigarbhā*) innermost chamber of a hut called the 'womb of the womb' (*garbhagarbham*)" (White 1996: 26). Rebirth follows a sequence of embryonic and infant development after the body is violently purged and cleansed. Regeneration begins after hair, nails, teeth, and skin have all fallen off, at which point, as Anantacharya puts it, "[the patient] is a ghastly sight" (quoted in White 1996: 27).

Ghastliness aside—and oozing fluids, wriggling worms, and dangling, rotting skin is certainly that—I would suggest that at the point in time when the body is most radically decomposed, it also is in a state of absolute perfection. If sexuality need not be "sexy," it then also is possible that, beauty aside, "perfection," too, is in the eye of the beholder, and something that is not at all keyed to an aesthetic ideal. All *dhātu* transubstantiation has ended, all flow of substance has stopped, and although the physical body may look to be in pretty bad shape, the material mass is in perfect balance. As described by Suśruta, it is from this perfect balance that the new, immortal man is born:

> The visionary man who makes use of the king of plants, Soma, wears a new body for ten thousand years. Neither fire nor water, neither poison, blade nor projectile, are powerful enough to take his life. He gains the strength of a thousand well-bred, sixty-year old, rutting elephants. . . . He is as beautiful as the god of love, as attractive as the second moon. He is radiant, and brings joy to the heart of all creatures. (Wujastyk 1998: 176)

One can focus on a number of features that characterize the new man. He is virile, physically powerful, and magnificently beautiful. Beyond this, I think his immortality is defined by the fact that once he is born he does not change; the substances of his body do not metabolize and are completely contained—at least in theory. It is on this level that celibacy, defined as the retention of semen, can be said to homologize with the embodied virility of the new man, who is energized with the power of *ojas*. He has become the supporting structure alone, apart from nourishment. He does not need to "control himself," since his body is not subject to transformation over time. In other words, the new man has a celibate body—in the sense that his semen does not flow—but can engage in sex without risk of deterioration, because his body is not constituted of substances that change.

VĀJĪKARAṆA: IMMORTALITY, SEX, AND VIRILITY

Rasāyaṇa therapy only really makes sense insofar as it anticipates the final and penultimate branch of classical Ayurveda—*vājīkaraṇa,* the "science of sexual potency." *Vājīkaraṇa* literally means "turning a man into a stallion," with all that suggests in terms of vigor, stamina, size, and so forth. As we shall see, however, this is only a small part of the picture. Other things matter much more than pleasure and masculine self-definition through that kinetics of sex as an act; more than the simple—and simplistic—correlation between vigorous, long-lasting sex and powerful masculinity.

As with most of the classical branches of medicine, and certainly *rasāyaṇa,* the paradigmatic patient for *vājīkaraṇa* therapy is a king, and sexual potency and vigor—controlled and regulated, to be sure—is cognate with dynastic, political power and the quality of rule. In this respect it is important to use the *Kāma Sūtra,* composed in the late classical period, as a point of comparative reference for understanding an ideological framework within which medically enhanced sexual potency is classified, categorized, and theorized structurally. The *Kāma Sūtra* defines the ways and means of sex, romance, and love, clearly indicating what is good, appropriate, and inappropriate for a king and his wives and courtesans to do in relation to one another. What celibacy—and the power derived thereby—is to the institution of renunciation (*sannyāsa*), virility is to the practice of politics and statecraft (*artha*). In this configuration the eternal youth of the virile king signifies the divinity of his person and the moral authority of his rule, just as the celibacy of the ascetic signifies his detachment from the world and his transcendental power.

A theory of *ojas* makes very good sense in terms of the logic of semen retention manifest in celibacy and the institution of asceticism. This has, almost exclusively, been the focus of the extent scholarship, and an ascetic paradigm has been proposed as central to the history of ayurvedic theory (Zysk 1991). But with regard to the stallionlike virility of a sexually active king—either in the person of the king himself or the mass of modern young men aspiring to an ideal of potency—*ojas* in particular, and the general theory of longevity reflected in ayurvedic science, is highly problematic. The idea of *ojas*—the essence of essence—creates the embodied paradox of virility. Once developed and medically enhanced, virility, as an expression of masculine power manifest in the act of sex, undermines that power and produces impotence, weakness, and premature death. Ayurveda resolves the paradox structurally and theoretically by linking *rasāyaṇa* and *vājīkaraṇa* in sequence (White 1996: 26) Given that sequence—one thing after the other—is a function of time, it is only a paradox from the perspective of those of us who are mortal.

But *rasāyaṇa* and *vājīkaraṇa* are linked together more directly in a very important way that has everything to do with procreation rather than the embodiment of immortality. One of the most striking features of *vājīkaraṇa* is not so much the image of a stallionlike man who has endless stamina but the concern of Caraka and others with the quality of his semen, and the obvious link between it and a directly related, but a very different kind of, immortality. Here is Caraka in the first chapter of *Cikitsāsthāna* after having distinguished therapies that promote strength and immunity in the healthy from those that alleviate disorders:

> *Vājīkaraṇa* . . . is that which produces lineage of progeny, quick sexual stimulation, enables one to perform sexual act with women uninterruptedly and vigorously like a horse, makes one charming for the woman, promotes corpulence, and infallible and indestructible semen even in the old persons, renders one great having a number of off-springs like a sacred tree branched profusely and commanding respect and popularity in society. By this one attains eternality based on filial tradition here and hereafter along with fame, fortune, strength, and corpulence. (1.1.9–12. Sharma 1992: 4)

The erstwhile king may have sex like a stallion but he does so in order to be transformed into an eternally self-generating banyan tree. Thus in a very important sense, *rasāyaṇa* and *vājīkaraṇa* are both about embodied perfection and immortality. To think of stallionlike sex as an end in itself is to completely miss the point. And it is a very easy point to miss, given that sexuality and the kinetic pleasure of sex has focused so much attention on the relationship between those engaged in the act, as the act has come to signify so much about masculinity and femininity in general. The question of reproduction—what the sex you have produces, and how the sex you have affects the production and combination of sexual fluids in discrete bodies—has become one of elemental biology rather than an issue that is linked to sex and sexuality. In some sense, sex and sexuality dissociated from reproduction, political power, and world renunciation have transformed the incipient tension between celibacy and virility—as this is reflected in Ayurveda—into a modern paradox.

GUPT ROG CIKITSĀ: HAVING YOUR *OJAS* AND EATING IT TOO

This tension between "asceticism and eroticism"—which is otherwise reflected in, and significantly made sense of, by a broad range of Hindu mythology (O'Flaherty 1973)—became particularly problematic in colonial and postcolonial India, when masculinity was politicized in the context of the nationalist movement (Alter 1992; Nandy 1983; Rosselli 1980; Sinha 1995). Just as celibacy was transformed into a "science of gendered public health" in the first half of the twentieth century, similarly a new, specialized branch of medicine called *gupt rog cikitsā*, sex therapy, lit. secret disease treatment, developed during the same period of time (see Amrohavi n.d.a., n.d.b., n.d.c.; Chatursen 1977, 1997; Gautam 1983). In essence, *gupt rog cikitsā* combines elements of *rasāyaṇa* and *vājīkaraṇa* to produce a science of sexual potency. The history of this development may be clearly and unambiguously inferred from the discourse on celibacy (see Hiralal 1983; Saraswati 1982; Shastri n.d.a, n.d.b). Advocacy for celibacy in the 1920s and 1930s developed, at least in part, as a critical, conservative response to the growing commercial market in sexual enhancement therapy (Alter 1994). It is clear that this history is linked to systems of medicine other than Ayurveda, namely, Siddha alchemical medicine and various permutations of Tantric medicine (Jaggi 1973), as both of these are explicitly and less self-consciously concerned with sex. Nevertheless, Ayurveda's concern with sex and "sexuality" is an important framework within which to study the history of sex therapy, precisely because of the way in which the relationship between immortality and virility is worked out in theory.

There are many different dimensions to *gupt rog cikitsā*, but in most general terms it may be understood as a cultural response—inconclusive and somewhat inconsistent, to be sure—to a post-Enlightenment colonial discourse on sexuality in general, the perceived self-image of effeteness, and the feminization of masculinity reflected in celibate asexuality in particular. Gandhi is simply the most well-known figure who, in the eyes of his detractors, embodied weakness in his advocacy for abstinence. The *gupt rog cikitsā* literature that deals with aphrodisiacs may be read as an antidote to the flaccid politics of nonviolence. In any case, in simple terms the discourse about and practice of celibacy confirms and conforms to the notion that sex is debilitating. For its part, the discourse about and practice of virility enhancement resolves the physiological problem of sex—or at least a key aspect of it—but contributes to the "problem" of sex as such. Similarly, celibacy solves the problem of sexual physiology but produces a body that is ambiguously virile. The paradox emerges as a consequence of immortality being factored out of the scenario. It is only the immortal king who can have his cake and eat it too, so to speak.

Linked to this is the particular way in which sexuality is articulated in the context of Indian modernity. As the word *gupt* (hidden) would suggest, sexuality has become a matter of prudish silence and secrecy; something that cannot and should not be spoken about openly in public. At the same time a whole discourse has been generated that is based on titillation—the oblique suggestion of precisely that which should not be spoken about directly. Ironically, titillation, which is about the oblique eroticism of the body, disconnects sex from physiology—the natural urge for semen to flow, for example—while linking sex to the body of sensual arousal, where orgasm is the only feeling that counts. When sex is linked to physiology, orgasm can be understood to homologize transcendence and immortality, even though it is also understood to be relatively unhealthy, relativity being a key factor here. But when orgasm is the be-all and end-all of sex, when sex is understood to be a pervasive force in the domain of the culture at large—instead of being discretely one of the four aims—then ejaculation can be understood to be mortally and categorically pathological.

Clearly there are any number of examples from the epic literature of saints and sages—not to mention gods—who are aroused to the point of ejaculation by unmitigated lust or passion. Similarly the *Kāma Sūtra* describes acts of sexual congress that are designed to enhance sexual pleasure in orgasm. In this context it is easy to understand that the whole purpose of *vājīkaraṇa* therapy is to enhance masculine sexual potency, in terms of stamina, control, and the quality of semen ejaculated. But in practice—and in the literature—it is very important to note that *vājīkaraṇa* is clearly linked to self-control. As Caraka, among others, makes clear, the stallionlike men produced by *vājīkaraṇa* therapy must be *nityam ātmavān*, completely self-possessed. Unto itself, sexual potency produces nothing, or at least nothing but momentary pleasure. But sexual potency combined with self-control produces the time-bound analog to immortality—virtue, wealth, public acclaim, and strong and healthy children. It is on this level of self-controlled moderation that celibacy and virility can be understood to be the same, even though their orientation to the problem of embodied immortality is somewhat different, as is their orientation toward sex. Celibacy works outward, so to speak, from a principle of absolute abstinence—and an ideal of arrested flow—to the act in moderation. Virility works inward, so to speak, from a principle of absolute potency—and an ideal of endless flow—to the act in moderation. One might say that absolute celibacy and immortal virility make sense as ideals in the cosmic domain of transcendence, but here and now in the material, time-bound world, the ideal must be an ideal of moderation. And to understand the value of moderation, it must be understood as an ideal rather than as a less-than-ideal compromise.

It probably has never been an easy ideal to live up to, but most certainly moderation is not an ideal that one would associate with modernity, either in India or elsewhere. Everything is in excess, even self-control. This is clearly reflected in the self-help virility literature, which is designed to enable the dedicated male reader to maximize everything, both in terms of the act—that is, length, hardness, stamina, and the number of orgasms, both for himself and his partner—and the product of the act, namely, healthy sons. Although many virility clinics may well advertise their services in terms of curing problems of impotence, semen loss, and most definitely infertility, in much of the literature there is a clear if somewhat an oblique emphasis on the maximization of pleasure. What I mean by the apparent contradiction of being both "oblique" and "clear" is that a desire for more and better sex may well be regarded as an end in itself, but it usually is framed in the literature—at least in the prefatory remarks made by a number of authors—as a means to having more sons. Consider here some examples, with the desire for more sons in the back of your mind:

> Take one gram of roasted *suhāga*, three grams of *bhimsen kafur*, three and a half grams of honey and massage it on your penis. Doing this will cause the woman to discharge [word in English] quickly. (Amrohavi n.d.a.: 20)

> Take six grams of *kapur rasa* [liquified edible camphor], fifteen grams of *ghongchā*, fifteen grams of *hafām*, twenty-five grams of *malkingni*, twenty-five grams of *ghapure* seeds, twenty-five grams of the root of the white *kaner* and the amount of *til* [sesame] oil that you need. Grind and sieve all of the ingredients and soak them over night in the oil. In the morning put the oil in a glass bottle. Taking out the amount you need, massage it all over your penis, except on the glans at the tip. Then wrap your penis in a *pān* leaf. By massaging the medicated oil into the penis it becomes stiff, powerful, long, and hard. This has particular benefits for those who masturbate and those who are impotent (Amrohavi n.d.a: 48). With this [aphrodisiac] semen is made potent, firm, and strong. It is the most effective tonic for getting rid of all problems linked to semen. The body becomes fit and energized. (Gautam 1983: 33)

> The juice of ginger and onions if taken every day after having had sex restores the vitality of youth. Onions promote feelings of desire, produce semen, and enable a man to last a long time before ejaculating while engaged in sexual intercourse. (Amrohavi n.d.b.: 33)

Thus most of the literature on virility is contextualized by a broader discourse on sexuality that is somewhat narrowly construed in terms of desire, pleasure, and masculine strength and identity rather than by a discourse on medicine and health, even though the question of virility is clearly medical in form and content. The principle is that aphrodisiacs enhance sexual potency as an end in itself, and an end that can be reproduced, pharmaceutically, time after time. This, then, is a clear case of the medicalization of sex. And this should be understood as categorically different from the "sexualization" of health and medicine—in terms of physiology and flow—which is, I think, closer to what is manifest in the ayurvedic corpus.

The development of celibacy followed a similar trajectory during the twentieth century, although it was not so much medicalized during this time as turned into a therapy designed to treat the illness of modernity, including, of course, the modern desire for virility and sexual potency, independent of all else. The two discourses fed off one another and are intimately, if paradoxically, linked together. Along these lines Amrohavi's ambiguous statement about how massaging the penis with oil can be "particularly beneficial" for those who masturbate perfectly reflects the paradox in the relationship between celibacy and virility.

The medicalization of sex in the context of ayurvedic *gupt rog cikitsā* fuses and confuses the goal of *rasāyaṇa* with the goal of *vājīkaraṇa,* wherein modern analogs of *soma,* such as the nearly ubiquitous *chyavanprash,* function as tonics that produce youthful energy to enhance sexual potency. A preliminary survey of some of the literature indicates that most books include a chapter on tonics that can restore youth and sexual potency, the former being, in most cases, almost synonymous with the latter. Graphically this is represented by the cover art on three books: *Sambhog Samrāṭ Banāne Wale Oṣadiyaṭ* [Herbs That Will Give You the Sex Drive of an Emperor](Amrohavi n.d.a), *Gupt Rog Cikitsā* [Therapy for Sex Problems] (Gautam 1983), and *Brahmacarya ke Anubhāv* [Guidelines for Maintaining Celibacy] (Shastri n.d.) On the cover of the first is an illustration of a powerfully built young man wrestling with a lion, and on the covers of the other two are illustrations of young men flexing their muscles in the pose of modern body builders. Although the first one is devoted exclusively to aphrodisiacs, the second one to both aphrodisiacs and the treatment of sexual dysfunction, and the third to celibacy as a cure for the involuntary loss of semen, each one makes an explicit connection between potency, power, virility, and youth. The focus is on having your *ojas* and eating it too.

Here the ambiguity of what *ojas* really is—*dhātu, upadhātu,* or an entity unto itself—plays into the modern mystique of the mysterious, magical aphrodisiac and the fantastic decoction recipes found in some contemporary Hindi publications. It also plays into the endless—and self-mimetic—debate about whether or not *soma* is a real plant, and whether or not if that plant can really be found *rasāyaṇa* therapy might just really work. This may not be *gupt* (hidden), but the endless search for the undiscoverable truth produces intense mystery. And mystery is, in a sense, an analog to secrecy, and it is secrecy that enshrouds sex in the *sotto-voce* discourse of sexuality.

PAHALWANS: THE EMBODIMENT OF THE PARADOX ITSELF

As I have pointed out elsewhere (Alter 1992), wrestlers in contemporary India are preoccupied with the problem of sex and the retention of semen, as sex and semen are directly linked to a lifestyle devoted to the development of "bodies of one color." These bodies are tremendously strong, thick, solid, and well balanced. With a body of one color a wrestler gives elemental, substantial form to moral virtue and high ethical standards and seeks to command social respect. From the vantage point of many wrestlers, sex is anathema, precisely because their moral physiques are produced and maintained through both the production and the retention of semen as a substance that imparts vital energy. In a direct and an explicit way, they view themselves as embodying the *ojas* they work so hard to produce. However, *ojas* is linked to semen, and this presents problems with regard to the containment of sex and the energy and power linked to sex.

In many ways the production and retention of semen in the context of the wrestling gymnasium is linked directly to ayurvedic principles, if not to ayurvedic therapy as such. Although in the gymnasium there is relatively little reference to *vāta* (wind), *pitta* (bile), and *kapha* (phlegm), wrestlers talk at great length about *guṇa* strands and the way in which their lifestyle is designed to produce the perfection of *sāttvik* (subtle purity) radiance as against the kind of *tāmasik* (coarse dullness) torpor that might otherwise be associated with a regimen involving such intense physical exercise and monumental consumption. A great deal of attention also is given to the question of digestion, a wrestler's strength being measured in terms of his ability to digest vast quantities of food and "cook"—by heat generated through exercise—the *rasa* of this food. Internal cooking contributes to the production of embodied power. Therefore, the daily health regimen of the wrestler—which involves careful attention to a range of imponderables such as sleeping position, dental hygiene, defecation, urination, and bathing—along with his diet—ghee, milk, and almonds, measured in liters and kilograms—fits directly with a theory of *dhātu* transubstantiation in general. Significantly, it also fits with the logic of *vājīkaraṇa* aphrodisiacs.

Many of the aphrodisiacs described by Caraka include milk and ghee. For example, the whole third quarter of the relevant chapter (*Cikitsāsthāna* 2.3.1–31) is devoted to tonics made from the milk and ghee of cows fed on the leaves of black gram. Although in many cases various specific herbs, roots, and fruits are added to milk, and are said to be semen- and bulk-promoting, one formula states, simply that "one who desires indestructible semen should use milk boiled with semen promoting vitaliser[s], bulk-promoting and glactogogue [drug that increases milk supply] drugs separately[,] and [add to this] wheat flour along with ghee, honey, and sugar" (*Cikitsāsthāna* 2.3.6, 7. Sharma 1992: 4). Another indicates that ten grams each of eleven different substances "should be boiled in 2.5 liters of milk that is diluted with half its volume of water until only the original volume of milk remains. This milk should be filtered. On taking it after adding honey, ghee, and sugar even though [one is] seventy years old [one will] get large progeny and [will be] exhilarated sexually like a young man (*Cikitsāsthāna* 2.3.8-10. Sharma 1992: 44).

To the best of my knowledge almonds are not referred to very extensively, if at all, by Caraka and Suśruta, but it seems very clear that in the context of the wrestler's diet almonds are crushed and mixed into milk—to which ghee is subsequently added—to make a tonic that is the structural and substantial analog of an aphrodisiac. This makes sense, since the wrestler is trying to produce indestructible semen. The key difference is that the wrestler drinks his tonic not only with no intention of having sex but with the intention of not having sex at all. He takes what can be classified as an aphrodisiac to be strong and celibate. As one might guess, this leads to an embodied paradox.

The production of semen to produce physical strength, as well as to produce and reproduce a kind of power that is understood to be beyond the range of normal, has probably been integral to the art of wrestling for a long time. In ways that still need to be further studied, there is a high degree of thematic and theoretical overlap, in terms of embodied practice, between wrestling, yoga and Tantra, and Ayurveda. If the paradigmatic patient in the ayurvedic literature is the king, then there is also an important way in which the wrestler represents—and in some instances is—the king's body (Alter 1992). He gives physiological form to political power.

Significantly, however, the emphasis on hypermasculinity in the discourse on wrestling is clearly a modern phenomenon linked to the perceived "emasculation" of the princely states, and their rulers, during the colonial era, particularly after 1857 (Alter 2002). Biographies of famous wrestlers of this period clearly seek to construct an image of hypermasculinity. The idea that a wrestler should count the number of exercises that he does in the thousands, if not tens of thousands, and measure his consumption of ghee and milk in terms of liters and liters, if not whole canisters—and thereby become like a bull or an elephant, if not a stallion—represents a degree of nervousness among many about the need to counteract the effects of having been cast in the role of the effete colonized subject.

There also is an important class component to this nervousness, as well as a sense of refracted history, since it is largely middle-class men writing in the latter part of the twentieth century about illiterate peasant wrestlers in the nineteenth, who emphasize the way in which these wrestlers embodied phenomenal power based on their absolute celibacy, the largess of their royal patrons, and their fantastic ability to exercise and eat almost endlessly. In an interesting way the image of the wrestler in these accounts reflects the kind of quest for perfection and immortality found in Suśruta's description of the post-*rasāyaṇa* new man. For wrestlers training in the late twentieth century, an over-the-top image of impossible perfection in the nineteenth century produces a high degree of anxiety about the limits to which the human body can be pushed, and the need to push those limits ever farther—particularly as concerns celibacy and the production and retention of semen.

It is noteworthy that in the medieval literature on wrestling, most clearly reflected in the *Mānasollāsa* (Srigondekar 1959) and *Mallapurāṇa* (Sandesara and Mehta 1964), there is a detailed emphasis on diet, exercise, and celibacy. The primary concern in these texts, however, is with balance and a kind of calibrated accommodation between regimen and the physiological characteristics of the particular wrestler engaged in his own specific regimen. Celibacy is recommended, but more in terms of the recommendation in the *Caraka-Saṃhitā*, which idealizes moderation rather than an extreme. In other words, the exaggerated concern that all wrestlers have come to have with the production and retention of semen must be understood within the context of a narrow history in which celibacy has become linked, problematically, to impotence, and to the weakness associated with impotence in both literal and metaphorical terms.

The problem of impotence, weakness, and emasculation that took shape during the colonial era has become an important feature of the critical stance that wrestlers take toward what they characterize as modernity. In the discourse that is concerned with the development of the wrestler's moral physique, the problem of eroticism and sensuality looms very large, particularly with reference to Indian cinema. Wrestlers who advocate strict celibacy view the sensual climate of modern India as being extremely unhealthy. They contrast their own bodies of one color with the weak, emaciated, unhealthy bodies of young men who spend their time in idle recreation going to movies, drinking tea, eating fried, spicy food, and, in general, doing things that will cause their semen to flow. And most certainly—contra-Caraka—not in terms of any "natural urge" on the part of the semen itself to do so. In this case it is clearly the young men whose hands and minds are thought to be out of control and in need of suppression. Wrestlers also criticize these young men for both having to resort to *gupt rog cikitsā* to find a cure for what ails them—usually impotence and the involuntary discharge of semen—and for further eroticizing their sexuality by going to seek treatment through *gupt rog cikitsā*, a case in which it is not so much that you are damned if you do and damned if you don't, but that you are doubly damned if you do, because the cause and effect are the same thing. The flow of semen causes the flow of semen, and so *gupt rog cikitsā* as a solution is also precisely the problem.

In this regard it is interesting to note that modern young men who are thought to be obsessed with sex to the point of chronic semen loss are described in terms that are very similar to those used by Caraka to describe the man who has no progeny, that is, the man who is impotent and sterile:

> A man alone without progeny looks like a tree having only one branch, shadeless, fruitless, and foul smelling. He is [like] a dried up pond, a non-metal [object] that [is made to look] like metal, and chaff made into the human form. The childless man should be regarded as unstable, naked, vacant, having one sense organ and inactive. (*Caraka-Saṃhitā Cikitsāsthāna.* 2.1.16–19. Sharma 1992: 36)

The image of the foul-smelling, shriveled, straw man—and he is most certainly that!—with one pathetic branch and one sense organ might fit well within a Freudian framework of analysis. However, the symbolism here is not so much phallic as arboreal. The man with one branch stands in contrast to the sexually potent banyan treelike king who lives forever through his many children, the heirs to his kingdom. Clearly it is the number of branches that matters in this imagery, and not the size of any one, as might be the case if the imagery—and symbolic point of reference—were different. A man without children is like a tree that is on the verge of drying out, losing all of its branches and then becoming rotten wood.

In this respect the modern discourse on wrestling is at the opposite end of the spectrum from the modern discourse of *gupt rog cikitsā*. The popular literature that reflects this discourse explains how one can, as one pamphlet puts it, "outlast a woman," "maximize one's pleasure," and "make one's penis long, thick, and stiff." It also explains how to "stay young and healthy forever," how to "make oneself young again," and how to "make one's semen thick and rich" (Amrohavi n.d.b). But wrestling is only at one end of the spectrum if the spectrum is envisaged—paradoxically—as a circle, something like the ouroboros snake with its tail in its mouth.

Both wrestling and *gupt rog cikitsā* can be understood in this way from the vantage point of a kind of patient who has become, in the context of modern scholarship, as paradigmatic and as distinctively stereotyped as the king in the ayurvedic corpus. He is, following Carstairs (1958), Obeyesekere (1976), Kakar (1981, 1990), and Edwards (1983), as well as others who have written more narrowly on the culture-bound syndrome known as *dhat*, the putative everyman of modern India. He is a man who is sick because he has lost his semen on account of having had too much sex, on account of masturbation, on account of his semen leaking out during urination, and on account of experiencing "night fall" through dream stimulation. He is a man caught in a vicious cycle wherein semen loss, and the fear of semen loss, produces intense anxiety that further causes semen to be weakened, watered down, and drained off. In his grounded mortality, as well as his paradigmatic status, he is the mirror opposite of the kingly, ayurvedic new man, as well as the "poor cousin" of a king for whom time is the ultimate risk factor. This is the king who embodies what White refers to as the "ontological disease" of *rājayakśma*, or royal consumption.

> According to both medical and literary convention the king who allows himself to become debauched in the clutches of too many passionate women also falls prey to "royal consumption": as a result his kingdom, sapped of all its *rasa*, withers and dies . . . His *rasa*, his vigor, his semen completely dried up, [he] must perform a *soma* (which is both a name for and the stuff of the moon, the *rasa* par excellence) sacrifice in order to restore his lost *rasa*, and so the cycle begins anew. (White 1996: 24)

The cycle begins anew, and it is virility that causes a loss of virility that makes the world go round. In this postcolonial era, when the "kingdom is sapped of all its *rasa*" and has withered and died, modern celibacy, on the one hand, and modern *gupt rog cikitsā*, on the other, seek to provide definitive solutions to a problem that is, and will continue to be for all time, ongoing and cyclical. The problem is, quite simply, that the fact of death is coded in the very substance of life.

REFERENCES

Alter, Joseph S. 1992. *The Wrestler's Body: Identity and Ideology in North India.* Berkeley: University of California Press.

———. 1994. Celibacy, sexuality and the transformation of gender into nationalism. *Journal of Asian Studies* 53:1: 45–66.

———. 1995. The celibate wrestler: Sexual chaos, embodied balance, and competitive politics in North India. *Contributions to Indian Sociology (n.s.)* 29:1–2: 109–31.

———. 1996. Gandhi's body, Gandhi's truth: Non-violence and the bio-moral imperative of public health. *Journal of Asian Studies* 55:2: 301–22.

———. 1997. A therapy to live by: Public health, the self, and nationalism in the practice of a North Indian yoga society. *Medical Anthropology* 11: 275–98.

———. 1999. Heaps of health, metaphysical fitness: Ayurveda and the ontology of good health in medical anthropology. *Current Anthropology* 40: S43–S66.

———. 2000. *Gandhi's body: Sex, diet, and the politics of nationalism.* Philadelphia: University of Pennsylvania Press.

———. 2002. Nervous masculinity: Consumption and the production of gender in Indian wrestling. In *Everyday Life in South Asia,* ed. Diane Mines and Sarah Lamb, 132–45. Indianapolis and Bloomington: Indiana University Press.

Amrohavi, Alizaha. n.d.a. *Sambhog Samrāñ Banāne Wali Oṣadiyañ.* Delhi: Medical House.

———. n.d.b. *Stri-Puruṣa Gupt Rog Cikitsā.* Delhi: Medical House.

———. n.d.c. *101 Sambhog Shaktivardhak Yog.* Delhi: Medical House.

Aṣṭāṅgahṛdaya of Vāgbhaṭa: The Book of Eight Branches of Ayurveda. 1999. Translated by Vaidya Asha Ram et al. Delhi: Sri Satguru Publications.

Babb, Lawrence A. 1983. The physiology of redemption. *History of Religions* 22: 293–312.

Caplan, Pat. 1987. Celibacy as a solution? Mahatma Gandhi and brahmacharya. In *The Cultural Construction of Sexuality,* ed. Pat Caplan, 271–95. London: Tavistock.

Caraka-Saṃitā: Agniveśa's treatise refined and annotated by Caraka and redacted by Dṛḍhabala—Text and English Translation. 1992. Edited and translated by Priyavrat Sharma. Varanasi: Chaukhamba Orientalia.

Carstairs, G. Morris. 1958. *The Twice-Born.* London: Hogarth Press.

Chatterjee, Partha. 1993. *Nationalist Thought and the Colonial World: A Derivative Discourse.* Minneapolis: University of Minnesota Press.

Chatursen, Acharya. 1977. *Yauvan or Svasthya Vijñān.* Delhi: Anupam Pocket Books.

———. 1997. *Nar-Nari: Kām Vijñān.* Delhi: Sadhana Pocket Books.

Cohen, Lawrence. 1995. The pleasures of castration: The postoperative status of Hijras, Jankhas, and Academics. In *Sexual Nature, Sexual Culture,* ed. Paul R. Abramson and Steven D. Pinkerton, 276–304. Chicago: University of Chicago Press.

———. 1998. *No Aging in India: Alzheimer's, the Bad Family, and Other Modern Things.* Berkeley: University of California Press.

Daniel, E. Valentine, and Judy Pugh, eds. 1984. *South Asian Systems of Healing.* Leiden: E. J. Brill.

Das, Rahul Peter. 2003. *The Origin of the Life of a Human Being: Conception and the Female according to Ancient Indian Medical and Sexological Literature.* Delhi: Motilal Banarsidass.

Edwards, James. 1983. Semen anxiety in South Asian cultures: Cultural and transcultural significance. *Medical Anthropology* 7:3: 51–67.

Eliade, Mircea. 1969. *Yoga: Immortality and Freedom.* Princeton, NJ: Princeton University Press.

Fausto-Sterling, Anne. 2000. *Sexing the Body: Gender, Politics and the Construction of Sexuality.* New York: Basic Books.

Filliozat, Jean. 1964. *The Classical Doctrine of Indian Medicine: Its Origins and Greek Parallels.* Delhi: Munshiram Manoharlal.

Foucault, Michel. 1990. *The Uses of Pleasure: The History of Sexuality, Vol. 2.* New York: Vintage Books.

Furth, Charlotte. 1999. *A Flourishing Yin: Gender in China's Medical History, 960–1665.* Berkeley: University of California Press.

Gautam, Chamanlal. 1983. *Gupt Rog Cikitsā.* Bareilly: Sanskrit Sansthan.

Gonda, Jan. 1952. *Ancient Indian Ojas, Latin *Augos, and the Indo-European Nouns in -Es-/-Os.* Utrecht: NVA Oosthoek's Uitgevers Mij.

Gupta, Charu. 2001. *Sexuality, Obscenity, Community: Women, Muslims, and the Hindu Public in Colonial India.* New Delhi: Permanent Black.

Hiralal. 1983. *Brahmacārya Vivāha-ke Pahale or Vivāha-ke Bād.* Unnav, Uttar Pradesh: Jan Swasthiya Prakashan.

Jaggi, Om Prakash. 1973. *Yogic and Tantric Medicine: History of Science and Technology in India, Vol. 5.* Delhi: Atma Ram and Sons.

Jolly, Julius. 1977. *Indian Medicine.* Eng. trans. by C. G. Kashikar. Delhi: Munshi Ram Manohar Lal.

Kakar, Sudhir. 1981. *The Inner World: A Psycho-Analytic Study of Childhood and Society in India.* New Delhi: Oxford University Press.

———. 1990. *Intimate Relations: Exploring Indian Sexuality.* Chicago: University of Chicago Press.

Laqueur, Thomas. 1990. *Making Sex: Body and Gender from the Greeks to Freud.* Cambridge, MA: Harvard University Press.

Leslie, Julia. 1994. Some traditional Indian views on menstruation and female sexuality. In *The History of Attitudes to Sexuality,* ed. R. Porter and M. Teich, 63–81. Cambridge, MA: Cambridge University Press.

Lynch, Owen. 1990. The mastram: Emotion and person among Mathura's chaubes. In *Divine Passions: The Social Construction of Emotion in India,* ed. Owen Lynch, 91–115. Berkeley: University of California Press.

Marglin, Frédérique. 1985. *Wives of the God-king: The Rituals of the Devadasis of Puri.* New Delhi: Oxford University Press.

Marriott, McKim. 1990. *India through Hindu Categories*. New Delhi: Sage Publications.

Nanda, Serena. 1990. *Neither Man nor Woman: The Hijras of India*. Belmont: Wadsworth Publishing.

Nandy, Ashis. 1980. *At the Edge of Psychology: Essays in Politics and Culture*. Delhi: Oxford University Press.

———. 1983. *The Intimate Enemy: Loss and Recovery of Self under Colonialism*. New Delhi: Oxford University Press.

Obeyesekere, Gananath. 1976. The impact of Ayurvedic ideas on the culture and the individual in Sri Lanka. In *Asian Medical Systems*, ed. Charles Leslie, 201—226. Berkeley: University of California Press.

O'Flaherty, Wendy Doniger. 1973. *Asceticism and Eroticism in the Mythology of Siva*. Oxford: Oxford University Press.

———. 1980. *Women, Androgynes, and Other Mythical Beasts*. Chicago: University of Chicago Press.

———. 1987. *Tales of Sex and Violence: Folklore, Sacrifice, and Danger in the Jaiminiya Brahmana*. New Delhi: Motilal Banarsidass.

Parry, Jonathan. 1985. *Death and Digestion: The Symbolism of Food and Eating in North Indian Mortuary Rites*. Man (n.s.) 20: 612–30.

Rao, S. K. Ramachandra. 1987. *Encyclopedia of Indian Medicine, Vol. 2*. Bombay: Popular Prakashan.

Roland, Alan. 1988. *In Search of Self in India and Japan*. Princeton: Princeton University Press.

Rosselli, John. 1980. The self-image of effeteness. *Past and Present* 86: 121–48.

Sandesara, B. J., and R. N. Mehta. 1964. *Mallapurāṇa*. Baroda: Oriental Institute.

Saraswati, Swami Yogananda. 1982. *Brahmacārya Rakshā He Jīvan He*. Alwar, Rajasthan: Ramji Lal Sharma.

Selby, Martha Ann. 2005. Sanskrit gynecologies in post-modernity: The commoditization of Indian medicine in alternative medical and new age discourses on women's health. In *Asian Medicine and Globalization*, ed. Joseph S. Alter, 120–31. Philadelphia: University of Pennsylvania Press.

Shastri, Kaviraj Jagannath. n.d.a. *Brahmacārya-kā Anubhāv*. Delhi: Dehati Pustak Bhandar.

———. n.d.b. *Brahmacārya-ke Sādhana*. Delhi: Dehati Pustak Bhandar.

Sinha, Mrinalini. 1995. *Colonial Masculinity: The "Manly Englishman" and the "Effeminate Bengali" in the Late Nineteenth Century*. Manchester: Manchester University Press.

Srigondekar, G. K. 1959. *Mānasollasa*. Baroda: Oriental Institute.

Srivastava, Sanjay. 2004. *Sexual Sites, Seminal Attitudes: Sexualities, Masculinities, and Culture in South Asia*. New Delhi: Sage Publications.

Urban, Hugh. 2003. *Tantra: Sex, Secrecy, Politics, and Power in the Study of Religion*. Berkeley: University of California Press.

Wadley, Susan 1975. *Shakti: Power in the Conceptual Structure of Karimpur Religion*. Chicago: University of Chicago Studies in Anthropology, No. 2.

White, David Gordon. 1984. Why gurus are heavy. *Numen* 33: 40–73.

———. 1996. *The Alchemical Body: Siddha Traditions in Medieval India*. Chicago: University of Chicago Press.

Wujastyk, Dominik. 1998. *The Roots of Ayurveda: Selections from Sanskrit Medical Writings*. New Delhi: Penguin Books.

Zimmer, Heinrich Robert. 1948. *Hindu Medicine*. Baltimore, MD: Johns Hopkins University Press.

Zimmermann, Francis. 1987. *The Jungle and the Aroma of Meats: An Ecological Theme in Hindu Medicine*. Berkeley: University of California Press.

Zysk, Kenneth. 1991. *Asceticism and Healing in Ancient India: Medicine in the Buddhist Monastery*. Oxford: Oxford University Press.

———. 2002. *Ratiśāstra and Ratiramaṇa. Text, Translation, and Notes*. Leiden: E. J. Brill.

CHAPTER 11

Ayurveda in Modern India

Standardization and Pharmaceuticalization

MADHULIKA BANERJEE

Ayurveda in modern India has developed in response to the various challenges that were posed by modern medicine when it came to India through British colonialism. These challenges were: the ready availability of mass-produced medicines (unknown to medical practice elsewhere in the world); a continuous output of information regarding the large number of new medicines for various ailments that were on the market; and, most of all, the efficacy of the new medicines as compared to the old. This competition required responses on different fronts—production, marketing, and research—and produced very interesting developments in Ayurveda that transformed it radically. One of the transformations was the standardization of medicines in accordance with the principles of mass production, in exactly the way that had come to characterize modern pharmaceuticals. This is manifest in both the production processes and lines of research toward modernization. Beginning at the end of the nineteenth century, the developments continue till today.

The standardization of ayurvedic medicine production is radically influencing the internal structure and epistemology of this knowledge system. This results in what we call the "pharmaceuticalization" of Ayurveda, where it is reduced to becoming merely a supplier of pharmaceutical products. The adherence to new criteria of evaluating the efficacy of medicines set by the expectations of biomedicine substantially changes the character of these medicines: ayurvedic pharmaceuticals become indistinguishable from any other pharmaceutical. They neither continue to carry the distinctive marks of their original knowledge system nor require their specific context to be effective. Thus the capacity of Ayurveda to be able to pose an "alternate" system is being gradually eroded. This is not just a problem for the internal world of Ayurveda but for the development of medicine for humankind, because it results in the shrinking of the medical knowledge base available as against expanding it. In order to counter this, I propose at the end of this chapter alternative perspectives to production and research.

The process of standardization in manufacture posed difficulties peculiar to Ayurveda. Unlike other "traditional" or "herbal" systems of medicine, Ayurveda has a very advanced, and organized pharmacology spelled out in the classical texts. This required the modern manufacturer to "translate" these detailed instructions on the method of making medicines. These methods needed to conform to the requirements of large-scale manufacture and to create legitimacy in the market. The "translation" in each of these instances involved a complex reorientation and transformation from the long-established forms and norms being followed in this line. This change was controversial on several counts. First, the forms of ayurvedic medicines were more varied than the table-syrup-capsule regimen of allopathy and unfamiliar to both modern market and practitioner. The dilemma of the modern ayurvedic manufacturer was therefore to determine whether the forms should be maintained, or should be changed to conform to the modern stereotypes. Second, there was no way of knowing whether the proper procedures were being followed in the new manufacturing processes. Third, by the time these medicines were being mass-produced, "scientific" norms such as randomized clinical trials to recognize the efficacy of new medicines were already being pushed for in the dominant pharmaceutical market. There was no established parallel to this in ayurvedic practice that could have been used as its own term of reference. So what it used initially was the evidence of efficacious history, indicated in the long use by the *vaidya* and deep faith of the patients. But this was not enough for the modern market and the new consumers. The power of modern science invited all to view these claims as fraud. But these arguments and counterarguments have now traversed a long path. There is no longer an offensive on the part of "science" as opposed to grand posturing on the part of "tradition." I propose to offer a summary of those positions as well to understand where this issue stands today.

RAW MATERIALS, MAINLY MEDICINAL PLANTS

Ayurvedic medicines are combination drugs, composed of mainly herbs, minerals, and metals. The traditional pedagogy and practice of Ayurveda instilled in all *vaidyas* knowledge of medicinal plants and other inputs into the medicines they would prescribe and be required to make themselves. But in modern manufacture, using this knowledge for large-scale supplies is the biggest difficulty, particularly true for plant and herb components. Identification, place of purchase, and the surety that the observation of the specified times for picking (including those of day, month, and season) have been met determine the expected levels of efficacy and action to be available from the plants. When the exact requirement is not met, it also may become necessary for those responsible to make decisions about locating and purchasing the possible substitutes. Thus a combination of detailed knowledge of pharmacognosy, pharmacy and market management, and the organizational skill of coordination with the other divisions of the firm would be required for this purpose.

One very important aspect must be considered in light of this: The quality of these supplies has deteriorated sharply due to increasing demand for medicinal plants, as more and more mass manufacturers enter the market. This is inevitable, because of the range and diversity of materials required in different parts of the country, by different concerns, at all times. While the market for this has expanded rapidly, the technological response to the problems of this situation has been unable to keep pace. The market of raw materials for traditional medicines remains unwieldy within the unorganized sector. The big industries visualize their responsibility to begin only when the material reaches their premises, and not before. Hence, the standardization of raw materials—of herbs in pristine or part-treated stages—is one dimension of the production process that remains at the level of discussion most of the time. The manufacturers' assumption that they are not responsible for the standardization and quality control of the raw materials in fact has a negative impact on them, since it compromises the credibility of their product. Because of heightened demand for ayurvedic products, however, suppliers are able to demand high prices for their non-standardized raw materials. This pushes the market average up and disadvantages the smaller buyers.

PRODUCTION PROCESS

Ayurvedic texts specify the making of medicines in great detail. Most of the medicines are compound drugs, which means two things. First, a number of inputs go into the making of medicines. Second, the order and specificity of each process are of the utmost importance. A number of processes are used, including preparing decoctions, pulverizing, powdering, drying in the shade, drying in the sun, and keeping a preparation in an earthen vessel beneath the ground for a length of time. From a modern manufacturing perspective, these processes appear time-consuming and very labor-intensive. Therefore, the most important question was what kind of mechanization would make it both economically viable and least harmful in terms of the sanctity of the processes? It entailed a number of steps at the research and analysis levels, including successive scaling, where the tenability of the method of the laboratory is tested out before being accepted by the production unit.

The account of how this took place in Dabur is indeed a classic example. The founder, Dr. P. C. Burman, actually initiated and executed this process for the company. Until the late 1940s, Dabur's medicines were being manufactured by hand, following the processes prescribed by the accepted texts. As the size of the company grew, it meant more space for more unwieldy tools, and more workers were required, posing a major management problem. A combination of both of these factors, therefore, led the company to opt for mechanization and to move away from their place of origin. Burman systematically approached the process of mechanization of ayurvedic medicines. He began by locating those texts/*granths,* which were considered both by *vaidyas* and the government the most important and most legitimate. He then set to translate and analyze them. For this purpose he had employed *kaviraj*s/*vaidya*s, who translated the Sanskrit to Hindi or English. Chemists then helped him analyze the physical and chemical dimensions of what was occurring when the prescribed processes of the texts were carried out.

In terms of the actual mechanization of processes, the most important governing condition was the availability of approximate machinery to fulfil the requirements of the processes. Given that machines available in the market were originally designed to meet very different needs, it was possible to arrive at the closest approximation only with great difficulty. For this, Burman turned to the help of qualified engineers, whom he had employed for this very purpose. It took him close to fifteen years to complete the mechanization processes to cover the entire range of medicines that Dabur had undertaken to produce.

The modernization of Dabur's manufacturing process illustrates clearly the hegemonic character of modern technology as well as the influence of the economic conditions under which they were adapted and adopted. When the scale of production increased, the logical option seemed to be mechanization, because that was the dominant ideology of production at the time, as was centralized production. Dabur's factories today are a shining example of a modern pharmaceutical company—gleaming clean, with uniforms for workers and the soft hum of machines. This company has invested hard to set and maintain standards of a very clean, efficient environment of production and has been in the forefront of a campaign with the government to articulate and pass a code for good manufacturing practices, to be followed by all traditional medicine manufacturing companies. Such a certification is certainly an incentive for those who do maintain standards of production.

QUALITY CONTROL OF THE FINAL PRODUCT

The principal issues in the standardization of the quality of ayurvedic medicines are those of safety and efficacy. This is part of what is now a worldwide debate on complementary and alternative medicine, taken up in all seriousness in Europe and the United States. In India, academia, government, and industry have engaged with this issue for at least the last fifty years, ever since new methods of clinical evaluation of medicines (i.e., controlled clinical trials and randomized clinical trials) became a part of legal requirements for production and marketing in the dominant pharmaceutical industry. Initially, both government and industry were convinced that if Ayurveda were to survive either as a recognized knowledge system or as an industry, it had no choice but to be proven efficacious by these trials as well. But there were two major problems—both CCTs and RCTs are very expensive to undertake, and incompatible in terms of the parameters of testing. Thus many doubts were expressed and especially over the latter, evoking further changes in policies and approaches. Industry struggled with product development and government over bringing scientific research and Ayurveda closer so that science was responded to without compromising the basic parameters of the knowledge system. It is a long and complex story, but in this part I will try to summarize it. This will then help clarify the current debates on these issues, especially the European and American responses.

In the modern pharmaceutical industry, any medical intervention usually has to go through seven stages to be transformed from a "promising report" to the status of a "medical innovation"—professional and organizational adoption, public acceptance and state endorsement, observational reports, the randomized clinical trials, and professional denunciation (McKinlay 1981: 374–411). Coming as it does, almost at the end of the process, clinical trials are the crucial legitimizing factor for the medical intervention in the market.

The most widely followed are the double-blind clinical trials, but they are not without controversy. One of the issues considered is the comparative merits of historical trials, or other techniques of testing efficacy, which also begs to ask the question of the final purpose of the trials as reflected in the conduct and questioning of the trials themselves.

Feinstein (1985) has criticized many clinical trials because they forsake outcomes that are clinically relevant but difficult to measure, such as the amelioration of pain or improvement in the quality of life and favor instead less subjective end points that are easier to measure but that may be of questionable clinical relevance.

The issue of the costs of conducting clinical trials vis-à-vis the benefits derived from them leads to doubts about conducting them in the first place. The standard justification of statistical rigor is questioned on the basis of the enormous costs involved, particularly when they are expected to reiterate equivalence of efficacy in comparable drugs. This latter has not always been found to be clinically and scientifically justifiable, and the critics are not hesitant to point out that the real beneficiaries are possibly industry and manufacturers. As Cox (1998) argues, "In a world facing uncertainties about the relative merits of alternative forms of health and social care and education, how should we write a history of fair comparisons between groups receiving different alternative interventions? And in such a history, how should we account for how and why people in previous times have appealed to chance to deal with uncertainties in judging therapeutic efficacy?" However, the fact remains that it forms the basis for the license for the manufacture of biomedical products.

The most important issue in evaluating ayurvedic medicines is that the synergy in the complex formulation between the active ingredients as opposed to the activity of one principle (the formula in allopathy) is what makes the medicine "work." How is this synergy to be measured or even approximated? It would be logical to assume that the assessment of any medicine in terms of its effectiveness in the treatment of disease has to follow the method of diagnosis and line of treatment particular to the system of knowledge from which it stems. But the protocols of the trials themselves are designed according to known parameters of allopathic medicine and the indicators considered acceptable to it. Thus clinical trials of traditional medicines have been conducted on the protocol design of allopathic medicine. Interestingly though, in India, this has been a contested position, there being differences in the approaches of industry and academia, as well as government research organizations such as the Indian Council of Medical Research (ICMR).

One of the most powerful arguments was made nearly thirty years ago, by a doyen of Ayurveda in modern times. Pandit Shiv Sharma argued that Ayurveda and modern medicine have different concepts of "standardization" (1979: 42). He scorned "those who twist and torture ayurvedic concepts to distort their meanings until they can be . . . misinterpreted to be *absolutely* identical with the allopathic concepts" (ibid., emphasis in original). He argued that the meaning of standardization is "strictly confined to the *chemistry* of the drug. It does not cover *uniformity of action on the patients*, . . . If one labours under the belief that a chemically standard drug has a standard therapeutic effect on every patient, he is obviously living outside the world of clinical practice. . . . The patient is a non-standard, and unstandardisable entity. And so are his reactions to standardised drugs" (ibid., emphasis in original). He was proposing a difference in the terms of analysis, something that has only now gained currency again, though by no means part of the mainstream dominant thought process yet. What is important to note here though is that it is only up to this point that there is any attempt to grapple with or question theoretical precepts of the standardization processes handed down by biomedicine. Thus nonindustry institutions have come up with alternative methods of evaluating efficacy. A very significant group of deeply knowledgeable traditional physicians has carried forward this debate in a very serious and worthy manner. They have taken care to also learn the form and substance of modern medical learning and then to engage in a dialogue with it to enable a better understanding on both sides of each other's knowledge. Equally significant, modern-trained scientists in India, with the best credentials in their field, also have undertaken this exercise. Their work has yielded some remarkable counterpoints that have considerably enriched the debate. Unfortunately, neither popular nor scientific media in the world or even in India bothers to hear these voices, and the common person then has to assume that they do not exist. This is why I believe that the debate over traditional and modern medicine appears static, old-fashioned, and even suspect to the mainstream West. In the next part, I present a summary of just two such efforts.

COUNTERPOINTS FROM SCIENTIFIC RESEARCH IN INDIA

One important initiative was taken in a leading hospital in Mumbai since the early 1990s and another by the Government of India's ICMR, also in the last fifteen years or so. The latter has had a significant impact on the World Health Organization's perspective on herbal medicines as well. The Department of Pharmacology, KEM Hospital, Mumbai, and now the same Department at the BYL Nair Hospital, Mumbai, have been the site of one of the most fascinating experiments in facilitating the communication between Ayurveda and science in recent years. Led by visionary pharmacologist Dr. S. Dahanukar, who studied Ayurveda under a traditional teacher after she was already a practicing pharmacologist, a series of pharmacological studies on ayurvedic drug action was initiated. Dahanukar's example was followed by a host of other academics, both trained in mainstream and ayurvedic medical disciplines, to engage in cross-system communication toward the pursuit of what should rightfully be the aim of every person engaged in medicine—the amelioration of pain and illness. In an event with a remarkably reflexive name, Update Ayurveda, she sought to bring together practitioners of Ayurveda and those of biomedicine in order to discuss the progress of this exercise. Held every three years in Mumbai, it has now become a site of debate and communication of a unique kind. While the scientific value of this exercise, by the participants' own observation and admission, is growing stronger every year, more importantly, the respect with which both constituencies are able to address each others' questions is remarkable in itself. At the same time, much of the doubt, defeat, and defiance that characterizes Ayurveda's response to modern science is evident as well—but this is a site of negotiation, precisely the kind that is sorely needed everywhere and between biomedical science and all other forms of medical knowledge.

The ICMR has taken up research in traditional medicine in the validation of traditional knowledge in the areas of diabetes, filariasis, benign hypertrophy of the prostate, coronary artery disease, cancer, HIV/AIDS, and so on, the fingerprinting of selected herbal preparations, agrotechnology of selected plants for various clinical trials (e.g., *Picrorhiza kurroa* and *Pterocarpus marsupiam*), and the development of new molecules from plant sources. What is important, however, is not so much these specifics of areas but the methodology for undertaking clinical evaluation of ayurvedic medicines (rather, all kinds of traditional medicines of India) in order to validate them. A remarkable scientist, Professor R. Roy Chaudhury, has led the initiative for this and offered a whole new methodology resulting from his experimental research. At the beginning of the program in 1984, eight areas of intervention in which the Indian Systems of Medicine (ISM) could provide effective intervention were identified: treatment of anal fistula by a medicated thread, viral hepatitis, urolithiasis, diabetes mellitus, bronchial asthma, filariasis, kalaazar, and wound healing. Initiated in 1984, it was a unique, multidisciplinary program of controlled, randomized, double-blind multicentered trials of a few selected medicinal plants in a few selected disease conditions.

Six innovative changes in conducting this program made it very different from any of the others done before. (1) Specialists from different systems of medicine, including allopathic, came together to select the remedies to be tested. (2) Multicentered protocols were again prepared jointly with experts from the different systems of medicines and experts from different disciplines such as clinical pharmacology, pharmacology, clinical medicine, toxicology, and biochemistry all working together. (3) Once protocols were finalized, they were strictly adhered to, the details coordinated by a Central Biostatistical Monitoring Unit of the ICMR set up at Madras. (4) All of the centers for clinical evaluation were at centers of modern allopathic medicine and were conducted by clinicians and clinical pharmacologists. (This was the point that emphasized the expertise required for the specificities of the clinical trials that would legitimize the drugs being tested far more than ever before). (5) The emphasis was on the clinical evaluation of herbal remedies already in use, implying that most trials were human trials to begin with, while toxicological, pharmacological, and biochemical studies in animals would be carried out as and when deemed necessary. This directly applies the principle of "long association" or "cultural use" that the European Union (EU) is currently struggling to apply to legislation. These trials distinguish themselves by including this in the fundamentals of the research itself. (6) All work on pharmacognosy and the standardization of herbal remedies and placebos was carried out at the Advanced Center of Standardization, Quality Control and Formulation, at the University Department of Pharmacy, Punjab University, Chandigarh. In spite of this, Chaudhury admits, "Sometimes it is impossible to reconcile differences in approach—what is done then is to develop a protocol on the areas of agreement. One problem which arises is that Ayurveda approaches, theoretically at least, health in a holistic manner and bases its treatment on promotive health behaviour, diet, exercise and then medicinal plants: however in these trials only *the clinical efficacy of the medicinal plants is being evaluated*" (Chaudhury 1992: 5, emphasis added).

Chaudhury argues further that the controversies, challenges, and problems that arise when carrying out clinical trials of plants with medicinal properties can be appreciated better if viewed against, (1) a background of the historical use of medicinal plants, (2) the past experience in screening such plants for pharmacological activity and (3) an understanding of some of the relevant concepts of the indigenous systems of medicine where plants have been traditionally utilized.

The issue of standardization is being addressed in the network of Indian traditional medicine research centers by one of four advanced centers, with a specific mandate to develop new standards. The other centers are dedicated to (1) statistics, placebos, and analysis; (2) pharmacological studies, and (3) translating basic research into product development. The network also has a scientific advisory group, ten expert groups, and ten groups involved in implementing clinical trials. Chaudhury emphasizes that double-blind, randomized clinical trials (RCTs) are not the only valid methodology, and that single-blind and open trials also can be helpful in some circumstances.

On the issue of the basic concepts that underlie traditional medical systems, Chaudhury has pointed out that in many systems the concept itself determines efficacy, citing Ayurveda and Unani medicine as examples. In both of these systems, there are three main body/personality types or temperaments, of which at least one predominates in every individual. Certain medicines may be unhelpful or even deleterious to individuals with a particular predominant temperament: for example, *Momordica charantia,* a plant used to treat diabetes, should not be given to patients with the ayurvedic *vāta* constitution. Clearly this factor should be taken into account when selecting patients for clinical trials if the results are to accurately reflect the efficacy of a given medicine as it would be prescribed by an ayurvedic practitioner.

Chaudhury uses the example of bronchial asthma to illustrate that the ayurvedic approach to disease has, in many cases, a more detailed stratification and is more complex than the biomedical approach. Other ayurvedic concepts that can potentially influence efficacy include the combination of plant components and the vehicle used to deliver the phytomedicine (such as honey, butter, ghee or molasses). In a combination medicine, one plant component may contain the "active" ingredients, while, for example, another enhances its activity or stimulates the patient's immune system, and a third substance reduces the toxicity of the second. It also is recognized that the vehicle can accelerate, slow, enhance, or oppose the effects of active substances, and these are all issues that often are overlooked in designing trials. Finally, Chaudhury identifies eight tenets for the evaluation of plant-based medicines.

When all is said and done in this radical and bold line of research, however, Chaudhury identifies a very important shortcoming—that of product development. Once the traditional knowledge of Ayurveda is validated in the preceding way, the research will have far-reaching legitimacy—much more than any other kind of research being done on Ayurveda. But unless they are transposed into "products" that will be prescribed by all kinds of doctors and be consumed by all kinds of patients, the fruits of the research will not be in evidence in the larger community for which it was meant. Even when the government does so much of the hard work and spends so much money, industry has not taken on the responsibility of "product development." Two kinds of excuses are offered: one, that it is too expensive and time-consuming to be ultimately profitable; two, the fear that the market of buyers and consumers is more willing to accept the criteria of allopathy as valid and the challenge to have them accept an alternative may again be too cumbersome. Industry has methods but is loathe to make the necessary investment, with an eye only on short-term profits. Thus very good work just lies there in the labs and goes to waste. What is most disturbing about this process of standardization is that it is unidirectional—the established market alone decides the target language. And the measure of the success of translation is in the sales figures. So the new products the industry comes up with are invariably on the lines of protocols of the trial that can only accommodate Ayurveda in form and not in substance. This is what leads to what we call "pharmaceuticalization," and it needs to be countered at all costs.

STANDARDIZATION AFTER GLOBALIZATION

In the last ten years or so, there has been a great change in the international climate on "herbal medicinal products," with a fast-growing market of nearly US$7 bn. This has meant that the markets in these countries are flooded with herbal products—putting a dent in the dominant pharmaceutical market, which wields enormous power over the governments of Europe and the United States. So the latter have responded with great alacrity in the last decade, and all of the issues that have been wrestled with in India are now being taken up in these countries. The perspective naturally is rather different from those being pursued in India. The fundamental issue there is of establishing the scientific basis, or the lack of it, so that consumers have reliable information about the products and are paying for those that have passed stringent tests for safety and efficacy. While the dominant approach is to apply the same tests to these medicines and products as to all other pharmaceutical products, there are also others approaches from both the United States and Britain. The National Institute of Medical Herbalists exemplifies this different approach. Margaret Whitelegg, one of its most active researchers, argues, "Even if hundreds more trials were performed along orthodox lines we would not necessarily be substantially nearer to defining non-conventional medicine adequately" (1997: 1). In another article, she states even more forcefully, "Rather than take on board the far-reaching changes demanded by a real shift, the strong pressure to intellectual conformity to cognitive norms inclines the orthodox to move into the alternative world with the existing paradigm intact. Hence it assesses the alternative by orthodox criteria, subjects remedies and therapies to objective scientific scrutiny, absorbs what will fit, redefines what cannot initially be readily explained, and rejects the remainder as 'unscientific' (1998–1999: 3).

What seems then to be the need of the hour is to return the science of medicine to the social realm and encourage a dialogue between the sciences and social sciences on the gamut of issues discussed. It is important to initiate this dialogue by asking the fundamental question again: For whom is the process of standardization?

The medical herbalists referred to earlier also are seriously engaged in looking for another set of methods to evaluate these medicines by considering the practice as a whole, rather than just the drugs. St. George recommends, "The starting-point for such a research strategy is the real world of herbal medical practice, which could be made explicit through regular reviews of case histories by groups of herbalists. Such group meetings would have three objectives: (1) to establish a regular, on-going clinical audit process; i.e. a systematic, critical review of the quality of herbal practice by practitioners themselves, in order to identify areas for improvement; (2) to provide the empirical data necessary for a critical analysis of the nature and practice of herbalism as compared to orthodox medicine (briefly touched upon above); and (3) to facilitate the establishment of a clinical database that can be used by a much wider group of herbalists as a research tool for more extensive in-depth clinical evaluations of particular problems or specific herbal remedies" (1999: 2).

Whitelegg argues, "The genuinely alternative paradigm provides a more human centered science in which subjectivity is valued, other knowledge accepted and uncertainty and ignorance admitted. It is not expert led but encourages a collaborative generation of knowledge. Public inclusion and empowerment in a healing context can lead to a deeper and more permanent healing experience. The essence then of alternative shift can be expressed as lying in the acknowledging of uncertainty and contingency" (1998–1999: 4). And it leads St. George to confidently claim, "Herbal medicine, then, is already on the road to the new holistic paradigm. The research and development strategy it chooses should therefore take it further down this road, rather than trying to drag it back to the road of biomedicine" (1999: 2).

With this kind of support from newer quarters, particularly located in the developed world, Ayurveda can gain confidence. It no longer needs to be anxious to be proven equal to biomedicine, having to abandon its holistic perspective on treatment and becoming increasingly drug centered. No longer does the research enterprise of Ayurveda have to sacrifice the experiential to the textual parameters of medicine. Combining the efforts of the last twenty years with these new developments, Ayurveda need not any more be integrated solely in the terms of biomedicine but in terms negotiated with biomedicine in which it truly exchanges knowledge, with a sense of self-respect for its own. It is possible to achieve this without there being a confrontationist stance, by viewing the process as a different set of terms of integration. No longer is it necessary to see this exercise as a "modern medicine" versus "complementary medicine," "modern science" versus "traditional science," but a collaboration with a view to enhancing the benefits of medical knowledge for humankind.

REFERENCES

Anderson, R. 1992. The efficacy of ethnomedicine: Research methods in trouble. In *Anthropological Approaches to the Study of Ethnomedicine*, ed. M. Nichter, 1–17; Montreaux, Switzerland; Philadelphia: Gordon and Breach Science Publishers.

Ayurvedic Interventions for Diabetes Mellitus: A Systematic Review. 2001. Summary, Evidence Report/Technology Assessment: Number 41. AHRQ Publication No. 01-E039 (June). Rockville, MD: Agency for Healthcare Research and Quality. http://www.ahrq.gov/clinic/epcsums/ayurvsum.htm.

Banerjee, M. 1998. The long road to Khari Baoli: Environment discourse and the market for medicinal plants. Presented at *Crossing Boundaries*: the 7th Annual Conference of the International Association for the Study of Common Property (June).

Bodeker, G. 2002. Following tradition into the future: The role of indigenous health systems. Presented at *Providing New Healthcare, World Congress of Ayurveda* (October 1–3), Kochi.

Bodeker, G., R. Jenkins, and G. Burford, eds. 2001. *International Conference on Health Research for Development (COHRED)*. Bangkok: Liebert.

Chaudhury, R. R. 1992. *Herbal Medicine for Human Health*. New Delhi: WHO.

Cox, D. C. T. 1998. Histories of controlled trials. In *Controlled Trials from History*, ed. I. Chalmers, I. Milne, and U. Tröhler, at http://www.web.archive.org/web/20001219124000/www.rcpe.ac.uk/controlled_trials/intro.html.

Efficacy of Interventions to Modify Dietary Behavior Related to Cancer Risk. 2000. Summary, Evidence Report/Technology Assessment: Number 25. AHRQ Publication No. 01-E028 (November). Rockville, MD: Agency for Healthcare Research and Quality. http://www.ahrq.gov/clinic/epcsums/dietsumm.htm.

Etkin, N. 1988. Biobehavioural approaches in the anthroplogical study of indigenous medicines. *Annual Review of Anthropology* 17: 23–42.

Feinstein, A. R. 1985. *Clinical Epidemiology: The Architecture of Clinical Research*. Philadelphia, London: Saunders.

Garlic: Effects on Cardiovascular Risks and Disease, Protective Effects against Cancer, and Clinical Adverse Effects. 2000. Summary, Evidence Report/Technology Assessment: Number 20. AHRQ Publication No. 01-E022 (October). Rockville, MD: Agency for Healthcare Research and Quality. http://www.ahrq.gov/clinic/epcsums/garlicsum.htm.

Government of India. 1999. (August). *Good Manufacturing Practices*. Ministry of Health and Family Welfare, Department of Indian Systems of Medicine. New Delhi.

Kleinman, A. 1980. *Patients and Healers in the Context of Culture: An Exploration of the Borderland between Anthropology, Medicine, and Psychiatry*. Berkeley: University of California Press.

Leslie, C., ed. 1976. *Asian Medical Systems: A Comparative Study*. Berkeley: University of California Press.

Leslie, C., and A. Young, eds. 1992. *Paths to Asian Medical Knowledge*. Berkeley: University of California Press.

McKinlay, John B., ed. 1981. *Health Care Consumers, Professionals, and Organizations*. Cambridge, MA: MIT Press.

Miller, L. G. 1998. Herbal medicinals: Selected clinical considerations focusing on known or potential drug-herb interactions. *Archive of Internal Medicine* 158: 2200–11.

Nandy, A., ed. 1993. *Science, Hegemony, and Violence*. New Delhi: Oxford University Press.

Nichter, M. 1992. Ethnomedicine: Diverse trends, common linkages. In *Anthropological Approaches to the Study of Ethnomedicine*, ed. M. Nichter, 223–59. Montreux, Switzerland; Philadelphia: Gordon and Breach Science Publishers.

Planning Commission. 2002. Task Force on Conservation and Sustainable Use of Medicinal Plants, New Delhi.

Sharma, Pandit Shiv, ed. 1979. *Realms of Ayurveda*. New Delhi: Arnold-Heinemann.

St. George, D. 1999. Research and development in herbal medicine: Biomedical research or new paradigm? *European Journal of Herbal Medicine*.

Uberoi, J. P. S. 1979. *The Other Mind of Europe*. New Delhi: Oxford University Press.

Vickers, A., and C. Zollman. 1999. ABC of complementary medicine. *British Medical Journal* 319 (October 16): 1050–53.

Waldram, J. B. 2000. The efficacy of traditional medicine: Current theoretical and methodological issues. *Medical Anthropology Quarterly* 14:4: 603–25.

Whitelegg, M. 1997. An alternative science for herbal medicine. *European Journal for Herbal Medicine* 2: 1–7.

———. 1998–1999. Patient steps to greener medicine: A personal view. *European Journal of Herbal Medicine*.

CHAPTER 12

Practicing Ayurveda in the United Kingdom

A Time of Challenges and Opportunities

SEBASTIAN POLE

It is called Ayurveda because it tells us which substances, qualities, and actions are life enhancing, and which are not.

—*Caraka-Saṃhitā, Sūtrasthāna* 30.23

INTRODUCTION

I am writing this from the perspective of a practicing herbalist and as a grower, importer, and manufacturer of organic ayurvedic medicinal herbs. It is an overview of the challenges and opportunities facing the ayurvedic community as Ayurveda takes root outside of India and confronts Western medical practice, herbal legislation, and other herbal traditions with particular reference to the situation in the United Kingdom at the beginning of the twenty-first century.

As Ayurveda spreads throughout the world, it is facing many challenges to the traditional ways in which it has been practiced. These challenges, stirring the winds of the ayurvedic community, are legislative, environmental, educational, clinical, and cultural. It is a time to act or be acted upon, meaning that the ayurvedic community must speak up and express its needs, otherwise it will face legislation over which it has no influence.

There are a number of challenges to the global ayurvedic community, beginning with the fact that the Indian authorities themselves regard Ayurveda as a second-rate medical system with a poor professional standing. This results in a weak image projected from its native country to the rest of the world.

One of the challenges to the globalization of any knowledge system is to "translate" its epistemology and to make it acceptable to different cultures. Ayurveda has difficulties on two counts here: one is that it embeds and is embedded within cultural traditions that are different from those in the rest of the world, potentially causing conflict when they mix with other cultures with different agendas. The other is the difference of epistemology between Ayurveda and Western medical science. These are not just in competition but are often in conflict with each other. The lack of evidence-based research and clinical trials that are the touchstones of the Western scientific paradigm hinders its acceptance by mainstream medical institutions and practitioners. Though there are many respectable research institutes in India, many of the clinical trials that are carried out in them are not available in easily accessible journals, and some do not meet rigorous research standards.

A set of different problems arises from most ayurvedic practitioners' lack of environmental awareness about the pressures that harvesting herbal medicines from the wild is placing on the supply of herbs. Increased popularity of herbal medicine as a whole is resulting in increased fears about safety issues. This in turn is leading to further legislation regulating the prescription and sale of herbal remedies. For example, legislation in the United Kingdom threatens to ban the use of certain medicinals such as Vidanga (*Embelia ribes*). Many *bhasmas* (oxidized metallic and mineral preparations) that are often considered the mainstay of internal treatments are illegal in Western countries such as the United Kingdom and the United States.

The environmental pressure on many species used in ayurvedic remedies is serious. For example, Chandan (*Santalum album*) and Kushta (*Saussera lappa*), which are wild and cannot be easily cultivated, are in increasing demand in domestic and international markets. They are fast becoming endangered species.[1]

There also are pressures on the educational front, as different countries struggle to define legally how complementary and alternative medicine (CAM) as a whole can be practiced.

Whether we like it or not, Ayurveda comes under this CAM umbrella. The standards of education are being set so that a portion of traditional education is being excluded, while new practical elements are being included. Then, after qualifying as a practitioner, challenges to implementing the traditional teachings of Ayurveda begin immediately. These center around the expectations of the client and the practicality of many of the procedures. This forces many ayurvedic practitioners to revitalize traditional methods of practice to ensure that their busy clients can comply with the recommendations.

Although a long journey lies ahead, I believe that this is a very exciting and positive time for Ayurveda to experience a renaissance. As a collective group, it means optimizing every opportunity for furthering the wisdom and healing potential of Ayurveda.

CHALLENGES AND OPPORTUNITIES FACING THE AYURVEDIC COMMUNITY

Legislative: Herbal Regulation Resulting in Loss of Pharmacopoeia

Regarding herbal legislation, it is the duty of any legislative body to protect the general public from harm and to promote safety. European Union herbal medicine legislation presents a challenge to every traditional medical system, which will have a major impact from production to supply. The serious threat to the practice of Ayurveda occurs when laws prohibit a herbal species or animal and mineral products from entering a country. There can be a variety of reasons for this, including toxicity and potency, as is the case with Vidanga (*Embelia ribes*) and Mercury. This means practitioners are forced to find alternatives to these banned substances.

At present, the following traditionally used ayurvedic herbs are banned for use under the 1977 Medicine Order:

Betel nut (*Areca catechu*)
Vidanga (*Embelia ribes*)
Kutaja (*Holarrhena antidyserentica*)
Pomegranate bark (*Punica granatum*)
Sarpagandha (*Rauwolfia serpentina*)
Vishamushti (*Strychos nux vomica*)

The following have restrictions on dosage:

Somalata or Ephedra (*Ephedra vulgaris*): 600 mg (MD) 1800 mg (MDD)
Dhattura (*Datura stramonium*): 50 mg (MD) 150 mg (MDD)

Such legislative challenges can disrupt the tradition of Ayurveda. For example, Vidanga, an indispensable herb that is currently banned, is required in a large number of formulations and cannot be replaced with another herb. It is incumbent upon the ayurvedic community to challenge such legislation with scientific data that will be of use to any committee evaluating the safety of medicines. In the United Kingdom, the Traditional Medicines Evaluation Committee has been set up by experts in the field of herbal medicine to communicate accurate and technically valuable information to the Medicines regulatory body. This enables the regulatory body to make informed decisions.

Though often valid in its intention of promoting safety, the law must understand the ways in which herbal medicines are prepared, prescribed, and dosed. We are far beyond the generality that because herbs are "natural" they are therefore "safe." Ayurveda is safe not because the herbs are natural but because only after having arrived at a correct ayurvedic diagnosis would certain herbs be prescribed. A diagnosis is based on an assessment of the patient's constitutional balance (*prakṛti*), digestive strength (*agni*), and tissue integrity (*dhātu*), as well as the patient's expression of a particular disease (*vyādhi*). This will result in a patient-specific treatment strategy that then results in a patient-specific prescription. Herbs should not just be dispensed on a disease-by-disease basis. They are only given when the individual patient with a particular pattern resulting in a specific diagnosis requires it. In this way, Ayurveda is considered a medical system that optimizes safety.

The various ayurvedic pharmacopoeias state that there are many remedies that must be prepared in a certain way, used up to a specific dosage, and only prescribed when the patient's pattern requires them. In Ayurveda, single-herb prescriptions are comparatively uncommon; rather, it is generally considered that the synergy between herbs in a formula reduces potential toxicities. Many herbs are "purified" by the process of *śodhana*, which may involve boiling the main ingredient with certain herbs or grinding the herbs with other detoxifying ingredients. For example, the potential allergenic effect of *Guggul* (*Commiphora mukul*) (see Murray 1995) is removed by decocting it in *Triphala* (*Emblica officinalis, Terminalia chebula, Terminalia belerica*), *Vasaka* (*Adhatoda vasaka*), milk, or *Nirgundi* and *Haridra* (*Vitex negundo, Curcuma longa*).[2] The determining factor in safety is the dosage of each ingredient. The herbs are prescribed within safe dosage limits that have been learned over centuries of practice. The ayurvedic community needs to communicate these safety mechanisms already contained within ayurvedic literature to the relevant legislative bodies.

Environmental: Overharvesting of Valuable Species Reducing Pharmacopoeia

Overharvesting certain species is reducing the pharmacopoeia of herbal medicine the world over. In January 2004, Alan Hamilton, a plant specialist at the World Wildlife Fund, released a paper on the threat to the herbal community faced by the indiscriminate overharvesting of medicinal herbs (Hamilton 2004). In this paper he notes that approximately 75 percent of all herbs that are used in herbal medicine come from the wild. He also stated that 50,000 species of herbs are used as medicines around the world, and that 10,000 of these, a staggering 20 percent, are endangered. The reasons for this can be reduced to pressures placed on the indigenous plant populations. But let us examine in more detail why there is a threat to herbal medicines.

It is estimated that the ayurvedic pharmacopoeia includes upward of 1,250 species with approximately 300 of these in regular demand. In India and Sri Lanka, in excess of 90 percent of herbal material used in Ayurveda comes from the forests, mountains, and plains.[3] That is a heavy burden for nature to bear. Similar pressure exists in other parts of the world, with 80 percent of species coming from the wild in China and up to 99 percent in Africa.[4] And as global population increases, there is increased pressure on natural habitats. At the same time, global demand has skyrocketed in the last decade, with demand increasing by 10 to 20 percent each year.

One of the social factors connected to the medicinal herb trade is that wild harvested herbal medicines offer a valuable source of income to financially pressured, low-income communities. Related to this is the difficulty in monitoring herbal collection. While there is an increase in the field-based cultivation of medicinal herbs, there is relatively little cultivation of herbal medicines. Pioneering companies such as Maharishi Ayurveda and Pukka Herbs are involved in managing cultivation projects in India and Sri Lanka.

Some examples include the following:

- *Yaṣṭimadhu* (*Glycyrrhiza glabra*), or licorice, grows all over the world. A large portion of that global supply has historically come from China and Turkey. Licorice has been in demand for years as a soothing *pitta* reducing anti-inflammatory. Its popularity and lack of controls on harvesting mean that Turkey is now suffering a shortage of wild licorice.[5]
- *Jatāmānsi* (*Nardostachys jatamansi*), or Indian spikenard, only grows in the Himalayas between 3,500–5,000m altitude and is highly valued for its aromatic *vāta*-calming properties. Apart from its limited growing habitat, it also takes three years to grow to full maturity, and it has been thoroughly plundered to the extent that it has been listed on the CITES list as a species to be protected from international trade unless it has been cultivated.

Some herbs are harvested from the wild because, first, that is where they naturally grow and, second, because they often require specific habitats that are contradictory to cultivation. In addition to that, herb prices are actually very low, so there is a lack of incentive for farmers to grow herbs, as they can receive a greater income from conventional food crops. Wild herb harvesting, on the other hand, is a relatively accessible source of income to people without land or a regular job. In the higher altitude region of Nepal, virtually all families harvest herbs, the value of which can translate into 15 to 30 percent of their income.

Another reason for wild herb harvesting lies in the demands of the market: Some authorities consider herbs grown in the wild more potent. This is reflected in their higher price; for example, wild American ginseng (*Panax quinqufolium*) in China commands up to 30 percent more remuneration to the collector than the cultivated variety.

The problems related to wild harvesting could be addressed in a number of ways.

1. The World Health Organization released its recommendations for Good Agricultural Collection Practices (GACP) in April 2004. These should be implemented into law on a national level.
2. The WHO and TRAFFIC implemented the Convention on International Trade in Endangered Species of Wild Fauna and Flora in 1975.[6] This offers some protection to threatened species on an international level. Its findings also should be included on a national level.[7]
3. Governments could include sustainability clauses in legal documents to ensure that the supply of herbal medicines is sustainable.
4. Cultivation could be encouraged to ensure that extra burdens on the wild are reduced.
5. Sustainable wild harvesting projects could be established. This involves working with the plant collectors, liaisoning with government officials, and establishing a relationship with the forest department.
6. A crucial part of sustainable wild harvesting is the use of Wild Collection Plant Monographs. This idea has been drawn up by Klaus Duerbeck, a consultant of Swiss Import Promotion Programme (SIPPO) (a Swiss environmental consultancy), and implemented successfully in Europe. A resource study is carried out to determine which species thrive in a given area, what the population density is, what needs to be harvested, and when and how regularly crops can be harvested without damaging resources.

7. Practitioner organizations could implement regulatory codes requiring that practitioners do not use certain banned or endangered herbs. An authorized supplier scheme could be set up to audit suppliers of ayurvedic herbs to ensure that they are meeting the correct standards of good manufacturing practice, batch traceability, and correct species identification.[8]

8. I strongly believe that certification is needed to protect the future of herbal medicines. This certification would inform the consumer if these herbs have been sustainably grown and harvested. At present, organic certification offers one solution to the lack of an international kitemark, and this is the route I support by having products certified by the Soil Association (UK). If one buys uncertified products, then there is a high chance that they come from an unsustainably harvested source.

A wise path would be to follow the example of the *Vṛkṣāyurveda* (The Science of Plant Life), a sixteenth-century text by Surapāla: "Knowing this truth one should undertake planting of trees, since trees yield the means of attaining *dharma* (life duty), *artha* (wealth), *kama* (pleasure), and *mokṣa* (enlightenment)."

Trade: Poor Product Quality Threatening Integrity and Image

Many products entering the European Union market from Asia do not meet certain production standards or customer expectations. These products threaten the image and safety of Ayurveda if they are not presented professionally. The threat is that they do not meet EO good manufacturing practice requirements. There is also the issue of label claims that are currently illegal without a product license. The name of the product should just list the name of the main herbal ingredient without reference to treating any system or disease. Most products from Asia do not meet these requirements. This gives the industry a poor image in the eyes of the enforcement agencies.

The entire herbal industry is being shaken up by new legislation pertaining to manufacturing procedures ensuring that a more repeatable process is in place. This will inspire confidence in suppliers and government regulatory agencies alike that certain necessary safety procedures are in place for producing traditional herbal medicines effectively and safely. The new directive regulating herbal medicine in the European Union is known as the Traditional Herbal Medicines Products Directive, which is an attempt to control the safety of herbal products in an effort to protect consumers. It introduces Traditional Medicine Product Licenses allowing for the use of functional claims based on traditional use. These are potentially very expensive but will offer opportunities for the safe and reliable supply of ayurvedic products whose use is described accurately.

The United Kingdom has the Ayurvedic Trade Association (ATA), which is a pan industry organization set up by Pukka Herbs, Vedic Medical Hall (Himalaya), Maharishi Ayurveda Products, and Indigo Herbs to oversee the quality of ayurvedic products available in the United Kingdom. Acting as a pressure group to represent the needs of the ayurvedic community to the Medicinal and Herbal Products Regulatory Agency (MHRA), the government-appointed agency to oversee the legislation and enforcement of all medicines, the ATA has been a strong representative for the interests of the ayurvedic pharmacopoeia in a hostile environment. It has set standards for quality-control procedures based on the WHO's recommendations, European Pharmacopoeia, and British Herbal Pharmacopoeia pertaining to good manufacturing practice, microbiological testing, heavy metal testing, pesticide testing, species identification, batch traceability, and product recall. It continues to lobby the government on important issues such as the use of animal products such as ghee, milk, and honey to be acceptable as part of traditional herbal medicinal products.

A further challenge to the future of Ayurveda is the production of many of the traditionally prepared medicinals. Because of the new legislation in the European Union, all traditional herbal medicines prepared outside of it will have to meet certain quality and safety requirements that will require verification by the particular regulatory agency of each member state. This means that the manufacturing factory will have to be inspected for compliance with European Union's GMP. This is a serious threat to using traditional ayurvedic medicines outside of India:

- The cost of paying for an inspector to visit and carry out an official inspection in India will be prohibitive in relation to the demand for some of these highly specialized remedies.
- The lengthy procedure required for manufacturing many remedies, such as *guggulūs, ārishtas, āsavas*, and *chyawanprāsh*, will make their manufacture outside of India complicated and costly.

The ayurvedic community needs to adapt to these realities and possibly consider a return to using more simple *churṇas* and *kaṣāyas* and even new methods of prescription (at least to Ayurveda) to using tinctures.

Community Politics: Lack of Cohesiveness among Practitioners

At present (2003), in the United Kingdom, there is a lack of unity among ayurvedic practitioners to present Ayurveda in a cohesive manner to the regulatory authorities. This gives an image of a disorganized system of medicine and a profession in disarray. Thankfully there has been a move toward greater unity among ayurvedic practitioners and bodies, which started when the Ayurvedic Medical Association formed a General Council of Ayurveda with the Maharishi Ayurveda Practitioners Association. This positive development received further impetus with the founding of the Ayurvedic Practitioners Association in March 2005, uniting the aforementioned groups and adding more members to them. This has unified the ayurvedic community in the United Kingdom and has given rise to increased optimism that the ayurvedic community can be represented by a cohesive body.

While it is very important that an open debate takes place among medical practitioners to discuss standards of education, codes of conduct, ethics, standards of pharmacy, dispensing practice, reporting schemes, and so on, it is also important to communicate with other medical professions and government agencies with a cohesive voice reflecting a democratic consensus. As far as I understand it, this is not happening in India, the United States or the United Kingdom. This should change if Ayurveda is to earn a reputation of a respectable, professional body of medical practitioners.

In the United Kingdom, the European Herbal Practitioners Association has forged the way for all traditional medical systems practicing with natural plant, animal, and mineral medicinals to pursue a path of statutory self-regulation (SSR). This means that practitioners will be self-regulating, and that the title "herbalist" or "Ayurvedic practitioner" will be protected as legal terms only usable by qualified and registered practitioners.[9] Herbal practitioners will be self-regulating with regard to membership, educational standards, ethics, continuing professional development, finances, and disciplinary actions. This is a very positive step for all herbal practitioners and will give the community a voice that is respected by the government and yet autonomous to its own needs.

Educational: Lack of High-Quality Ayurvedic Education in the United Kingdom

In order to build a strong body of practicing ayurvedic professionals, the education needs to be of a university level, and it needs to be widely available. At present in the United Kingdom, there is one university offering a theoretical degree resulting in a BA (Thames Valley), and another offering a full BSc has just started (Middlesex University and the College of Ayurveda). Further integration is required, with training being based on the traditional medical model while also incorporating modern sciences, toxicology, research methodology, and clinical practice.

Further support for raising the standard of education will come from experienced practitioners and teachers from India, utilizing the skills of practitioners versed in the Western lifestyle in a clinical setting as well as greater communication with the academic community and its pioneering work in translating ayurvedic texts.[10] The United Kingdom and other countries teaching Ayurveda must create a professional environment in which high-quality clinical practice can take place so that students are familiar with the needs of their clients in the particular environment in which they will be practicing.

While the ayurvedic community in the United Kingdom is still immature, it is making positive progress.

Cultural: Lack of Public Awareness

Ayurveda is an Indian system of medicine with concepts that are alien to European culture. The practice of *panchakarma* itself is quite challenging for many Western temperaments, while the practice of *vamana* (therapeutic emesis) is culturally taboo in the United Kingdom. Promotion of its principles requires skilfull transmission that will engender confidence and trust in its profound and effective healing techniques. Ayurveda has a great opportunity here because it offers so much in the way of individual empowerment and life-skills coaching. Learning simple daily seasonal and lifestyle tips that can enhance health is at the root of ayurvedic wisdom. Its ability to help prevent disease as well as to alleviate the pain and discomfort of chronic diseases is at the forefront of its medical fame. These tools together offer a great deal to a Westernized culture that is craving self-awareness and personal responsibility.

Opportunities

The overall opportunity for Ayurveda is that in meeting the aforementioned challenges it will raise itself to a respected medical system that is recognized by all sectors of the global medical and patient community as a professional system of medicine that is based on traditional values while also meeting the needs of modern times. Its reputation as a system of medicine that is clinically effective, patient sensitive, and economically viable will spread. This increased popularity will fulfil its intention of enhancing life and alleviating illness.

NOTES

1. Trade in specimens of these species is permitted only in exceptional circumstances. Species not necessarily threatened with extinction but in which trade must be controlled in order to avoid utilization incompatible with their survival: *Papra* (*Podophyllum hexandrum*) and Red Sandalwood, or *Rakta candana* (*Peterocarpus santalinus*). These often are accepted if they come from verifiable cultivated sources. The following two species that are protected in at least one country, that have asked other Convention on International Trade in Endangered Species of Wild Fauna and Flora (CITES) parties for assistance in controlling the trade: *Jatāmānsi* (*Nardostachys jatamansi*) and *Kutki* (*Picrorrhiza kurroa*).

2. *Ayurvedic Formulary of India* (Indian Department of Health 1976).

3. This figure is based on comparative harvesting figures available from China and Europe, where greater levels of herbal medicinal production occur; see Schippmann et al. (2002).

4. See Schippman et al. (2002); Williams (1996: 12–14). Also see Hamilton (2004).

5. Plantlife International Report *Herbal Harvests with a Future* (January 2004).

6. For TRAFFIC, see http://www.traffic.org. This organization "works to ensure that trade in wild plants and animals is not a threat to the conservation of nature."

7. The Convention on International Trade in Endangered Species lists the flora and fauna that are regulated for trade. It divides the species into three categories. I only list the relevant ayurvedic species that I have found.

8. The Register of Chinese Herbal Medicine already does this in the United Kingdom.

9. The precise nomenclature of these titles was not finalized as of August 2004, as the Department of Health is still in consultation on the matter of SSR.

10. See Meulenbeld (1999–2002) and Wujastyk (1998) as examples of objective academia furthering the understanding of Ayurveda.

REFERENCES

Dutta, R., and P. Jain. 2000. CITES listed medicinal plants of India. An identification manual. TRAFFIC-India, WWF-India.

European Herbal Practitioners Association. 2004. Consultation document.

Hamilton, A. C. 2004. Medicinal plants, conservation, and livelihoods. International Plants Conservation Unit, WWF-UK, *New Scientist* (January 8).

Indian Department of Health. 1976. *Ayurvedic Formulary of India.*

Meulenbeld, G. J. 1999–2002. *A History of Indian Medical Literature*. Groningen: Egbert Forsten.

Murray, M. T. 1995. *The Healing Power of Herbs.* Rome: Prima Health.

Murthy, K. R. Srikantha, trans. 1998–2001. *Bhāvaprakāśa of Bhāvamiśra.* Krishnadas Ayurveda Series 45. Varanasi: Krishnadas Academy.

Schippmann, U., D. J. Leaman, and A. B. Cunningham. 2002. *Impact of Cultivation and Gathering of Medicinal Plants on Biodiversity: Global Trends and Issues. Inter-Department Working Group on Biology Diversity for Food and Agriculture.* Rome: FAO.

Traditional Herbal Medicines Products Directive. 2004.

Vines, G. 2004. *Herbal Harvests with a Future.* Towards sustainable sources for medicinal plants. Plantlife International. The Wild Plant Conservation Charity.

WHO. 1998. Quality control methods for medicinal plant materials.

Williams, V. L. 1996. The Witwaterrand muti trade. *Veld and Flora* 82: 12–14.

Wujastyk, Dominik. 1998. *The Roots of Ayurveda: Selections from Sanskrit Medical Writings.* New Delhi: Penguin Books.

CHAPTER 13

Cultural Loss and Remembrance in Contemporary Ayurvedic Medical Practice

MANASI TIRODKAR

This chapter explores the reasons—both direct and indirect—an increasing number of urban Indians utilize ayurvedic medicine in the contemporary globalizing landscape. By describing the effects of globalization on society, on health care, on health and, ultimately, on its treatment, I am suggesting that there is a systematic "cultural forgetting" in the name of globalization and modernization in urban India, and that contemporary ayurvedic treatment aims to aid people in "cultural remembering."

CONTEMPORARY AYURVEDIC PRACTICE

In this section I outline four categories of contemporary ayurvedic practice—traditional, modern, commercial, and self-help—as I had hypothesized them before I began my research. I have conceived of these categories based on popular writing on alternative medicines and conversations with consumers and practitioners. Here I envision the progression of ayurvedic practices as lying on a continuum that begins at the traditional category and reflects a progressive modernization of the system. In reality, these categories do not exist as neatly as I have conceived of them, either theoretically or practically. Rather, the ways in which these categories intersect and overlap appropriate a "web" more than a continuum or "map."

Traditional ayurvedic practices would entail the methods of diagnosis and treatment laid out in Sanskrit medical texts (the *Caraka-Saṃhitā* and *Suśruta-Saṃhitā* and others). Traditional practitioners would ideally be trained in *guru-śiṣya* style (i.e., pupilage), ashram-based settings, or in some sort of oral tradition. As a criterion, traditional practitioners would *not* be trained in formal (government or privately owned) institutional settings. Traditional practitioners would not employ the use of modern devices such as stethoscopes, lab tests or X-rays. They use the eightfold examination method, which involves examination of the pulse,[1] tongue, face, hair/nails, stool/urine, palpation, percussion, and inquiry. Traditionally they would mix herbs and other medicines for a patient personally, or they would pass on the job to a "compounder" to mix the prescribed amounts of medicines. Today, increasingly, such practitioners also might write a prescription for a compound that has been manufactured by a pharmaceutical company. These medicines might be either traditional compounds using recipes from the texts (*granthayokta*), or proprietary—one that has been concocted by the pharmaceutical company based on basic clinical trials and reports.

Modern practices involve methods of biomedical diagnosis as well as ayurvedic diagnosis. Modern practitioners have been trained in ayurvedic medical colleges that are currently the norm for ayurvedic training. They have earned a Bachelor of Ayurvedic Medicine and Surgery (BAMS) degree, which takes five and a half years to complete. A select few have done an additional three years of training to complete an M.D. in one of the eight branches of Ayurveda[2] or other specialties, such as panchakarma or pharmacology. In these colleges, ayurvedic doctors were taught to use not only pulse diagnosis, which is the primary diagnostic method in the classical tradition (according to *vaidya*s I met), but also a stethoscope to diagnose illnesses. Modern practitioners thus make regular use of modern technology such as X-rays, lab tests, blood pressure gauges, and stethoscopes in their practices. Several of them, especially in hospital settings, also wear a white coat, which is a symbol associated with Western medical knowledge (Kleinman 1988). They are taught not only to prescribe herbal and mineral powders but also injections and antibiotics. Modern practitioners rarely mix medicines for their patients—they generally only prescribe prepared medicines from pharmaceutical companies. These doctors tend to prescribe more proprietary medicines that medical representatives tell them about, along with free samples, glossy brochures, and attractive commissions on orders. The emphasis in the modern model is on the treatment of specific symptoms and illnesses as opposed to illness prevention.[3]

Commercial ayurvedic practices, also known as health spas and rejuvenation centers, offer primarily health-promoting services such as oil massages, nutritional counseling, and other relaxation therapies. Practitioners of these therapies generally have a certificate, diploma, or license in the services they offer. In the 1970s, as a reaction to the perceived harshness of biomedicine, the ayurvedic tradition began to take the form of an all-natural, "nonviolent" alternative. For example, bloodletting, emetics, and purgatives (methods of cleansing a patient's humoral system by causing vomiting and evacuative enemas) have been mostly eliminated from the array of ayurvedic treatments in many contemporary Indian and Western ayurvedic practices. The near elimination of these treatments has given way to an emphasis on massage "treatment." Gradually the emphasis on gentler treatments has led to the widespread perception of ayurvedic procedures as luxurious commodities rather than necessary, and sometimes unpleasant, treatments (Zimmerman 1992). There is hardly any diagnosis involved in the commercial model. Treatment is based on the current perceived state of the body (for example, "I feel stressed"), and there is generally no prescription (except perhaps to come back for another herbal oil massage!). The emphasis in the commercial model has shifted away from illness prevention and treatment and lies more on rejuvenation (Cohen 1998). Thus the sites of "commercial" ayurvedic practices are health spas and resorts that provide extensive massage, stress management, and rejuvenation packages. Many resorts have Web sites and quote their prices in rupees as well as U.S. dollars, indicating that their target clientele is largely foreign.

Ayurveda-based "self-help" practices include the voluntary use of books, Web sites, and bottled ayurvedic "medicines" available over the counter in pharmacies. Toward the self-help end of the spectrum, the practitioner practically disappears. A person diagnoses his or her own constitution, imbalances, and symptoms and treats them with herbs and natural supplements that are available without prescriptions over the counter or on the Internet. Prominent figures in the self-help "movement" include Deepak Chopra, who has popularized the concept of "perfect health," which is based on ayurvedic principles, and Maharishi Mahesh Yogi, the founder of Maharishi Ayur-Veda, who has popularized Transcendental Meditation, as well as an array of ayurvedic health-promoting herbal treatments (Sharma, Triguna, et al. 1991; Skolnick 1991). In the self-help and alternative health sections of mainstream bookstores, one can find books such as *Ayurveda: The Science of Self-Healing* (Lad 1984) and *Perfect Health* (Chopra 1991). These books contain chapters, such as "Determining the Individual Constitution," that allow consumers to diagnose their own constitution and imbalances.

Alternatively, consumers will go to a pharmacy and ask a sales representative or store owner what the best treatment would be for their symptom, illness or disease. Store staff will always oblige, despite the fact that most of them have no formal knowledge in pharmaceuticals, much less ayurvedic medicines. Most of the staff I met in ayurvedic pharmacies simply learned what was good for certain symptoms from the labels of medicine bottles and prescriptions for patients for whom they had already provided medicines.

WHO USES IT AND WHY?

Ayurveda is used by everyone from the lowest classes to the highest classes, including celebrities and politicians. Who uses which type of Ayurveda, though, is a different matter. It is in the sociology of the utilization that the story of Ayurveda's modernization and globalization gets complicated. It is in this aspect that the ultimate reality of ayurvedic practice resembles a complex web rather than a neat line or map.

From the aforementioned description of traditional Ayurveda, I have intended to portray the *common* perception of traditional ayurvedic practitioners. One can picture an old physician sitting cross-legged or on a low stool on the floor of a mud hut with a thatch roof. One can imagine the pungent smells of brewing decoctions and stewing oils. Several foreign students of Ayurveda go to India in search of "traditional" practitioners. What they are looking for is "authentic" practice—whatever that may be. Perhaps they are looking for a mystical character—the old physician sitting cross-legged on the floor, who can close his eyes and divine a diagnosis upon simply feeling the pulse of a patient. In the minds of these tradition seekers, the traditional practitioner exudes his knowledge—it travels around him like a halo or an aura. It is primarily the magical diagnostic capability of the *vaidya* that distinguishes the "authentic," therefore, "traditional," practitioner from the rest—the modern ones, the commercial ones, and any other existing imposters. The people who come to him for help would be, perhaps by default, lower-income, lesser-educated villagers because, again, the image of the traditional practitioner is of one who lives in a rural area, in the forest, on the edge of civilization.

There is some truth to this mental image I have constructed here of the traditional practitioner in the village hut brewing potions and powders to treat his patients. The truth lies partially in his diagnostic abilities and knowledge of pharmacopoeia and medicines. The practitioner does in fact have a deep and complex ability to diagnose, especially based on traditional methods such as pulse, observation, and palpation (of the body). However, he acquires this knowledge from years and years of experience, and not divine power, as some people with a more New Age interest in Ayurveda would have it (both urban Indians and Westerners). There are, however, two caveats to this general observation: (1) the divine association with abilities is attributed to the increased sensitivities of the practitioner's touch gained through extensive meditation, and (2) few practitioners claim to derive their diagnostic capabilities from divine sources besides only meditation, although they do not fit the rest of the traditional model.

Today's urban traditional practitioner is more sophisticated than the mud-hut-dwelling character I have just described. He practices in a proper concrete clinic in the city. Some practice in small rooms in the midst of inner-city concrete dwellings. I visited one such place, and although I did not meet the practitioner, despite visiting on many occasions, I saw many people camped out in the alley waiting for him. From what I heard, this practitioner, a bonesetter who used only two herbal plasters to heal all muscular and bone problems, made his own plasters from herbs he collected himself on the hillsides in the country. His clientele included some upper-class, educated people (such as those I talked to), as well as middle-class people and lower. He charged very little money for his consultations. One of the patients I talked to reported that he visited this practitioner because he had chronic back problems and was in a situation once that he could not move—his back was bent in a curved position. He could barely walk when he went to this clinic, and the practitioner, seeing him in pain, immediately applied his paste to his back and told him to keep it on for at least a day. The next day, the patient, a middle-age man, was pain free and could walk. He had been avoiding surgery, which is what the allopathic doctors had told him was the solution to his chronic back problems.

Another persistent stereotype of the traditional practitioner is that he is the successor to generations of ayurvedic knowledge. Thus he has acquired knowledge orally from his father and grandfather and follows in a *tradition* of Ayurveda. A few such third- and fourth-generation practitioners I met had acquired their knowledge from their forefathers, but they very much resented being called "traditional." As far as they were concerned, they had been formally educated in a college and were therefore "modern" practitioners. These same practitioners, however, insisted on making their own decoctions and oils and mixing powders or pastes for their patients. They rarely prescribed ready-made medicines from pharmaceutical companies, despite the insistence and repeated visits from medical representatives offering tempting incentives to prescribe their medicines. The type of clients that visit these practitioners falls into two categories: (1) patients of their fathers or grandfathers who continue in the lineage with the son because they have faith in the familial tradition, and (2) others who have heard of the practitioner from friends, relatives, or other public sources (such as newspaper or magazine articles). The clients draw from all socioeconomic classes. Those from lower and lower-middle classes tend to come either because they are clients of the family, or because they have run out of all other options for treatment (allopathic, surgical, and other ayurvedic). Others tend to come via a recommendation from friends or relatives, generally because they are fed up with allopathic medicine or have chronic illnesses for which they have exhausted other options. It must be said that the practitioners who come from a tradition of Ayurveda tend to be comparatively expensive for their consultations and treatments because they have not only a reputed household name but because they claim their medicines are made from the purest and highest-quality ingredients. In general, it is more expensive to prepare medicines on a small scale rather than in a large-scale manufacturing unit, because cutting, grinding, and stirring materials and preparations manually require much more time, effort, and energy expenditure of clinic employees. Pharmaceutical companies generally have large automated machines that cut down on labor charges for manufacturing.

This leads me to describe the modern practitioners. As I have previously described, modern practitioners make regular use of biomedical technology in their diagnosis and pharmaceutically manufactured medicines that they either dispense or prescribe. They are generally located in private urban clinics or hospitals. Most practitioners will work a combination of hospital or joint practice and private practice. Some who work in hospitals enjoy the benefits of institutional affiliation, such as teaching medical students, accessing resources such as libraries and computers that they may not otherwise have, and working on research projects. The clients who come to them in institutional settings are generally from the lower-middle or lower classes,[4] because medicines and treatments (such as massage and panchakarma) are heavily subsidized by the government or the foundation that owns the outpatient clinic. As a rule, government-funded hospitals tend to exhibit abysmal conditions in terms of cleanliness, resources, and space. Institutions run by private foundations are generally cleaner and better staffed.

Clients who come to the private clinics are mostly middle class or higher because they can afford consultation and treatment fees. They also can generally afford the pharmaceutically prepared medicines that tend to be several times the cost of powders mixed at home in raw form. Lower-middle and lower-class clients who come to these clinics usually come upon a recommendation from a relative or friend. I regularly saw doctors examining and treating these patients on a sliding scale because they could not afford the regular fees. I also observed such doctors accommodating clients' wallets by giving them cheaper medicines. For example, a bottle of pharmaceutically prepared decoction (tea) that lasted about a week would cost around Rs. 70. The amount of raw material required to make that much decoction would average one-tenth of the cost of the bottle. Several doctors I met increased their regular lower-middle and lower-class clientele by gaining reputations for making such accommodations.

Commercial centers—day spas and health resorts—are frequented by exclusively upper-middle class, upper class, and foreign clientele. These are well-educated people who are generally employed in well-paying professions such as business, fashion, acting, or art. They are likely to have seen one of the self-help books I described earlier, or at least an article on a self-help guru in a magazine or newspaper before coming for treatment. Many of them are from different cities, coming for a relaxation and rejuvenation vacation break. Many want help for chronic problems such as back pain, obesity, and constipation, as well as the break from the "fast life," hence the visit specifically to a "health" resort, and not just any vacation resort elsewhere.

Pharmacies are frequented mostly by middle, lower-middle, and lower-class clients who want to avoid consultation costs with doctors in clinics and hospitals. The rest of the clients, across all classes, come with prescriptions from doctors. Pharmacies are staffed by salespeople who may or may not have any formal pharmaceutical knowledge, as I described previously. Even if they do, their diploma or degree will more than likely be in "modern" (i.e., allopathic/biomedical) pharmacology, because there are no existing diploma or degree programs for ayurvedic pharmacology. Most people who work behind the counters in urban ayurvedic pharmacies are required to be literate in English and at least one Indian language, such as Hindi or Marathi, and efficient at handling cash transactions. At one particular pharmacy I observed, the only person who might contest a prescription was the owner. Contesting a prescription entails a process of knowing when a dose of a medication that is prescribed might be too much for a given person (based on age, gender, and condition of the patient). The owner of this pharmacy had a business background and could only identify a "funny" prescription because of his twelve years of experience in the business. It was especially important to identify such prescriptions for metal- and mineral-based preparations, which if taken in high or otherwise unregulated doses can lead to fatal side effects (Saper et al. 2004).

When asked why they use Ayurveda, several reasons are cited by patients in clinics and spas. In all types of clinics, the four main reasons people give for turning to Ayurveda are (1) allopathy has failed them, (2) it "cures from the root," (3) it is "all natural," and (4) there are no side effects. In the section that follows on modern health care, I elaborate on the issues surrounding the current state of allopathy. When people cite "cures from the root" as a reason, they are drawing on propaganda from doctors who tell them that allopathy provides only symptomatic treatment, and that illnesses will recur because of this. In contrast, patients are told that although Ayurveda takes longer to be effective, it cures the disease or illness from the root and thus reduces or eliminates the chances that it will recur. Ayurveda is said to cure illnesses from the root because it entails prescriptions for lifestyle and diet that might contribute to ill health. Ironically, the initial treatment for a patient's illness will be symptomatic, because in today's market, patients have become consumers, and they demand immediate relief for their problems. As a side note, I would estimate that less than 50 percent of patients who come for an initial consultation return after a couple of weeks. Many patients tend to be noncompliant with rigid medicinal and dietary regimens. Alternatively, they complain that it is not effective after a couple of weeks and will drop the treatment or look for another practitioner.

The reasons ayurvedic medicines are "all natural" and have "no side effects" go hand in hand. Many patients are willing to give ayurvedic medicine a try because they do not believe it will harm them. It can either work in a positive way or not have any side effects (adverse effects) at all. Many do not realize that the extensive instructions for time of day (before or after a meal) and accompaniments (milk, ghee, honey, water) are arranged so as not to cause side effects. When they are ignored or neglected, as they frequently are, side effects can occur, such as acidity or headaches, or an increase in symptoms. The other aspect of the "all-natural" claim is that with the increasing pharmaceuticalization of Ayurveda, it is not uncommon for synthetic content to be found in pharmaceutically produced medicines (Saper et al. 2004). In addition, medicines are increasingly sold in the form of coated tablets and capsules for easy palatability by the patient. These coatings and coverings also are often made of synthetic materials, including mixtures of sugar, gums, polyvinyl, and cellulose derivatives (see http://www.eurotherm.com). This demonstrates that both of these reasons for the use of Ayurveda are more beliefs than present realities.

Other reasons people cited for using Ayurveda were: (1) they thought that "diagnosis is more accurate," (2) it "works better for chronic ailments," (3) the "healing works more because of faith than physiology," and (4) "It is the oldest thing from our culture . . . the science is complete, there is no question." The perception that diagnosis is more accurate is based largely on a mysticism related to Ayurveda, that practitioners have a "sixth sense" or almost divine ability to perceive a diagnosis beyond what is obvious and observable in the Foucaultian sense. The aspect of ayurvedic practice that most lends itself to such perceptions is examination of the pulse. Especially in the now-popularized Westernized/global Ayurveda, a practitioner is often deemed to be inauthentic in some way if he or she does not perform an examination of the pulse. However, diagnosis based entirely on the pulse is a dying art and is rarely, if ever, taught in ayurvedic colleges (as told to me by current students and recent graduates of the BAMS degree). Most practitioners will examine the pulse to get an idea of imbalance in the *doṣas*, or humors, but not to actually diagnose a condition.

The reason that it "works better for chronic ailments" can be seen from the fact that most of the patients with chronic ailments have exhausted all other options for treatments. This line of thought is related to the previously elaborated belief that Ayurveda "cures from the root." A related point of interest is that practitioners frequently refuse to treat acute and infective illnesses because the illness has progressed too far for the medicine to be effective in curing it from the root.

In general, faith in the doctor and the system of medicine is considered the foundation of healing and good health. Skeptical patients are generally scorned by practitioners to a certain degree. After such patients have left the room after their consultation, I have frequently heard a doctor say, "That person will never get better."

The cultural history of colonization and current trends in globalization have lent themselves to an increase in the degree of scientific and rational thought, so much so that a few patients will come to a practitioner for medicines and proceed to ask about the exact mechanisms of the chemicals, and how long it will take to heal. Doctors will frequently respond with "have faith rather than asking such questions." Some patients see the lack of scientific evidence as the failure of indigenous and traditional medical systems. However, at the point in their illness at which such patients show up at the doorstep of an ayurvedic doctor, they usually are out of all other options and desperate to be healed. Their faith, if they had any, has already been shaken, because nothing else has worked, and they are frequently spent of monetary resources if they are middle class or lower.

The reference to culture as the context for the source of Ayurveda is most relevant to my position in this chapter. Several people draw on the fact that Ayurveda "is the oldest thing from our culture . . . the science is complete, there is no question." These are people who doubtless have "faith." These are people who remember, or who perhaps never forgot, their culture. It is difficult to say whether these patients have succumbed to the negative effects of globalization and are now experiencing recourse to their culture, or whether they were staunch believers and consumers of their cultural heritage from the beginning.

MODERN HEALTH CARE

In the health care arena, allopathy, or Western biomedicine, has been the norm for the past 100 years due to colonial influence. At least 80 percent of the people I interviewed turned first to allopathic medicine when they did not feel well. Allopathy is regarded as a modern treatment that acts fast and is convenient. Most medicines are available as pills or capsules, and they act immediately. By many, an injection is still regarded as a powerful and quick cure for pain or any other illness (Nichter 1996).

Most middle-age and younger people are of the pill-popping variety. They do not want to take the time to heal themselves. For example, they eat shellfish, even though they are allergic to it, by taking an antidote, and they eat spicy and oily foods, even though they have stomach problems afterwards. Instead of eating healthy foods that do not cause these stomach problems, they resort to the Western methods of treating the symptoms with a pill. One comment that a number of doctors made to their patients during the consultations was, "You eat for your tongue and not your body." What they mean is that people eat for pleasure more than for their health or to care for their stomachs and bodies, and that they do not listen to their bodies when they are suffering. I observed diabetics eating sweets because they believed that their pills would counteract the sugar. Others with high cholesterol also ignored dietary restrictions on fried foods; they believed that their pills would counteract the fat.

Aggressive options for treatment, such as surgery, also are quite commonplace. Having an "operation" for some dubious reason is not uncommon. A lot of lesser-educated and lower-income people often do not even know why they are having these operations. The doctor told them to do it, so they do. People from lower incomes and with less education tend to defer to doctors' authority. Many people go into great debt to have such surgeries. Often the surgeries are not necessary, do nothing to alleviate the problem, or make the problem worse. The most common cases were patients who had surgery in their lower back/spine and for whom the surgery had either done nothing to alleviate the pain or had aggravated the nerve compression and numbness in their legs. Other common operations deemed unnecessary by ayurvedic doctors were heart bypass surgeries and hysterectomies. One unique case that sticks in my mind was that of an eighteen-year old young man who came to the clinic on crutches—he had only one leg. He had been diagnosed with bone cancer a few months earlier and a general practitioner, having detected a malignant growth on the thighbone, had mandated an amputation of the leg. The patient and his family, not knowing any better, had the leg amputated. The patient had come to the ayurvedic clinic for weight loss and general weakness. During the first consultation and examination, the ayurvedic doctor discovered the beginning of another malignant growth on the pelvic bone. The doctor commented to me later that the man did not need to have his leg amputated, and that the general practitioner he had originally seen was incompetent at best. The patient started radiation for the tumor as well as ayurvedic medicines for general health shortly thereafter. This was one of many cases I observed in ayurvedic clinics where allopathy had allegedly failed these patients. Ultimately they returned to what they knew has existed for several centuries but had not utilized: Ayurveda.

About 90 percent of patients I interviewed admitted that they turned to Ayurveda after they had exhausted all allopathic options. Some had even tried other nonallopathic options, such as homeopathy and naturopathy, before trying Ayurveda. People's anxiety about Ayurveda stemmed from their fear of being restricted from their pleasures such as meat,[5] alcohol, cigarettes, and sweet, fatty, or spicy foods, all of which are considered detrimental indulgences. One comment made by a patient I interviewed (thirty-two year old, male, software engineer) sums up this sentiment when I asked him if he followed the prescribed diet: "I don't follow the diet. . . . If you follow that you end up starving!"

MODERN DISEASE ETIOLOGY

A number of doctors pointed out to me that among the recent culprits in today's digestive problems are pizzas and burgers (i.e., the consumption of a new style of fast foods). The main components of these foods are bread, cheese, and tomato sauce, and meat in some cases. The first three foods are all fermented and classified by Ayurveda as sour, and they are said to inherently foster acid production in the body. Incidentally, none of these foods is native to the subcontinent. In particular, food coming from the central-western region of India (Maharashtra, where I conducted my research) does not contain many fermented foods because of the climatic conditions (humid on the coast, arid inland, hot all around). In India, there is a strong emphasis on eating foods that are native to the region, and regional cuisines are distinctly different depending on the availability of local produce and grain. Patients who do not adhere to local diets are often told that they should. For example, patients who come from South India (Kerala and Tamilnadu) tend to eat a diet heavy in fermented and sour foods, such as tomato-based soups (*rasam*) and *idli/dosa* (which is made from dough made of fermented ground rice and lentils). These patients are told to eat less fermented and sour foods because the climate in Maharashtra is not conducive to consuming these foods. As a side note, this scenario reflects a trend not only on an *inter*-continental global exchange but also in an *intra*-continental domestic exchange. The current boom in industries such as computer software programming and biotechnology has necessitated an increase in domestic mobility. One consequence is the transporting of food between regions, and the resulting incompatibility of foods from a particular regional culture and in a different climate.

Another cause for many current ailments cited by doctors was the "fast life" caused by advances in technology and modern conveniences. The irony of the "fast life" is that there are people who are immobile or sedentary because they use modern conveniences and amenities, as well as those who move around too much because of them (although these two types of people are not necessarily in exclusive categories). The first type of person tends to eat convenient and prepackaged foods, does not exercise or walk regularly, and watches a lot of TV. The second type of person commutes great distances to work, travels on scooters or motorbikes, and thereby stresses his or her body. Thus due to modern conveniences and modes of transportation, people do not get enough exercise, in addition to eating less healthy food. Many women are of the first type in that they tend to stay at home and lead relatively sedentary lives. Predictably, many men fall into the second type. However, an increasing number of women are coming into the second category, as more of them have high-tech jobs and juggle work, family, and household responsibilities.

STRATEGIES FOR CULTURAL REMEMBRANCE

Restoring Faith

Many of the patients I interviewed reported that they had used allopathy and it had not worked. As a last resort, they turn to Ayurveda. Ayurveda brings them *back* to their culture. Doctors often remind them to have faith in them, in the system, and in the universe, and that they will get better. This was especially true for patients who had chronic ailments or terminal illnesses (yes, they too were convinced they would "get better"). The doctors draw on patients' spiritual beliefs—even the patients who are not practicing Hindus will listen and accept this advice, because they are raised in a Hindu cultural framework. I am reminded of my interview with the skeptical computer techie who started to meditate because he had no choice but to believe—not believing was not getting him anywhere, and after years of using allopathic medicine, he had to try this.

One doctor whose entire practice is based on astrological and spiritual advice prescribes mantras, prayers, regular fasting, and temple visits. I asked him once what these spiritual prescriptions did to actually alleviate the patients' condition. He told me, "People have lost faith. And by making someone go to the temple every Monday for three months or saying a prayer every morning, they stop thinking about their lives and problems for just a few minutes. It makes them reflect on why they are doing what they are doing, and thereby restores their faith." Once they stop thinking about the problems they will open themselves up to being healed. This doctor's practice was more "traditional" (as opposed to "modern"), yet his treatments were geared to the people of today (i.e., common people in the modern world whose lives had been shattered or wounded because of the disintegration of their culture and loss of faith). Although most of the patients in this clinic were from the lower and lower middle classes, whose problems are generally different than those of the middle and upper classes, it seemed to me that the sources of the problems were largely social stresses related to their engagement with the rapidly changing modern world.

Home Cooking

Another approach to reminding patients of their culture was the prescription of a diet that drew on the strategic use of various spices, vegetables, grains, and lentils to aid in the treatment of an ailment. What I saw repeatedly during consultation and interviews is that many of the prescribed remedies, especially dietary suggestions, were a part of the patients' cultural framework already. Suggestions such as "Don't eat tomatoes or ginger because they are 'hot' foods and will increase the heat in your body and will therefore aggravate your acidity," and "Don't consume too much milk or yogurt because they are 'cooling' " and will increase the phlegm (*kapha*) in your body" were understood easily by patients. Patients did not have to learn what "heating" and "cooling" meant, or even which foods had these properties, because this is local cultural information.

Many people know a few basic home remedies but do not necessarily link them to Ayurveda or any organized medical system. For the most part, they do not use these remedies with any regularity or for prevention of illness. Many of the patients I interviewed saw "home remedies" as something quite different from and unrelated to Ayurveda, which is what they knew I was asking them about. Yet they acknowledge that these home remedies came from their mothers or grandmothers. One phrase commonly used to refer to home remedies was that they came from the "grandmother's little [herb] bag" (*ājībāī-chā batwā*). Conversations with doctors showed that many home remedies have originated from ayurvedic principles. For example, a pinch of turmeric in milk is drunk to fend off a cold. Turmeric has antiseptic properties, and because turmeric by itself is extremely potent and acidic, it is consumed in milk, which is an alkali medium. Another example is coriander—it releases gas and has cooling properties, so whole coriander seeds are soaked in water, and the decoction is drunk to alleviate gas.

I would suggest that home remedies are not regarded as something distinctly medical because they are so embedded in the cultural framework of these patients. The difference between "medical" and "nonmedical" lies in the systematic nature of the former and the lack thereof in the latter. Despite the fact that most of the home remedies are based in principle on Ayurveda, Ayurveda itself is considered a medical system, albeit an alternative one. "Medicine" in this sense may then be paradigmatic of foreignness. As I mentioned earlier, what is going on is that patients are being reminded of the preexisting contents and processes of a cultural framework that might have been lost or forgotten in the process of colonization, decolonization, and recolonization, or globalization.

CONCLUSION

In this chapter I have discussed current trends in contemporary ayurvedic practice with the intention of arguing that the use of Ayurveda by Indian consumers, patients, and clients entails a process of remembering cultural information. In some ways this is a process of reestablishing oneself in the local cultural paradigm, and in some cases extracting oneself from the global paradigm. For example, someone who is told to eat less fast food, commute less, if possible, and cook more hearty *khichaḍi* (rice and yellow split mung beans) and drink a decoction day and night to aid in digestive problems is forced to engage in more local cultural processes and less in the fast-paced global processes.

One of the drawbacks of the revitalization of indigenous cultural practices such as the use of ayurvedic remedies, practices that also include ethnic food, clothes, music, and media, is that they become aggressively commodified. The reintegration of contemporary cultural paradigms into daily living is far from smooth or tension free. On the contrary, these reestablished paradigms often remain superficial and exist as superimposed structures. However, it is only because they remain isolated and superficial that institutions such as health resorts and many contemporary meditation movements "work." The idea of a fast track to health (or nirvana, as the case may be) is incongruous with the original framework, which holds that it takes time to heal (or to achieve spiritual peace). The rapidity of change in every domain of society and culture is too great to facilitate the reintegration of classical traditions, either in theory or practice. Thus health care utilization in India will continue to be fractioned and pluralistic.

NOTES

1. I realize that pulse diagnosis is not included in the eightfold examination in the classical textual tradition, therefore, I assume that this might be specific to the region in which I did my fieldwork (Maharashtra), where ayurvedic practice is known to be a syncretism of northern and southern Indian traditions.

2. The eight branches are internal medicine, pediatrics (includes ob/gyn), exorcism, ENT/ophthalmology, surgery, toxicology/preventive medicine, geriatrics/rejuvenative therapy, and aphrodisiac/sexual therapy.

3. I am not suggesting here that "traditional" practice is completely focused on illness prevention. My point here is that there is a *distinct* lack of attention to prevention in the modern model of ayurvedic practice.

4. I am basing assessment of class on area of residence and socioeconomic status. These were determined by self-reported occupation and residence of the client/patient.

5. Ayurveda does not advocate complete vegetarianism, however more often than not meat is restricted because it is considered "heavy" and "hot" and therefore difficult to digest. These properties can lead to internal imbalance.

REFERENCES

Chopra, D. 1991. *Perfect Health: The Complete Mind/Body Guide.* New York: Harmony Books.

Cohen, L. 1998. *No Aging in India: Alzheimer's, the Bad Family, and Other Modern Things.* Berkeley: University of California Press.

Kleinman, A. 1988. *The Illness Narratives: Suffering, Healing, and the Human Condition.* New York: Basic Books.

Lad, V. 1984. *Ayurveda: The Science of Self-Healing.* Wilmot, WI: Lotus Press.

Nichter, M. 1996. *Anthropology and International Health: Asian Case Studies.* Amsterdam: Gordon and Breach Publishers.

Saper, R. B., et al. 2004. Heavy metal content of Ayurvedic herbal medicine products. *JAMA* 292:23: 2868–73.

Sharma, H., D. Triguna, et al. 1991. Maharishi Ayur-Veda: Modern insights into ancient medicine. *JAMA* 265:20: 2633–37.

Skolnick, A. 1991. Maharishi Ayur-Veda: Guru's marketing scheme promises the world eternal "perfect health." *JAMA* 266:13: 1741–50.

Zimmermann, F. 1992. Gentle purge: The flower power of Ayurveda. In *Paths to Asian Medical Knowledge*, ed. C. Leslie and A. Young, 209–23. Berkeley: University of California Press.

CHAPTER 14

Practicing Ayurveda in the Western World

A Case Study from Germany

ANANDA SAMIR CHOPRA

Ayurveda, which has long been an object of study for philologists and historians of medicine, has in the last two decades been perceived outside of India as a promising approach for the restoration and preservation of health. Indeed, a number of qualified people have begun to practice it in Europe and America. By describing a medical Ayurveda department in a German hospital, I will try to show how Ayurveda can be practiced as a medical discipline in a Western country. I will discuss not only the dynamics of practice but also the problems and perspectives related to such a practice. The discussion is based on my experience as medical director of the Ayurveda-Klinik,[1] an independent department in a German rehabilitation hospital, the Habichtswaldklinik, located in Kassel in central Germany. Many of the issues presented reflect not just my experience, however, but exist mutatis mutandis elsewhere in Europe and North America.

The Habichtswaldklinik is a hospital with about 350 beds. Apart from the Ayurveda-Klinik there are three departments in this hospital: the Department of Internal Medicine/Naturopathy, where patients are usually admitted for rehabilitation, the Department of Oncology, and the Department of Psychosomatic Medicine. The latter is at present the largest department in the Habichtswaldklinik. In the Department of Oncology, in addition to the usual allopathic therapies such as chemotherapy, a special emphasis is placed on alternative and complementary approaches, including mistletoe therapy and orthomolecular medicine. In the Department of Psychosomatic Medicine, too, conventional psychotherapy is combined with complementary and alternative approaches.

The Ayurveda-Klinik opened in April 1995 as an independent section in the Department of Internal Medicine, with the aim of offering authentic ayurvedic treatment as an alternative or a complementary mode of therapy. The facilities within the hospital, including the pathology laboratory and encephalograph (ECG), enable the physician to offer the best possible care for the patient while simultaneously providing the opportunity to assess the effects of ayurvedic therapy. This ayurvedic department is not a "wellness center"; patients usually come here to treat or prevent diseases. It also must be stressed that Ayurveda, as it is understood here, is not a spiritual discipline, nor is it "New Age Ayurveda."[2] Rather, it is a medical discipline in continuation of a centuries old tradition.

The Ayurveda-Klinik comprises a ward of approximately thirty beds, a "therapy floor," where the oil and sudation therapies are given separately to women and men (women are treated by women, men by men), and a special kitchen and dining hall, where lactovegetarian food is offered. In the last few years we have admitted between 500 and 700 inpatients per year and treated about 300 outpatients per year. This number, however, is steadily growing.

ON WHAT BASIS DO WE PRACTICE AYURVEDA IN A WESTERN ENVIRONMENT?

In my view, four factors must serve as a basis and an orientation for practicing Ayurveda in a Western environment.

1. *The ancient tradition as preserved in the four works ascribed to the so-called bṛhat-trayī (i.e., "the great triad" of Caraka, Suśruta, and Vāgbhaṭa).*[3] The practice of Ayurveda must adapt to this new environment. This is consistent with Jan Meulenbeld's observation that ayurvedic medicine in India is characterized by "a remarkable continuity of thought and practice"[4] in spite of constant culture change, at least in regard to fundamental concepts. In the Ayurveda-Klinik we view the ancient tradition as the central point of orientation for our necessary adaptation of ayurvedic concepts to new circumstances. Such processes of adaptation have precedents in, for example, Tibet or the southwestern part of India. The exact relationship between the classical texts and clinical practice may be a matter of controversy,[5] but it must be noted that ayurvedic medicine evolved from the basis of these texts. Commentators of past centuries and ayurvedic doctors of present times show us how the concepts of the texts can be related to actual practice.

For example, Dṛḍhabala, in his commentary on Suśruta, gives vernacular terms for plants or even anatomic structures (marking them with the expression *iti loke*).

2. *The great number of lesser-known ayurvedic treatises that followed the early classical texts.* As Ayurveda has always been a living science that has continually developed and changed over the centuries, we can and should make use of the vast body of ayurvedic literature produced after the texts of the *bṛhat-trayī*. The later ayurvedic works introduce new diagnostic procedures, as well as new diseases and therapies. Pulse diagnosis and tongue diagnosis, as described in the *Yogaratnākara*, are examples of new procedures that have become highly relevant for ayurvedic practice. For the past two centuries Ayurveda has been engaged in an encounter with Western biomedicine, and this has initiated further development in the ayurvedic tradition.[6] Such developments are reflected in ayurvedic medical literature.
3. *The current practice of Ayurveda in India.* This is especially important because most of us have learned ayurvedic medicine from members of the vast community of ayurvedic physicians in India. In the case of the Ayurveda-Klinik, ayurvedic medical concepts and the understanding of Ayurveda were shaped by three ayurvedic physicians from India: Dr. Jayaprakash Narayan and Prof. Paramesh Rangesh (Bangalore), who have often served as consultants in Kassel, and the respected Dr. Paresh Chandra Tripathi (Kolkata), who was the chief guide of the medical director of the Ayurveda-Klinik when he studied Ayurveda during a one-year-stay in Kolkata. All three advisors are ayurvedic doctors (BAMS.—Bachelor of Ayurvedic Medical Science), with a strong traditional background.
4. *The medical and social environment in which we live.* Western societies have their own sophisticated medical system that dispenses health care of the highest standard to everyone. It is in the interest of neither the patient nor the physician to ignore this. I firmly believe that we achieve the best results only if we stay in constant dialogue with modern medicine. This requires that the physician be adequately qualified. In Germany, at least, I am of the opinion that anyone practicing Ayurveda should be a physician with a qualification in modern medicine.

The ancient authors admonish us time and again to practice only after considering place, time, and the individual patient.[7]

Therefore, the practice of Ayurveda in Germany cannot be just a matter of copying ayurvedic therapy from India but rather a matter of intelligent "translation."

THE PRACTICE OF AYURVEDA AT THE AYURVEDA-KLINIK, KASSEL

Upon admission the patient's history is taken and a physical examination performed. Here, both the ayurvedic perspective and the perspective of modern medicine are taken into account as part of the diagnostic procedure.[8] In addition, laboratory tests may be performed, either in the interest of the patient or for research. On the following morning a pulse and tongue diagnosis is carried out at the patient's bedside. In performing all of these diagnostic procedures, we follow the standard ayurvedic system as it was taught to me by the three ayurvedic doctors mentioned earlier and as found in contemporary ayurvedic literature.[9]

Because we are housed in a modern German hospital, we must document both ayurvedic diagnoses and modern medical diagnoses. The first page of our six-page admission form will convey a graphic idea of our perspective (see Table 14.1).

Ayurvedic therapy usually includes detailed considerations and recommendations regarding dietetics (*āhāra-vihāra*), based on the results of the diagnosis. This refers to food habits as well as general dietetic recommendations as part of a treatment plan that might include exercise and oil massage. We counsel patients on all of these aspects of treatment when they conclude their course of in-house therapy. For outpatients who come to us for consultation, these recommendations are given at the end of the consultation. We are often surprised at the profound effects such supposedly simple recommendations can have on patients and their disease. For various reasons that I cannot discuss here, ayurvedic drugs play only a minor role in our daily practice.

PATIENT PROFILES

A study performed in 2002[10] shows that more than two-thirds of our patients are female, two-thirds are between forty-one and sixty-five years old, and almost two-thirds have completed higher education. This comparatively high level of education among our patients may be one reason they are usually intensely interested in Ayurveda and show a high grade of compliance with our therapy and recommendations. In this respect our clientele differs from the consumers of

Table 14.1. Admission Form

Habichtswaldklinik AYURVEDA

AYURVEDA SEKTION

AUFNAHMEBOGEN [Admission form]
(Ātura--parīkṣaṇa--patra)

Datum [date]:
Arzt [physician]:
Station [department]:

Name: ....

geb. [D.o.b.]: ....

Konstitution [constitution](*Prakṛti*):
Ungleichgewicht [disbalance](*Vikṛti*):
Puls [pulse](*Nāḍī—Parīkṣā*) am .... :
Zunge [tongue](*Jihvā*):
Allergien [allergies]:

Medikamente [medication]:

Diagnosen (*Roga*):

ayurvedic medicine in Germany, as characterized by Frank and Stollberg in their pioneering study, according to which patients did not show much interest in ayurvedic concepts.[11] Regarding socioeconomic characteristics, our patients are almost equally distributed into three main income groups (high, medium, and low). Stollberg has drawn attention to the fact that Ayurveda in Germany is founded on a migration of knowledge and not of persons, as in the United Kingdom.[12] This is confirmed by the fact that almost all of our patients are Caucasian, coming mainly from Germany or, to a much lesser extent, from the rest of Europe (Switzerland, Luxemburg, and other nearby countries). This situation applies to practitioners of Ayurveda as well. In Germany very few ayurvedic practitioners of Indian origin are found.

A statistical summary (see Table 14.2) of 417 patients (based on discharge reports) admitted in 2003 reveals the following ten disease patterns to be the most common (the second column gives numerical codes according to the International Classification of Diseases (ICD) [10th revision] as developed by the WHO).[13]

This enumeration does not imply that we can treat all of these conditions effectively. In the case of breast cancer, for example, patients usually come to us after having undergone allopathic therapies, including surgery, chemotherapy, and radiation. Their intention in coming to our clinic is to recover from the physical and psychological stress of both the disease and the therapy, and to improve their quality of life. Clinical medicine in general should include not only the healing of the disease but the healing of the whole person, which implies an attempt to improve the person's quality of life as much as possible.[14] More and more patients contact us before coming to the Ayurveda-Klinik to inquire whether we are able to treat their particular problem.

In the Ayurveda-Klinik, we mainly practice the so-called panchakarma therapy, following to a certain extent current clinical practice in India.[15] Two case studies follow. These are primarily meant to demonstrate that within panchakarma different individuals require different therapeutic combinations. The first one also shows that ayurvedic therapy is effective even when assessed by methods of modern medicine. This kind of evaluation serves as a tool for intercultural communication with physicians of cosmopolitan biomedicine, and may help gain general acceptance for Ayurveda in Germany. However, I must emphasize that in my view this is not a means to prove the validity of Ayurveda in general. This can only be achieved from within the system itself. In the present era of evidence-based

Table 14.2. 2003 Statistical Summary of Disease Patterns

Disease Entity	*ICD 10 Code*
Fatigue disorders,"burnout"-syndrome, stress-related fatigue	F 48/R 53
"Back pain," spondylosis	M 47/M 54
Essential (primary) hypertension	I 10
Insomnia (disorders of sleep)	G 47
Depressive disorders	F 32
Lipidaemias (elevated blood fats)	E 78
Congestive heart failure	I 50
Obesity	E 66
Arthrosis/Osteoarthritis	M 19
Breast cancer	C 50

medicine, the presentation of single cases such as this may seem preposterous. But let us not forget that our everyday clinical practice consists of single cases such as this, and evidence gained on large groups of selected patients is sometimes not very helpful in the treatment of the single individual.[16]

CASE STUDY 1: METABOLIC SYNDROME AND HYPERTENSION

The first case study involves a forty-seven-year-old male with a metabolic syndrome, a combination of obesity,[17] diabetes mellitus (type 2), and elevated blood lipids. In addition, he suffers from hypertension and is being treated for that with a conventional drug (75 mg. Irbesartan twice daily). From the ayurvedic point of view, this patient has a mixed constitution, a *pitta-kapha prakṛti* and is at present suffering from a *vāta* aggravation, as confirmed by pulse diagnosis. The disease entity presented here corresponds to *medoroga,* as described in the *Mādhavanidāna.*[18] The patient underwent a course of therapy for sixteen days based on the system of panchakarma. This included:

1. Preparatory procedures (*pūrvakarma*):
   Snehana ("therapy with oils and fats") with external oil massages and internal application of a specially prepared butter fat or ghee (*snehapāna*).

   Svedana ("sudation therapy"), in which the patient is made to sweat in a special steam bath.

2. Main procedures (*pradhānakarma*):
   Virecana, purgation with the help of laxative drug preparations.
   Bastikarma, application of specially compounded enemas.
   Nasya, nasal instillation of specially prepared herbal oils.

The exact course of therapy is shown in the Table 14.3.

Over the whole period of time, the diet was adjusted to the therapy.

On the second day the patient stopped taking his antihypertensive medication against the recommendations of the physician. At the end of this course of therapy the patient had lost about 9 kg of weight (about 20 lbs.) and had normal blood pressure without any medication. The effect of the therapy was assessed by laboratory investigations. Some of the more significant results can be seen in Table 14.4.

The patient's fasting blood sugar level had come down significantly, as had his serum cholesterol level and the level of serum triglycerides. In such a patient we may suspect some degree of fatty liver,

Table 14.3. Course of Therapy

Day:	1	2	3	4	5	6	7	8	9	10	11	12	13	14	15	16
Snehana: A. *Snehapāna* (internal application of ghee)		*	*	*												
B. *Bāhya Snehana* (external oil application)	*	*	*	*		*	*	*	*	*	*				*	
Svedana (sudation)				*			*									*
Virecana (purgation)					*											
Basti (enema)							*	*	*	*	*					
Nasya (nasal instillation)												*	*	*		

Table 14.4. Laboratory Results on Effects of Therapy

Parameter	*Before*	*After the Therapy*	*Norm*
Fasting blood sugar	170 mg/dl	93 mg/dl	< 100 mg/dl
Serum cholesterol	243 mg/dl	140 mg/dl	< 220 mg/dl
Serum triglycerides	253 mg/dl	68 mg/dl	< 100 mg/dl
Gamma-GT	36 U/l	23 U/l	< 28 U/l

and the development of the GGT, a liver parameter, shows that even in this respect there is marked improvement in a rather short period of time.

CASE STUDY 2: INSOMNIA

The second case study presents us with a completely different problem. This fifty-eight-year-old lady had been suffering from insomnia for two years. The problem started when her ailing mother, whom she had been taking care of, died. The woman had constantly refused any conventional medication for her insomnia, as she was an ardent follower of homoeopathy, but even the homoeopathic treatment could not help her. Apart from this she had some leucorrhoea (vaginal discharge), which had begun a few months before and did not respond to conventional therapy. She had had a history of chronic pyelonephritis about thirty years earlier, which had been treated successfully with homoeopathic therapy.

This patient stayed at the Ayurveda-Klinik for fourteen days, and in this case too we planned a course of therapy based on the panchakarma concept. This included an internal ghee application and a day of purgation. From day nine onward we did a series of *śirodhārā* (pouring a thin stream of warm oil on the forehead). In Table 14.5, the exact course of therapy is shown.

Until day thirteen nothing changed—the patient was still unable to sleep. But on her last day she greeted us in the morning with the news that she had slept from 11 p.m. at night till six o'clock a.m. for the first time in more than two years. This effect has been stable now for more than five years. From time to time I have had contact with this patient, and it was about six weeks after her therapy that she told me for the first time about her leucorrhoea. She had suffered from this for some months, but two days after she returned home from Ayurveda therapy the leucorrhoea stopped.

PROBLEMS AND PERSPECTIVES

Finally, I turn to some problems we encounter in the practice of Ayurveda in a Western environment. As mentioned earlier, I believe that these fundamental problems may be rather similar in other Western societies, although my experience is limited to Germany. The first problem is that Ayurveda is at present not covered by health insurance. Germany has a very comprehensive system of social security, of

Table 14.5. Course of Therapy

Day:	*1*	2	3	4	5	6	7	*8*	9	*10*	11	12	13	14
Snehana: A. *Snehapāna*		*	*	*										
B. *Bāhya Snehana*	*		*	*		*		*						
Especially: *Śirodhārā*		*							*	*	*	*	*	
Svedana				*										
Virecana					*									

which health insurance is a part. In practice this means, to put it very simply, that an average German goes to his or her doctor and may undergo sophisticated medical procedures without knowing what this service costs. Medical services are paid for by health insurance, and almost everyone is a compulsory member of a health insurance program, the fees being taken directly from one's income. As Ayurveda is normally not covered by health insurance in Germany, and is not part of the public health care system in other Western societies, treatment appears to be rather expensive for many people.

The second problem is that almost anything can be called "Ayurveda," a problem that to a certain extent also exists in India. Barbershops, beauty farms, meditation centers, and many others use the term *Ayurveda* rather indiscriminately. This makes it difficult to establish Ayurveda as a serious science in Germany. The third problem is that there is, until now, too little data acceptable to the modern physician on the clinical efficacy of ayurvedic therapy and too little information on what Ayurveda actually is. While I see a need for more clinical research on Ayurveda in Europe and North America, I am convinced that this research will only be meaningful if the ayurvedic perspective is included as well.

In sum, I believe there is a perspective for Ayurveda in the Western world. I have tried to show through the two case studies that Ayurveda can offer an alternative mode of therapy or complement conventional therapy in a sensible manner. Apart from this it can be observed that globalization, with all of its questionable developments, also broadens the horizon of patients and doctors. At present we have the opportunity to acquire knowledge about other cultures and their medical arts. Patients can quite readily learn about other forms of therapy that may suit them better than biomedicine. Indeed, these may sometimes offer help where current therapies fail, thus representing a broadened global vision that may turn into a boon for suffering humanity.

NOTES

This chapter developed from earlier papers that were presented and discussed in December 2003 at the Indic Health Workshop and in July 2004 at the Conference on Modern and Global Ayurveda in Cambridge, Great Britain. I would like to thank all participants for their comments and discussion, especially Prof. R. P. Das, who served as respondent to my paper in December 2003, and Prof. Charles Leslie, for his critical comments put forward to me in writing. All members of the Dharam Hinduja Institute for Indic Research, Cambridge, deserve credit for initiating and accomplishing such an important innovative project.

1. The German term *Klinik* denotes a hospital or a hospital department where patients are admitted and undergo treatment. This is different from the English usage of the term *clinic*, which usually applies to a medical institution where outpatients are treated.

2. Comp. Zysk (2001: especially 24): "Classical Ayurveda in India has consciously separated the medical training of Ayurveda from the spiritual and religious discipline of Yogic asceticism."

3. In the ayurvedic tradition, Agniveśa is said to be the redactor of the *Caraka-Saṃhitā* (Collection of Caraka), Suśruta is named as the author of the *Suśruta-Saṃhitā* (Collection of Suśruta), and Vāgbhaṭa is credited with the authorship of two important compendia, the *Aṣṭāṅgasaṃgraha* (Compendium of the Octopartite Science) and the *Aṣṭāṅgahṛdaya-Saṃhitā* (Collection of the Essence of the Octopartite Science). For more information on authors and works, see the indispensable work by Meulenbeld (1999–2002).

4. Meulenbeld (1995: 1). He continues: "When one reads Sanskrit medical texts from various periods, one cannot but be struck by a remarkable continuity of thought and practice, on the one hand, and equally remarkable changes on the other."

5. See Das (1993: especially 69ff).

6. For a concise account of this development see, for example, Sharma (1981: 567–83); for a critical assessment, see Leslie (1992).

7. See, for example, Caraka (Sū. 1.123): "He is to be known as the best among physicians who knows the application of combinations of these (herbal preparations) considering place and time after having looked at each person (individually): *yogam āsām tu yo vidād deśakālopapāditam/ puruṣaḥ puruṣaḥ vīkṣya sa jñeyo bhiṣag uttamaḥ//*.

8. This way to proceed, then, which is standard in modern medicine, also follows ayurvedic diagnostic procedure as outlined in the classical texts.

9. For diagnostic procedures in general, see Rāy and Tripāthī (1993), and for pulse diagnosis in particular, see Vaidya Tārāśaṃkara Miśra (1995 [1993]). However, both works rely heavily on traditional literature.

10. See Wiese (2002), who did an analysis of thirty patients of the Ayurveda Klinik, Kassel, with a semi-structured questionnaire. Her results correspond well to our subjective impression.

11. Frank and Stollberg (2002): "Most patients appeared highly indifferent to Ayurvedic knowledge, and this did not change during the course of treatment" (236ff.).

12. See Stollberg (2001).

13. An online version of the ICD code may be found on the WHO Web site http://www3.who.int/icd/vol1htm2003/fr-icd.htm.

14. Compare the well-known Sanskrit verse (*Bhāvaprakāśa* 6 [Miśra-prakaraṇam] 53, p. 168): *vyādhes tattvaparijñānaḥ vedanīyāś ca nigrahaḥ/ etad vaidyasya vaidyatvaḥ na vaidyaḥ prabhur āyuṣaḥ//* ("True and complete knowledge of the disease as well as alleviation of pain, this is the medical art of the physician; the physician is not the lord of life").

15. The most important work for reference, even for us, is H. S. Kasture's *Āyurvedīya Pañcakarma-Vijñāna* (Kasture 1993). R. H. Singh (1992) also gives a

short summary of clinical research with panchakarma therapy; see also Chopra (1998).

16. A critical article on the problem of individuality in evidence-based medicine in general has recently appeared in the *Journal of the German Medical Association* (see Niroomand 2004).

17. The patient weighed 111 kg. (244 lbs.), with a height of 1.85 m. (6 ft. 1 inch), resulting in a BMI (body mass index) of 32 kg/m^2.

18. *Mādhavanidāna* 34.

REFERENCES

Bhāvaprakāśa of Śrī Bhāvamiśra. 1993. Edited and with the Vidyotinī Hindī Commentary, Notes, and Introduction, by Brahma Śaṅkara Miśra. 5th ed., 2 vols. Varanasi: The Kashi Sanskrit Series 130.

Carakasaṃhitā by Agniveśa. Revised by Caraka and Dṛḍhabala, with the Ayurveda-Dīpikā Commentary of Chakrapānidatta. 1941. Edited by Vaidya Jādavji Trivikramjī Ācārya. 3rd ed., Bombay.

Chopra, Ananda Samir. 1998. Pañcakarma in Deutschland—Grundlagen, Praxis, Perspektiven. *Erfahrungsheilkunde—acta medica empirica. Sonderausgabe März* 47: 192–98.

———. 2003. Ayurveda. In *Medicine across Cultures: History and Practice of Medicine in Non-Western Cultures* (Science across Cultures: The History of Non-Western Science, vol. 3), ed., Helaine Selin, 75–84. Dordrecht: Kluwer Academic Publishers.

Das, Rahul Peter. 1993. On the nature and development of traditional Indian medicine. *Journal of the European Ayurvedic Society* 3: 56–71.

Frank, Robert, and Gunnar Stollberg. 2002. Ayurvedic patients in Germany. *Anthropology and Medicine* 9:3: 223–44.

Kasture, Haridāsa Śrīdhara. 1993. *Āyurvedīya Pañcakarma-Vijñāna.* 4th ed. Nāgpur: Baidyanāth Āyurveda Bhavan.

Leslie, Charles. 1992. Interpretation of illness: Syncretism in modern Ayurveda. In *Paths to Asian Medical Knowledge*, ed. Charles Leslie and Allan Young, 177–208. Berkeley: University of California Press.

Mādhavanidāna by Mādhavakara with the Commentary Madhukośa by Vijayarakṣita and Śrīkaṇṭhadatta and with extracts from Ātaṅkadarpana by Vācaspati Vaidya. 1986. Edited by Vaidya Jādavjī Trivikramjī Ācārya. Jaikrishnadas Ayurveda Series No. 68. Varanasi: Chaukhambha Orientalia.

Meulenbeld, G. Jan. 1995. The many faces of Ayurveda. *Journal of the European Ayurvedic Society* 4: 1–10.

———. 1999–2002. *A History of Indian Medical Literature.* 3 vols. Groningen: Egbert Forsten.

Miśra, Tārāśaṃkar. 1995 [1993]. *Nāḍī-Darśana. Bhāratīya cikitsā kendriya pariṣad dvārā svīkṛta evaṃ uttar pradeśa-śāsana dvārā puraskṛta.* Reprint of the 5th corrected ed. (Vārāṇasī 1993). Dillī (= Delhi): Motilal Banarsidas.

Niroomand, Feraydoon. 2004. Evidenzbasierte Medizin. Das Individuum bleibt auf der Strecke. *Deutsches Ärzteblatt* 101: A 1870–1874 (Nr. 26).

Rāy, Nimāi, and Tripāṭhī, Pareśa. 1993 [1st ed. 1986]. *Biśikhāra prathama adhyāya (āyurvvedīya chātropayoga)*. Kālikōtā (Calcutta): Āyurveda Vikāśa Maṇḍala.

Sharma, Priya Vrat. 1981. *Āyurveda kā vaijñānika itihāsa (Scientific History of Ayurveda)*. 2nd ed. Jaikrishnadas Ayurveda Series 1. Varanasi/Delhi: Chaukhambha Orientalia.

Singh, R. H. 1992. *Panca Karma Therapy (Ancient Classical Concepts, Traditional Practices and Recent Advances)*. Chowkhamba Sanskrit Studies CIV. Varanasi: Chaukhamba Sanskrit Series Office.

Stollberg, Gunnar. 2001. Asian medical concepts in Germany and the United Kingdom: Sociological reflections on the shaping of Ayurveda in Western Europe. *Traditional South Asian Medicine* 6: 1–9.

Suśrutasaṃhitā of Suśruta, with the Nibandhasaṅgraha Commentary of Śrī Dalhaṇācārya. Edited by Jādavji Trivikramjī Ācārya. Chaukhamba Āyurvijñān Granthamālā 42. Reprint: Varanasi: Chaukhamba Surbhāratī Prakāśan.

Wiese, Brigitte. 2002. *Zielgruppenanalyse von Nutzern Ayurvedischer Medizin bezogen auf die Ayurveda Klinik Kassel*. In *Ayurveda als Naturheilverfahren dargestellt an der Habichtswaldklinik, Kassel*, ed. Martina Ackermann, Ananda Samir Chopra, Uwe Herzog, and Brigitte Wiese, 42–58. Unpublished dissertation in management of social security, College of Commerce, Kassel, Hessische Verwaltungs- und Wirtschaftsakademie, Kassel.

Zysk, Kenneth G. 2001. New Age Ayurveda or what happens to Indian medicine when it comes to America. *Traditional South Asian Medicine* 6: 10–26.

CHAPTER 15

Ayurvedic Medicine in Britain and the Epistemology of Practicing Medicine in "Good Faith"

SUZANNE NEWCOMBE

This chapter attempts to elucidate the history of Ayurveda in Britain. However, serious practical problems arose when researching this subject. The primary difficulty is Ayurveda's very contemporary nature in Britain. Practitioners and businesses are establishing and disestablishing themselves with enormous rapidity. The records of the ayurvedic organizations, for example, The British Ayurvedic Medical Council and the Ayurvedic Medical Association (UK), are scant and unavailable in public archives and copyright libraries. There is only sufficient material for historical comment where the practice of Ayurveda intersects with government policy interests and in instances where Ayurveda has captured the attention of the popular press.

A particular episode that did create a significant paper trail was a 1991 trial for professional misconduct brought by the British General Medical Council (GMC) against two registered medical doctors practicing Maharishi Ayur-Veda on HIV-positive individuals. The press was involved first as a vehicle for reporting claims of the Maharishi program and later as commentators on the trial. In fact, the Maharishi Ayur-Veda (MAV) program was the only discussion of Ayurveda in the mainstream British press before the mid-1990s. Therefore, this case is particularly important, as it is the context in which ayurvedic medicine was first introduced to the anglophone majority in Britain. This event provides an interesting case study on the negotiation between alternative and biomedical health care epistemology in a specific situation. A description and analysis of these events form the most substantial section of this chapter. The overall exposition, however, is chronological.

THE BEGINNINGS OF AYURVEDIC PRACTICE IN BRITAIN

Some of the practices now associated with Ayurveda were practiced in Britain from at least the early nineteenth century. By 1814, an Indian, Dean Mahomet, and his Anglo-Irish wife, Jane, were offering "Indian remedies" for a variety of complaints. They had established a bathhouse in Brighton offering "Indian vapor baths" and "Shampooing with Indian oils." The "Shampooing" has similarities to an "ayurvedic massage" that one might receive today.

> [Shampooing] . . . consists of friction and extension of the ligaments, tendons, &c., of the body, the operation commencing by briskly administering gentle friction gradually increasing the pressure, along the whole course of the muscles; imperceptibly squeezing the flesh at the same moment: the operator then grasps the muscles with both hands whilst he kneads it with his fingers; this is succeeded by a light friction of the whole surface of the body . . . anointed with a medicated oil, . . . the muscles are then gently pounded with the thick muscle of the hand below the thumb. (Mahomet c.1997: 155–56)

Treatments described as specifically "Indian" were marketed for a wide range of ailments, including rheumatism, consumption, skin problems, and poor circulation (Mahomet c.1997: 169–71). Unusually, Mahomet's services were patronized by Kings George IV and William IV (173). While Mahomet was remarkable in his businesses' success and in leaving extant records, it is not impossible that there were others practicing similar techniques on a smaller scale during the nineteenth century. One rival Bath in Brighton was sometimes confused with Mahomet's in guidebooks, although it offered "Turkish" treatments (Mahomet c.1997: 170).

Immigrants of Indian descent in Britain were relatively insignificant numerically until after the Second World War; in 1955, it was estimated that 10,700 Indians or Pakistanis resided in the United Kingdom. However, by February 1960, that estimated number was 40,000 Indian-born immigrants alone (Desai 1963: 6). After this initial rush of immigration, restrictions for Commonwealth citizens came into effect from 1962 onward (Mason 1995: 27–30). Many of the immigrants were recruited to fill specific labor shortages, and a significant number of Indian qualified biomedical doctors came to work in the National Health Service (NHS). By 1987, however, almost 26 percent of all general practitioner doctors in Britain were born outside of the country, the majority originating from the Indian subcontinent (McNaught 1990: 34). Considering these strong ties with biomedicine, it is not surprising that Ayurveda did not make a significant appearance with the first increase in immigration.

Studies vary considerably in the extent to which it is estimated that British Asians consult practitioners of Unani and Ayurveda or self-medicate along their principles (Donaldson 1990: 247; Qureshi 1990: 95). Additionally, an idea of an unspecified "Indian medicine," rather than an understanding of Ayurveda, Unani, and Siddha as separate medical systems, continued in Britain until at least 1980 (Aslam 1979: 12). It seems that the British Asian practitioners of Ayurveda did not organize in a way that was visible to the anglophone population until the second half of the 1980s (see the final section of this chapter for more details). However, a systematic survey of the Indian-language papers in Britain might reveal more information about the practice of Ayurveda among ethnic communities than is presently available.

For some small circles of the anglophone population, an idea of Ayurveda has been percolating into public consciousness since at least the 1970s. The School of Economic Science has at times formed an informal networking center for individuals interested in Ayurveda. But it has never taken any formal initiatives relating to ayurvedic medicine (Skelcey 2003). The SES was founded in 1938 to explore questions relating to economic justice. It was later influenced by the thinking of Ouspensky and Gurdjieff, as well as Maharishi Mahesh Yogi, although no formal ties with organizations related to these individuals remain. From the mid-1960s the SES has seen itself as a "new spiritual movement" aligned with the Advaita Vedānta tradition (Barrett 2001: 266–76). From the 1970s some well-known practitioners have had loose associations with the SES, finding a sympathetic interest and a client base (Skelcey 2003). However, this activity has never made national headlines and is therefore hard to document.

It is often imagined that yoga groups have a particular interest in ayurvedic medicine. While this may be true in comparison to the general population, organizational discussions of Ayurveda within these groups have tended to be minimal. Ayurveda undoubtedly informs aspects of the Iyengar tradition: Geeta Iyengar, daughter of B. K. S. Iyengar, is qualified as an ayurvedic doctor (*Iyengar Yoga Jubilee* 2002: 44), and Mira Mehta, who has been influential in the growth of Iyengar Yoga in the United Kingdom, has studied and written on Ayurveda (Mehta 2002). However, it is only mentioned occasionally—and usually in passing—among the Iyengar publications in Britain (e.g., *Dipika*). British students of yoga teacher T. V. K. Desikachar also have expressed some interest in Ayurveda, though this has likewise not been focused or continual (Harvey 1988). The Sivananda organization in Britain occasionally hosts lectures on Ayurveda and workshops on the subject, particularly on ayurvedic cooking. While British practitioners of "postural" yoga (De Michelis 1995, 2004) might have some familiarity with the term *Ayurveda* and have perhaps experienced an "ayurvedic massage" in India, the majority of practitioners probably continue to be unsure of what Ayurveda entails.

There is, however, a longstanding interest in diet and alternative health care options among yoga practitioners. While shiatsu, reflexology, and the Alexander technique are regularly featured in advertisements and articles within the *British Wheel of Yoga* journals, Ayurveda is remarkably absent (*Yoga* and *Spectrum*). Where it does appear, it is within the context of an "alternative health supermarket" of many different complementary and alternative approaches to health. It is worth considering that a working understanding of Ayurveda cannot be obtained as easily as that of some of the other alternative and complementary therapies. This and the paucity of visible, competent, and respected ayurvedic physicians serving the English-speaking community can account for the relative neglect of Ayurveda compared to other alternative therapies. However, a very recent (post-1995) explosion of ayurvedic-related businesses might begin to change this relative stagnation.

THE CONTEXT OF MAHARISHI AYUR-VEDA'S ENTRY IN BRITAIN

Possibly the first mention of Ayurveda in the UK national press came in December 1986, with the headline "Healthy mind plea—Doctors call for NHS adoption of a system of natural medicine associated with Transcendental Meditation." The article goes on to claim that Ayurveda (as revived by Maharishi Mahesh Yogi) is based mainly on preventative herbal preparations and "the belief that 80 percent of ill health is psychosomatic in origin" (Wainwright 1986). This was eventually followed by a number of other articles in both the local and national press testifying to the profound benefits of Maharishi Ayurveda (e.g., Harley 1989; Waters 1989). Although advocating a form of medicine that was new to mainstream Britain, the call was directed to a well-established, popular base for alternative and complementary health care.

Interest in alternatives to biomedical treatment has always been present in Britain to varying degrees (Porter 2000). The late 1970s and early 1980s saw the establishment of a number of professional organizations relating to "holistic health" in Britain. Patronage by high-profile figures such as Prince Charles did much to raise their respectability during this time. But simultaneous to this growing interest in holistic health was the perception of a crisis in biomedicine and the NHS in particular (Power 1991: 60–61). Public dissatisfaction with the NHS rose dramatically during the 1980s. In 1983, 25 percent of the British population was "quite" or "very dissatisfied" with the NHS; by 1990, these responses reflected 47 percent of the population (Bosanquet 1992: 213). While dissatisfaction came from a variety of origins, not the least of which was a perceived chronic underfunding of the health service during this period (Webster 2002: 151), confidence was being specifically eroded by the AIDS crisis.

The British tabloid press picked up the story of an epidemic known as the "gay plague" in 1983, an incurable disease that could easily spread to the heterosexual population ("Watchdogs in 'gay plague' blood probe," "Alert over 'gay plague' "). It took several years before accurate information reached the public. As an *Observer* retrospective recounted, the first (1986) public health campaign was largely counterproductive: "Before the campaign, 5 percent thought there was a vaccine against AIDS; after it, 10 percent did. Before, 10 percent believed the infection could be spread by sharing eating and drinking utensils—[after] this had risen to 14 percent" (AIDS: The First 20 Years 2001). However, the second public health campaign, backed by 20 million pounds, was more effective in raising awareness and providing accurate information. The number of British persons affected by AIDS in the mid-1980s remained small; in 1988, some 1,000 people had been diagnosed with AIDS, and around 50,000 had been diagnosed as HIV-positive (Weeks 1988: 10). However, the sense of panic loomed large in public consciousness (Wellings 1988: 84).

Compared to the perceived size of the public health problem, the medical establishment's ability to treat HIV and AIDS appeared inadequate. The first effective treatment was announced in 1987 to great fanfare (Weeks 1988: 11). The efficacy of azidothymidine (AZT) was established with one major trial published in the *New England Journal of Medicine*. At the end of six months, only one patient in the AZT group was dead, while there were nineteen deaths among the placebo group (Fischl et al. 1987). The clinical trial was stopped early, because it was thought to be unethical to deny the patients of the placebo group a better chance of survival. However, the good news was not altogether unambiguous. In the same issue of the *New England Journal of Medicine*, a second article, immediately following, raised serious issues on the side effects and general toxicity of the AZT treatment (Richman et al. 1987). These side effects were recognized to include liver damage, nausea, fatigue, headaches, and anemia. For those living with the condition, and their loved ones, there was little peace of mind, or the possibility of a return to good health, due to the drug's extreme side effects.

The possibility that a "holistic" system of medicine, treating the entire person without the damaging side effects of biomedical pharmaceuticals, could make an important contribution to the health of

AIDS patients seemed obvious to those involved with Maharishi Ayur-Veda. After a February 1989 press conference called by the (Maharishi) World Medical Association for Perfect Health at the Charing Cross Hotel, entitled "Stop using modern medicine: Start using Maharishi Ayur-Veda," a number of articles trickled into the press. The Southampton *Southern Evening Echo* ran two articles in late 1989 that indicated that Maharishi Ayur-Veda offered a possible AIDS cure (Waters 1989; Jenkins 1989). Two doctors primarily associated with this project were qualified biomedical physicians Dr. Roger A. Chalmers and Dr. Leslie J. Davis, both British practitioners of Transcendental Meditation and enthusiastic proponents of the potential of Maharishi Ayur-Veda medical treatment.

Even though these two doctors would later be struck off the medical register due to behavior related to their treatment of AIDS patients, it is worth noting that the Maharishi organization had a clear marketing plan and a full-time public relations officer up until at least 1992 (Campbell 2004). Although the doctors were actively involved with making comments on the efficacy of MAV in the press, they did not initiate the press campaign. In fact, Chalmers claims that his name was used in media articles without his permission (Brennan and Hankey 2007). When Chalmers and Davis were brought before the GMC disciplinary council, their statements showed what appears to be a genuine faith in this alternative system of medicine. Indeed, recent interviews have shown that those who promote the Maharishi health care products continue to believe in the product's ability to effect a benefit to the whole person (Brennan and Hankey 2007; Whitley 2004).

THE EPISTEMOLOGY OF MAHARISHI AYUR-VEDA MEDICINE

Maharishi Mahesh Yogi first introduced Transcendental Meditation (TM) to Britain in 1960. The Beatles' brief association with Maharishi did much to raise the profile of TM, and the system of meditation it offered was widely known as an aid to relaxation during the 1970s—if not without controversy (Barrett 2001: 276–82). It is likely that Maharishi's work on Vedic medicine began around 1980 (Bodeker 1990: i). A few British doctors already practicing TM began studying Ayur-Veda with Maharishi in India in the early 1980s (Brennan and Hankey 2007; Hempsons 1991; Le Brasseurs 1991). But MAV formally entered Britain in late 1985 (Companies House No. 1941862 and No. 1954087). Outside commentators have noted that the introduction of Ayur-Veda, the TM Sidhi program, and other "Vedic sciences" to TM occurred after a period of decreasing initiations and a U.S. court case that ruled that TM was a religious technique that could not be taught in U.S. state-funded schools (Bainbridge 1997: 188–89, *Malnak v. Yogi* 1977).

The Maharishi's interest in Ayurveda also began not long after the World Health Organization officially recognized the important role that Ayurveda and other traditional systems of medicine have in providing health care for the global population (WHO 1978). However, Maharishi Mahesh Yogi is reported to have shown some of his followers a plan for the sequential introduction of subsidiary techniques and "Vedic Sciences" in the early 1970s; current members understand all new initiates to have been initiated at the appropriate time as part of a preconceived plan (Brennan and Hankey 2007).

For Maharishi, the project of helping the physical body through Vedic medicine is only secondary to laying the foundation for contact with "transcendental consciousness"—the principle that Maharishi considers the root of all phenomena. By letting the mind settle to its natural, undisturbed state through the technique of TM, it is believed that an individual's sense of well-being and physical health will improve (not to mention improving the well-being of others in the vicinity of the meditator by the meditation's beneficial effect on the underlying foundation of all matter [e.g., Hatchard et al. 1996]). Maharishi's organization believes that meditation is more effective than only treating symptoms with medicine, because meditation changes organic material at its "base." However, ayurvedic products are important within Maharishi's organization. Through the use of the Ayurveda, the natural energy of the body (*ojas*) should improve. This is an aid to the practice of allowing the mind to settle and can assist a practitioner in experiencing deeper experiences in meditation. For the followers of the Maharishi, true healing begins at a level deeper than the physical cells—it begins at the "Unified Field" of matter and consciousness.

DEEPAK CHOPRA AND THE IDEOLOGY OF MAHARISHI AYUR-VEDA (MAV)

The founding ideological treatise of MAV came in 1989 in the form of Dr. Deepak Chopra's (1989) book *Quantum Healing: Exploring the Frontiers of Mind/Body Medicine.* Chopra, an Indian-born biomedical doctor, then working from within the TM movement in the United States, expounded a justification for Maharishi's Vedic medicine based on theoretical physics and the concept of a "Unified Field" of consciousness that unites mind and matter. This book was a U.S. best seller and attracted the attention of many within the medical profession. In the words of Dr. Zamarra's *New England Journal of Medicine* book review:

> In a quantum interpretation, a patient's thoughts, emotions, and memories are more real than his cells, because thinking

> and feeling are the quantum fluctuations that give rise to all cellular processes. To support his highly provocative conclusion, Chopra aligns himself with Heisenberg, Eddington, and other quantum pioneers who flatly declare that "mind-stuff" underlies the physical universe and projects itself as matter. Healing, then, is a quantum event first, a mental one second, and physical only in its last stages. . . . However, the most original aspect of this book is its lengthy excursion into Ayurveda, the ancient medical tradition of India. In this "science of life," Chopra contends, a fully articulated model of the quantum-mechanical human body already exists.

It is precisely this mind/body medicine emphasis that Kenneth Zysk characterizes as "New Age Ayurveda" (2001). Significantly for Zysk's theory, Chopra's book was first published in Bantam's "New Age Books" series. Additionally, Maharishi frequently appeals to rediscovery of a *natural* and an *ancient* health care system. Both adjectives, liberally sprinkled throughout most MAV promotional literature, have assumed superiority to the modern and (by implication) "unnatural" biomedical treatments (Zimmermann 1992). Zysk also characterizes an equation of antiquity and naturalness to "truth" as characterizing this modern permutation of Ayurveda.

Chopra's ideas and personal charisma were very influential in the early days of MAV in Britain. He held at least one workshop at the Maharishi community in Skelmersdale, UK, and his books were regularly noted and quoted in Maharishi newsletters. He also designed the "Maharishi Natural Approach to Weight Loss" program, which was being marketed in Britain in 1991, as well as audiotapes and videotapes for this and several other programs (Law c.1990: 8; *Maharishi European Sidhaland News* 1990–1998 4(3):3, 4(5):3, 6(1): back cover; *Perfect Health News* 1991). Chopra's ideas have not changed significantly since he officially left Maharishi's movement in 1993, and his books continue to enjoy wide circulation (Baer 2003; Leland and Power 1997; Ross 1997). Conversely, although some of the preferred vocabulary has changed, Maharishi's movement is still working with essentially the same concepts elucidated in Chopra's early work.

In the preface to *Quantum Healing,* Chopra describes how Maharishi has rediscovered the "true" Ayurveda (i.e., the ability to cure patients through "nonmaterial" means). The essence of Ayurveda, according to Chopra, is this "nonmaterial" mind/body therapy, including "sound therapy." Chopra concludes his "Personal Introduction" with this poetic prose:

> Leaping across the void of time and space, surviving the waves of destruction that swallow up mankind, the ancient Vedic

> wisdom speaks to us with profound simplicity: In nature's perfect design, nothing ever dies. A human being is as permanent as a star; both are illuminated by the spark of truth. . . . I didn't need Ayurveda's knowledge to find out that doctors are battling against death. I needed it to find out that we will win. (1989: 7)

Appealing to dreams of personal immortality, Chopra's message is full of hope. This is more poetry than medical science. His book alternates between medical descriptions of the complicated and interconnected nature of human biology, particularly focusing on the body's ability to heal itself, and "miraculous" case studies of people apparently healing themselves through his mind-over-body approach.

Chopra describes in a vignette advising a doctor recently diagnosed with leukemia, but relatively asymptomatic, to imagine that he has a "mysterious disease" that would not necessarily be terminal. The doctor, despite his knowledge of the probable outcome of his diagnosis, found hope in this idea and physically felt better (1989: 212–14). This, among other methods, is part of treating disease as a mind-body problem, according to Chopra and Maharishi. There is obviously some value to treating the mental aspects of illness in such a way. But in what way do these anecdotal examples make a therapy "true"? And, if it is true, is it scientific?

In *Quantum Healing,* Chopra acknowledges that he "needed a way to make these techniques credible. People might dismiss them as faith healing; others would accuse me of selling false hope." Although he appears to acknowledge the validity of these critical perspectives, his confidence in the scientific value of his project is ultimately grounded on faith. Chopra continues: "I needed to show that this was a science in its own right. How to do that? It would come. Indian thought has always been grounded on the conviction that *Satya,* the truth, alone triumphs" (1989: 4-5). This argument is tautological. The system of Ayurveda taught by the Maharishi is true, therefore, it is scientific. Being true, it is not merely "faith healing" or "false hope."

Tautological statements can appear to accurately describe the world and in that sense to be "true." The ideas expressed in a tautological theory can be helpful for an individual or a society. But a tautological statement cannot be scientific. Truth and science are not synonymous. While modern notions of science can encompass many areas, science is generally associated with materialism, empirical observation, experimentation, falsification of theories, quantification, and a developed conception of proof (Engler 2003: 422). In the modern scientific community, the authority of assumptions—including those of what science *is*—is to some extent always contested (Chalmers 1982). Therefore, good scientific research must do more than simply conform to a fixed set of assumptions. Tautologies cannot be falsified or confirmed by empirical observation. Work supporting a tautology is simply providing support to a predetermined assumption. Although there is no universal account of what science is that is accepted by the entire scientific community, the premises of scientific knowledge remain epistemologically distinct from other forms of knowledge. I argue that the model of knowing the world presented in the Maharishi Ayur-Veda system during this period does not have the same epistemology as that of the general scientific and medical community.

Chopra's experience of "knowing" the "truth of Ayurveda"—"In nature's perfect design, nothing ever dies. A human being is as permanent as a star; both are illuminated by the spark of truth"—is essentially based on a mystical, gnostic insight. This knowledge is gained through the direct experience of TM rather than through observation of empirical phenomena or logical analysis. It might be true that in some way both human beings and stars are permanent. This "truth" can have a powerful motivating ability. And it is commonly assumed that such beliefs can initiate and encourage the body's ability to heal itself. But an assertion of the transcendental unity of all phenomena is not part of the same epistemological framework as modern science. There is simply no way to prove there is not a "Unified Field" of consciousness; there is no way to prove that both "human beings and stars" are not "illuminated by the spark of truth." The use of language is such that it is difficult to know what, precisely, the latter statement means. This kind of poetic truth cannot be incorporated into scientific epistemology. While the efficacy of specific therapies related to beliefs, prayer, and so on is regularly tested, these tests cannot actually affirm the underlying assumptions. For example, clinical trials of healing through prayer cannot determine if God is the agent of healing or if it is the subjects' belief in God (or even the belief in a positive outcome more generally) that inspires the healing (e.g., Hughes 1997; Ai et al. 2002).

Chopra's writing is compelling, but compellingly poetic and inspirational. The ability of the mind to inspire healing is a belief that enjoys considerable popularity alongside biomedicine all over the world, particularly in the United States (Baer 2003; Leland and Power 1997). It is a theory that can be held complementary to biomedical models of illness causation. Alternatively, it can be held as a system replacing the biomedical model. The MAV theories of health and wellness are unproblematic when used as a complement to conventional biomedical treatment—particularly when used as complementary therapy by those with both good health and a disposable income. But it became a very controversial theory when applied as an alternative treatment model to individuals suffering from HIV and AIDS.

THE INVESTIGATION OF MAHARISHI AYUR-VEDA

The event that led up to the prosecution of Drs. Chalmers and Davis began with the attempt to organize the workshop "Body-Mind and the Healing System: Towards a New View of AIDS: The Art of Unfolding the Healing Response through Maharishi Ayur-Veda, the Supreme Scientific System of Natural Health Care" (Campbell 1990a: 1). The doctors arranged for this workshop to be held at London Lighthouse, a venue known to support HIV and AIDS groups. Large advertisements were placed in *Capital Gay,* a weekly newspaper for homosexual men in the London area (Campbell 1990a: 2). Advertisements and glossy leaflets also were placed in the November 1989 newsletter *Body Positive,* an organization for people with HIV (Campbell 1990a: 3).

This obviously targeted marketing came to the attention of Mr. Michael Howard, then chief executive of Frontliners, a British organization for people with AIDS (Campbell 1990d: 2). While the homosexual population was the most affected by AIDS and desperately in need of relief, it also was the most informed and networked of all the social groups affected by HIV and AIDS. Howard contacted investigative journalist Duncan Campbell, then an associate editor of the *New Statesman & Society,* who had previously published exposés of fraudulent AIDS cures in that magazine and who had brought a doctor to trial in front of the GMC for a fraudulent AIDS treatment in November 1989 (Campbell 1990d: 2). Campbell then started the investigative processes that he eventually submitted to the GMC. But in the meantime the two major AIDS charities, the Terrence Higgins Trust and Frontliners, wrote to London Lighthouse asking it to cancel the booking of this "questionable" organization.

In response to the lobbying of these charities, London Lighthouse wrote to cancel the booking of the Maharishi organization's "Disease Free Society Trust" only nine days before the event, "in light of information that the organization was acting exploitatively towards people with HIV, ARC, and AIDS." The concerns of the Terrence Higgins Trust were laid out in a letter to Dr. Davis at the World Medical Association for Perfect Health. The trust reported that it had evidence of the sale of untested therapies to HIV-positive patients, the proffering of therapies by practitioners who were not qualified to offer therapies in the field of immunology, and the presentation in the press of unverified and anecdotal information claiming efficacy against HIV preceding the normal scientific process of peer-reviewed publication (Campbell 1990a: 9).

Additionally, the trust requested that all treatment that was experimental be provided free of charge to AIDS patients (Campbell

1990d: 12). While free treatment might sound like a heavy demand, the trust was primarily concerned with vulnerable people being asked to pay out large sums for unproven or experimental treatment. In fact, in a *Sunday Times* article, free Maharishi Ayur-Veda treatment had been offered as part of a trial study for HIV-positive individuals willing to forgo AZT treatment (Harley 1989). The risks involved in giving up a known effective treatment and using an untested product to treat HIV/AIDS was alarming in the eyes of the Terrence Higgins Trust. Responding to this letter, Davis appeared to acknowledge that the cost of treatment for people with AIDS was approximately £360 per month, and that several of the AIDS patients profiled in their case studies of Maharishi treatment had died (Campbell 1990d: 13). Therefore, Campbell continued his investigations, contacting a number of HIV-positive patients who had previously or were currently taking MAV products.

In particular, Campbell was distressed to note that the case histories of several patients were continuing to be circulated as success stories, without any "statement that the patients had in fact died" (1990d: 19). Campbell found that spokespeople for Maharishi Ayur-Veda had made claims that individuals diagnosed as HIV-positive may have even become HIV-negative (1990d: 30). Another of Campbell's key concerns was that the doctors treating HIV-positive patients did not clearly know the contents of the preparations they were prescribing (1990d: 14). On the basis of these concerns and other evidence, Campbell posted a letter of complaint on *New Statesman and Society* letterhead against Drs. Davis and Chalmers on April 5, 1990, to the GMC.

While the Maharishi organization was aware that Duncan Campbell was investigating their program of Ayur-Veda treatment for HIV-positive/AIDS patients, it was confident in the efficacy of its treatments. The doctors concerned did not see themselves as offering a specific treatment for HIV/AIDS but rather as using an ayurvedic model to promote the health of the whole person and correct all imbalances. From the Maharishi perspective, the targeted marketing of HIV-positive patients was simply an extention of normal treatment models to a population in great need. In particular, Mahrishi doctors believed that their Ayur-Veda treatment and worldview offered an opportunity for improving peace of mind and quality of life that the side effects of AZT and standard biomedical treatment at that time denied (Brennan and Hankey 2007).

THE GMC TRIAL

The General Medical Council was founded under the Medical Act of 1858, which established the dominance of the biomedical profession by restricting those who could legally claim the title of medical doctor (Porter 1999: 355–56). All individuals wishing to practice medicine as a doctor in the United Kingdom must be registered with the GMC, including foreign and visiting medical doctors. The main objective of the council is to "protect, promote, and maintain the health and safety of the public" (Medical Act 1983: 1A). The GMC has the power to remove doctors from the register who are considered unfit to practice medicine. A GMC caseworker will assess the claims and complaints made against a doctor. If the caseworker finds there is enough evidence to bring charges, then solicitors acting for the GMC Professional Conduct Committee continue the case against the doctor on behalf of those making the complaint (see http://www.gmc-uk.org). In Britain, the GMC is the official biomedical organization regulating biomedical doctors, and as such its opnions carry a great deal of authority both within the biomedical community and in general public opinion.

The case of Dr. Davis and Chalmers involving Maharishi Ayur-Veda treatment was brought in front of the GMC Professional Conduct Committee in 1991. Out of 1,087 complaints against doctors brought to the attention of the GMC in that year, only 126 (12%) of these cases were referred for formal disciplinary action. Erasure from the medical registrar (i.e., being "struck off") is the maximum penalty, and it is only imposed after serious consideration. In 1991, only twelve doctors were erased from the GMC registrar (GMC 1992: 16–23). Two of those erased were Drs. Leslie Davis and Roger Chalmers (Chalmers has since been reinstated to the registrar [GMC 2007]. This was not a decision that the Professional Conduct Committee made lightly.

It discusses the case specifically in its 1991 annual report under the heading "False Claims Concerning the Treatment of Patients Suffering from HIV, AIDS, and Related Conditions and Associated Matters." It considered as "proven" facts that the doctors had "insufficient knowledge, training or experience to engage in independent practice in the treatment of these conditions"; that there was "inadequate scientific evidence to support the use of therapies"; that they were "practicing the form of therapy without first conducting proper and approved clinical trials to assess the effects of the therapy on persons suffering from AIDS or HIV"; that "both doctors had acquiesced in the publication in the non-medical press of a number of articles claiming that this therapy could reverse the aging process"; that the doctors suggested patients stop using modern medicine; and that they had made "false claims on the value of the therapy." Additionally, it was considered proved that appropriate action was not taken when the doctors were notified that the condition of a particular patient suffering from AIDS had deteriorated after receiving treatment (GMC 1992: 23).

In expecting the doctors to know the contents of the pills they were prescribing, the Maharishi Ayur-Veda practitioners believe that the GMC was imposing a condition to which practitioners prescribing standard pharmaceutical products cannot conform (Brennan and Hankey 2007). While individual doctors might not be aware of the contents of their prescriptions, this information is easily accessible in biomedical databases; the contents of the Maharishi Ayur-Veda products were not listed in any such publicly accessible location. Additionally, pharmaceutical preparations have the support of professional biomedical consensus and pharmaceutical funding for clinical trials. It is very difficult to fund clinical trials for herbal products. Clinical trials are expensive, and there is little chance of recouping the costs by the creation of a patented drug at the end of the process. Herbal remedies can be perceived as competition to pharmaceutical hegemony. Some argue that the pharmaceutical establishment has, at times, behaved unethically to maintain its profit margins and to undermine competition from herbal and traditional medicines. It has been argued that the GMC case gainst Drs. Chalmers and Davis was an example of a kind of biomedical conspiracy to discredit natural health care (Walker 1993).

Initially the prosecution was interested in proving that the doctors were not qualified to offer the Ayur-Veda remedies they were prescribing (Wujastyk 2007). However, this line of argument soon became overshadowed by another issue. Analysis during the course of the trial revealed that some of the prescribed pills were contaminated by bacteria contained in human feces, a situation widely noted in the popular press while the trial was ongoing ("AIDS therapy 'contained feces' " 1991; Campbell 1991). The prosecution argued that this was due to processing with an impure water supply in India (Campbell 2004). If true, it would be an egregious lapse in medical judgment to offer to an AIDS patient any product that could be contaminated. However, Maharishi spokespeople described that upon cross-examination, it was admitted that it was possible that the patient himself had contaminated the pill with his own fecal material; the sample was taken from an open container, and the owner was suffering from severe diarrhea during the period he had been using the medications. Additionally, the Maharishi organization prides itself on its strict quality-control standards and random testing of all imported products to Europe. The Maharishi organization believes that negative press coverage on this issue during the trial biased the GMC Ethical Conduct Committee to an extent that it would have caused a mistrial in a civil or criminal court (Brennan and Hankey 2007).

In the conclusion to its decision, the GMC went out of its way to make clear that "*it was not the function of the Committee to assess the relative merits of differing forms of treatment or approaches to medicine adopted and practiced by doctors in good faith*" (1992: 23, emphasis in original). Institutionally, the Maharishi organization took the GMC comment on "good faith" as recognizing that Maharishi Ayur-Veda was outside of GMC jurisdiction. A Maharishi spokesperson emphasized that "the GMC made it quite clear that Transcendental Meditation and Maharishi Ayur-Veda were not in any way on trial or criticized" (Lines 1992). Strictly speaking, the GMC's jurisdiction only extends to the conduct of individual doctors. However, Drs. Chalmers and Davis were acting as national spokespeople for the Ayur-Veda program in Britain prior to the trial. So, in an important way, the ethics of presenting MAV to the British public *were* on trial. Significantly, the phrase "good faith" is open to several interpretations.

For the GMC, the issues of professional misconduct involved in the 1991 trial contravened the Good Medical Practice standards of Probity and Good Clinical Care (GMC 1998). This includes not publicizing positive results for new therapies in the popular press that had not yet undergone approved clinical trial, and not promising unproven results for experimental therapies. The GMC did not wish to prohibit scientific experimentation with alternative therapies. But, for the GMC, simple "faith" in an alternative system is not necessarily compatible with good medical practice.

By claiming that it cannot comment on treatments offered by doctors in "good faith," the GMC betrayed a confusion with the epistemological assumptions of modern scientific knowledge and those of "good faith." The epistemological assumptions of good medical practice for a registered doctor remain largely assumed and unarticulated in the write-up of the trial. However, while both faith and modern medical science provide ethical guidelines, their ways of discerning truth are fundamentally different. The phrase "good faith" can have radically different implications, depending upon one's perspective. Acting in accordance with good medical practice is not always compatible with providing treatment in which the doctor has "good faith."

The doctors practicing Maharishi Ayur-Veda clearly believed in what they were doing; as far as they were concerned, their actions were in "good faith." During the trial Dr. Davis was quoted as saying, "I am not ashamed to say I consider MAV a superior system of health care to modern medicine. If people taking modern medicine start to use MAV they can reduce their requirements and eventually not have to use modern medicine at all" (Mackinnon 1991). Especially when dealing with a theory of mind-body medicine, belief in this system could be considered a requirement of its efficacy. In the eyes of the GMC, the behavior of the doctors was not ethical, based on the assumptions of scientific epistemology. In the scientific framework, belief must take second place to a form of knowledge validated by the methodological procedures of empirical testing. But for Maharishi Ayur-Veda, the belief in mind-body healing is an essential part of the treatment paradigm itself.

The epistemological basis of Maharishi Ayur-Veda's claims of "truth" and efficacy is further obfuscated by a strategy of publishing reviews of its therapies in peer-reviewed medical journals. The Maharishi organization emphatically believed and continues to believe that its system is both true *and* scientific. The involvement of trained medical doctors within its programs adds "scientific" validity to that of the "pure," "natural," and "ancient" Indian wisdom. While no peer-reviewed articles have been published (at least to my knowledge) considering the effects of Maharishi Ayur-Veda on HIV/AIDS, a huge array of scientific literature deals with other aspects of Maharishi Ayur-Veda. Journals that have published peer-reviewed studies include the *International Journal of Neuroscience, Frontiers in Bioscience,* and *The American Journal of Cardiology* (Fields et al. 2002; Generloos et al. 1990; Nader et al. 2001). The bibliography of publications in biomedical journals can and does show efficacy of specific aspects of the MAV treatment programs (see also Maharishi International University 1990, 1998; Orme-Johnson and Farrow 1977). Although specific therapies can be shown to have good effects for certain physical conditions, this cannot validate or falsify the assumptions on which the Maharishi system rests. In its attempt to solve the perceived AIDS crisis, the Maharishi organization slipped from offering claims based on clinical trials to claims based on faith in the underlying assumptions of the Maharishi worldview.

RAMIFICATIONS AND OBSERVATIONS RELATING TO THE GMC TRIAL

Facing the results of the 1991 trial and the barrage of negative publicity, the response within the Maharishi Ayur-Veda program in Britain was twofold. First, there was an organizational denial of any misconduct. To this day, the Maharishi organization would prefer not to mention the trial at all. The event was ignored in the TM newsletter, *TM News*, although this journal regularly reports on MAV's successes and new initiatives. When I pressed the current manager of the MAV products department to comment on the trial, he called the results a "national shame and a lapse in the proper duty of the GMC." The organization itself sees the effects of the trial to be negligible: TM practitioners always made up the bulk of Ayur-Veda consumers, and they did not decrease their use of the products as a result of the trial (Whitley 2004).

However, it appears that the Maharishi organization has become more careful to preach the power of MAV to those who already share assumptions of its worldview (i.e., TM practitioners) rather than directly targeting the British population as a whole. Since the trial, the Maharishi organization has refrained from making unsubstantiated claims about its health care system—at least to those outside the TM community. Since 1991, the Vedic Health programs have barely been mentioned in the UK national press. The organization has continued to concentrate on the publication of articles testifying to the efficacy of MAV treatment in medical journals. Yet considering the institutional denial of any misconduct, as described earlier, and the inherent place of insight into the knowledge of the Unified Field, it is likely that the fundamental approach has changed little as a result of the trial.

Recent publication on Maharishi Ayur-Veda in the United States presents a more qualified exposition of Ayur-Veda's potential than was seen in the 1980s' literature. The claims for MAV's efficacy made in Hari Sharma and Christopher Clark's *Contemporary Ayurveda: Medicine and Research in Maharishi Ayur-Veda* (1998) are more in line with the results of clinical trials. However, Sharma and Clark are clearly calling for a paradigm shift from biomedical science to "the consciousness model," because a "truly satisfactory medical model must begin at the foundation of human experience," (i.e., the "Unified Field") (150). The theory of "The Consciousness Model of Medicine" is clearly laid out in Chapter 2 of this book. MAV has plenty of evidence to support its efficacy in specific areas and undoubtedly improves the quality of life for many—whether through the placebo effect or not is immaterial to efficacy. However, the ramifications of this model as applied to a seriously ill population exclusive of the biomedical model are not immediately apparent in this exposition. This makes meditation on the 1991 GMC trial of Drs. Davis and Chalmers all the more important for looking at the role of complementary and alternative medicine in modern British society.

Although it has a controversial origin and history, MAV is an important part of the contemporary understanding of Ayurveda in Britain and North America. It is misguided to describe MAV as distinct from "real" Ayurveda, as Stephen Fulder does in his 1996 *Handbook of Alternative and Complementary Medicine.* He singles out Maharishi Ayur-Veda as a "highly commercial venture . . . [that] should not be confused with real Ayurveda" (160). MAV claims inspiration and authority from the Vedas and ayurvedic texts. Although MAV tends to use "proprietary mixtures" rather than herbal mixtures prepared by the physician for each individual patient, this is true of many other forms of Ayurveda in Britain. Maharishi Ayur-Veda is an important part of the practice of Ayurveda in contemporary society, despite the ideological claims of those opposed to the system.

This overly simplistic understanding of the multifaceted nature of modern Ayurveda was echoed in the series of articles and letters in both the *JAMA* and *The Lancet,* published between 1990 and 1992, dealing with MAV. This series of publications was marked, above all, by polarized letters from Maharishi supporters or Maharishi detractors (Chalmers 1990; UK: Ayur-Vedic Medicine 1990; "Letters: Ayur-Vedic Medicine" 1990; Duncan Campbell 1990; Sharma, Triguna, and Chopra 1991; Correction—Financial Disclosure 1991; Skolnick 1991; Letters 1991, 1992). One *JAMA* article (Skolnick 1991) was so negative that Deepak Chopra sued the author for defamation, and the case was settled out of court (Leland and Power 1997). Chopra disassociated himself from Maharishi Ayur-Veda not long after the controversial articles in *JAMA* were published.

More generally, it is important to note that alternative systems of thinking about health and illness can be, and usually are, complementary to biomedical models of thinking. The Maharishi organization claims that it does not ask patients to abandon biomedical treatment options (Whitley 2004). Furthermore, the Maharishi organization in Britain strongly encourages fully qualified biomedical professionals to become involved in its alternative paradigm of conceptualizing health and health care. The 1989 request of HIV-positive patients to abandon biomedical treatment for free Maharishi products (Harley 1989) has not been repeated publicly. Both providers and consumers of Maharishi Ayur-Veda hold their "minority health beliefs" simultaneously with certain convictions about the efficacy of biomedical treatment and the validity of "scientific" criteria for evaluating treatments. Although this observation might seem obvious, this fact is often overlooked by the press—both popular and medical—in the search for a sensational story.

Another important observation is that whether or not an alternative way of thinking is perceived as a problem depends largely on the level of social responsibility taken for a given population. MAV only became the focus of a GMC trial because it had been marketing its therapy specifically to one of the most vulnerable and controversial groups in the late 1980s (i.e., HIV-positive homosexuals). When an alternative way of thinking about medical treatment remains largely in a population that is relatively healthy and well-off, there is little call for the intervention of public institutions. This is the situation of MAV and most other complementary and alternative medical traditions in Britain today. However, when the focus is on a population that is considered particularly vulnerable—whether children, the elderly, the destitute, or the critically ill—public pressure for government and professional bodies to intervene becomes powerful.

Following from this tendency, there is a tension between the freedom of belief and the need to protect the vulnerable from exploitation. The freedom of the general population to explore alternative health care treatment options comes at the cost that occasionally things will go wrong for the vulnerable. It seems as if several HIV-positive patients hoping for a cure from MAV may have died prematurely (Campbell 1991: 32–33, 42–44). However, the risk of not allowing minority beliefs to flourish could be that innovation or challenges to dominant theories would have difficulty emerging.

The results of the 1991 trial also came at the cost of destroying the livelihood and reputation of two doctors who showed integrity in their conviction of the health care they were providing. It is my impression that the Maharishi organization still does not fully comprehend why the doctors, practicing a therapy so obviously *true* and practicing in "good faith," should have been the subject of the GMC malpractice trial. Considering that belief in a mind-body cure is one of the primary tenets of Maharishi health care, an enthusiastic belief that MAV could offer a cure for AIDS is logical when seen from within the Maharishi worldview. The Maharishi organization is able to publish a bewildering array of peer-reviewed scientific articles testing elements of its treatment and providing claims to scientific validity. However, this literature only obfuscates the fact that the fundamental assumptions of Maharishi's teaching are based on a spiritual insight rather than on scientific epistemology.

This trial provides an interesting case study about how competing health care beliefs were negotiated. Among other things, it demonstrates that the epistemological basis of "truth" in medicine is not unambiguously rooted in what is generally considered the scientific model. While the different epistemological assumptions of biomedical science and faith-based approaches remain unarticulated, it is easy for both sides to become entrenched in their views. This typically creates a situation where one side calls the other "quacks," and the other side retaliates with blanket denouncements of the drug-company-funded biomedical profession.

Randomized controlled trials (RCT), which are often seen as the "gold standard" of assessing the efficacy of any therapy, do not provide much information on the assumptions that underlie an approach to therapy. The epistemology underlying a complementary treatment is worth greater discussion by the general population, medical practitioners, and social scientists alike. This might lead to more fruitful information about both real and perceived problems with specific health care theories and therapies. Patients and doctors would be better able to make informed decisions on treatment options if information on the risks, benefits, epistemological assumptions, and history of complementary or alternative treatments was more easily accessible.

CODA—AYURVEDA IN BRITAIN SINCE 1991

Since the Maharishi organization has removed itself from the public limelight, a number of ayurvedic organizations have attempted to gain dominance in Britain. It is with several different ayurvedic organizations that the British government is now attempting to find a consensus for a minimum standard of training required for an ayurvedic practitioner.

One ayurvedic organization that has been established a relatively long time and has achieved success in gaining the interest of the national press is the Ayurvedic Company of Great Britain, founded in 1989 by Gopi Warrier and associates. The company has the advantages of professionally trained business and marketing advisors and considerable financial backing. In recent years this group has hosted many events to raise awareness about the rigorous and regulated training of Indian-qualified doctors and to insist upon these qualifications in Britain. Associated with the company are the professional organizations The British Ayurvedic Medical Council (BAMC) and the British Association of Accredited Ayurvedic Practitioners (BAAAP). For several years, it ran a BA (hons.) degree in Ayurveda in association with Thames Valley University, and an attempt was made to initiate a degree program in association with Manipal University (Karnataka, India) in 2004 (D'Silva 1999; Warrier 2003). Currently this group is running a London-based BSc (hons.) in Ayurveda under the name the Manipal Ayurvedic University of Europe (MAYUR). It describes its degrees as awarded by the Manipal Academy of Higher Education.

From 1996, the major competition to the Ayurvedic Company of Great Britain was the Ayurvedic Medical Association (UK) and associated organizations. The Ayurvedic Medical Association (UK) (2002) was founded as a professional association for qualified Indian and Sri Lankan ayurvedic practitioners, offering malpractice insurance and a code of ethics. For a time, qualifications were offered by the College of Ayurveda (UK) in Milton Keynes, which advertised its association with the Gujarat Ayurved University and the University of Pune (College of Ayurveda [UK] 2002). However, the College of Ayurveda has now been disbanded, and the organizers of this program are now offering BSc and MSc courses on Ayurveda accredited by Middlesex University. Several other degree programs are currently being offered in Britain, either through correspondence or part-time courses (Ayurvedic Institute UK 2004; Ayurveda Institute of Europe 2004).

After the publication in 2000 of a House of Lords report on alternative medicine, the British government has sought to establish minimum standards for practitioners of all alternative and complementary therapies. Since the House of Lords Report, the Medicines and Healthcare Products Regulatory Agency (MHRA) (2004) has been holding meetings with representatives of organizations representing the various professionals that use herbal medicine in Britain. The Herbal Medicine Regulatory Working Group (HMRWG) estimated that there are approximately 1,300 herbal medicine practitioners who hold memberships with voluntary registrars in the United Kingdom; "the size of these registrars is approximately equal for the traditions of Western Herbal Medicine and Chinese Herbal Medicine/TCM. The numbers of practitioners of Ayurvedic Medicine are small by comparison" (HMRWG 2003: 4). The lack of agreement between the various ayurvedic organizations is perhaps less relevant to the fate of Ayurveda in Britain than it might seem; the more numerous Western and Chinese herbal practitioners are very likely to define a large part of any new regulation. Ayurvedic practitioners will be legally obliged to follow minimum standards and regulations set in consultation with these numerically more significant groups.

While there are probably less than 100 practicing ayurvedic practitioners in Britain, the new degree programs are turning out each year dozens of individuals who have an interest in practicing ayurvedic medicine. Meanwhile, ayurvedic businesses are establishing themselves at a prodigious rate. Before 2000, only sixteen companies with names beginning with "Ayur" (appearing to be involved in ayurvedic products or services) had registered with Companies House. However, between 2000 and 2004, thirty-one companies of this description were registered. But there is a high turnover within the businesses; between 2000 and 2004, eleven companies were dissolved from the registrar, and three others proposed removal (Companies House 2004). Some of these represent branches of established Indian companies opening branches in Britain, while others are new business ventures. While various ayurvedic organizations and businesses vie with each other in the emerging market, UK and EU legislation exerts external pressure.

During recent negotiations with the HMRWG, the ayurvedic organizations represented could not agree to minimum standards of education and training that would deliver threshold competency across the ayurvedic profession; therefore, the Indian and Sri Lankan High Commissions were additionally drawn in for consultation (HMRWG 2003: 7). The BAAAP and the BAMC were pushing for an additional 60 hours of Sanskrit, 60 hours of Ayurveda philosophy, and 1,000 hours of clinical training to what was accepted as minimum training standards by the other ayurvedic groups in Britain. Additionally, the BAMC and the BAAAP maintain that there should be regulation for Ayurveda that is distinct from herbal medicine generally (HMRWG 2003: 7).

While the statutory self-regulation proposals are ongoing, there are general regulations related to the sale and promotion of health products that restrict the practice of ayurvedic medicine in Britain

(Stone and Matthews 1996). Products "presented for treating or preventing disease in human beings or animals" require a medical license under European law (Medicines Control Agency 2001a: 5). While certain herbal products are exempt from licensing requirements, others may be sold as food, as in the 1968 Medicines Act (Medicines Control Agency 1996). Additionally, the use of certain herbal ingredients may be restricted to use by medical practitioners only, or prohibited from use altogether (Medicines Control Agency 2001b). The European Parliament passed a directive, also in March 2004, that took effect in October 2005. Rather than requiring clinical trials for herbal medicines, the directive allows for registration of products that have an established tradition of use within the European community. Many of the ayurvedic products currently on the market have appeared within Europe during the last fifteen years and may be required to produce supplementary documentation testifying to the safety of the product for human consumption (European Parliament 2004). The effect these restrictions have on the practice of Ayurveda in Europe has yet to be determined.

In the face of increasing governmental regulation, the Ayurvedic Practitioners Association (APA) was founded in 2005 to "establish Ayurveda as a distinct, relevant, and credible system of traditional medicine in the UK" (see http://www.apa.uk.com). This organization includes many members of the Ayurvedic Medical Association (UK) and recent graduates of the British Ayurveda degree programs. Practitioners of Maharishi Ayur-Veda have taken an active role in this organization and in negotiations with the government. The organization is taking an active role in unifying and professionalizing the variously qualified ayurvedic practitioners in Britain. It aims to include and support all of those with an interst in Ayurveda and to present a united front for negotiations with government regulation. The APA currently has a membership of about 100, with between twenty and thirty fully qualified practitioners (Hubbers 2007). While it is too soon to analyze the success of this venture, Ayurveda will increasingly be subject to more stringent governmental regulation as the numbers of those interested in Ayurveda continue to rise.

NOTE

1. The author wishes to acknowledge the financial support of the United Kingdom Arts and Humanities Research Council and Amherst College's Evan Carroll Commager Fellowship, which made this research possible. She also is grateful for feedback received when presenting information in this chapter at "A Celebration of Ayurveda," a conference held by the Ayurvedic Practitioners Association in London on January 27, 2007.

REFERENCES

Ai, A. L. et al. 2002. Private prayer and optimism in middle-aged and older patients awaiting cardiac surgery. *The Gerontologist* 42: 70–81.

AIDS: The first 20 years. 2001. *The Observer (London)* (June 3). http://www.guardian.co.uk/aids/story/0,7369,500773,00.html, accessed September 26, 2004.

AIDS therapy "contained feces." 1991. *The Guardian* (July 16). http://web.lexis-nexis.com/xchange-international, accessed February 22, 2004.

Alert over "gay plague." 1983. *Daily Mirror*. (May 2). http://www.web.lexis-nexis.com/xchange-international, accessed February 22, 2004.

Aslam, Mohamed. 1979. The practice of Asian medicine in the United Kingdom. Dissertation, University of Nottingham.

Ayurveda Institute of Europe. 2004. *Courses* (October 14). http://www.ayurvedainstitute.org/courses.html.

Ayurvedic Institute UK. 2004. *New Three-Year Diploma Course from January 2005*. (October 14). http://www.theayurvedicclinic.com/3course.html.

Ayurvedic Medical Association (UK). 2002. *Qualified Practitioners List*. November 17, 2003. http://www.natural-healing.co.uk/ayurvedic-medical-association-uk/practioners.htm.

Baer, Hans A. 2003. The work of Andrew Weil and Deepak Chopra—Two holistic health/New Age gurus: A critique of the holistic health/New Age movements. *Medical Anthropology Quarterly* 17: 233–50.

Bainbridge, William Sims. 1997. *The Sociology of Religious Movements*. London: Routledge.

Barrett, David. 2001. *The New Believers*. London: Cassell.

Barton, Laura. 2001. Health: Open to the elements: Ayurveda, one of the oldest medical systems in the world, is suddenly the next big thing in alternative health. Hollywood celebs and wealthy Brits are all talking about their "doshas." *The Guardian (London)* (March 22): 16.

Berridge, Virginia. 1996. *AIDS in the UK: The Making of a Policy, 1981–1994*. Oxford: Oxford University Press.

Bodeker, Gerard C., ed. 1990. *Maharishi Ayur-Veda: Documents, Scientific Research, Bibliographies, Letters of Recommendation*. Lancaster, MA: Lancaster Foundation.

Bosanquet, Nicholas. 1992. Interim report: The national health. In *British Social Attitudes, the 9th Report*, ed. Roger Jowell et al., 209–20. Aldershot: SCPR.

Brennan, Donn, and Alex Hankey. (Maharishi Ayur-Veda Representatives). 2007. Personal interview January 29.

Campbell, Duncan. 1990a. *Document Submissions to the General Medical Council*. London: Wellcome Library Western Manuscripts and Archives. MS 7967.

———. 1990b. Heaven on earth, Inc. *New Statesman* (September 28): 10–11.

——— 1990c. Letter to the General Medical Council. April 5. Personal files of Duncan Campbell. Brighton.

———. 1990d. *Statement to the GMC*. London: Wellcome Library Western Manuscripts and Archives. MS 7967.

———. 1991. Cult doctors struck off." *Capital Gay* (November 1): 4.

———. 2004. (February 26). Personal interview.

Chalmers, Alan F. 1982. *What Is This Thing Called Science?: An Assessment of the Nature and Status of Science and Its Methods.* Milton Keynes: Oxford University Press.

Chalmers, Roger. 1990. Maharishi Ayur-Veda. *The Lancet* 336: 1322.

Chopra, Deepak. 1989. *Quantum Healing: Exploring the Frontiers of Mind/Body Medicine.* London: Bantam.

College of Ayurveda (UK). 2002. *Prospectus 2002.* November 3, 2003. http://www.collegeofayurveda.com.

Companies House. 2004. *Register of Companies.* http://www.companieshouse.gov.uk, accessed October 2004.

Correction—Financial Disclosure. 1991. *Journal of the American Medical Association* 266: 798.

De Michelis, Elizabeth. 1995. Some comments on the contemporary practice of yoga in the UK with particular reference to British Hatha Yoga schools. *Journal of Contemporary Religion* 10: 146–56.

———. 2004. *History of Modern Yoga: Patanjali and Western Esotericism.* London: Continuum.

Department of Health. 2004. *Regulation of Herbal Medicine and Acupuncture: Proposals for Statutory Regulation.* London: DH.

Desai, Rashmi. 1963. *Indian Immigrants in Britain.* London: Oxford University Press.

Dipika: Journal of the South-East London Iyengar Institute. 1981–1984; *Journal of the Iyengar Yoga Institute (Maida Vale, London).* 1984–present.

Donaldson, Liam. 1990. Elderly Asians. In *Health Care for Asians,* ed. Brian McAvoy and Liam Donaldson, 237–49. Oxford: Oxford University Press.

D'Silva, Beverley. 1999. Instant karma. *Sunday Times (London).* August 8, p. 8.

Duncan Campbell. 1990. *The Lancet* 336: 1390.

Engler, Steven. 2003. "Science" vs. "religion" in classical Ayurveda. *Numen* 50: 416–63.

European Parliament. 2004. Directive 2004/23/EC of the European Parliament and of the Council of 31 March 2004 Amending, as Regards Traditional Herbal Medicine Products, Directive 2001/83/EC on the Community Code Relating to Medicinal Products for Human Use. *Official Journal of the European Union (OJ)* (April 30): L 136–85.

Fields, Jeremy Z., et al. 2002. Effect of multimodality natural medicine program on carotid atherosclerosis in older subjects: A pilot trial of Maharishi Vedic Medicine." *The American Journal of Cardiology* 89: 952–58.

Fischl, M. A., et al. 1987. 'The efficacy of azidothymidine (AZT) in the treatment of patients with AIDS and AIDS-related complex, a double-blind, placebo-controlled trial. *The New England Journal of Medicine* 317: 185–91.

Fulder, Stephen. 1996. *The Handbook of Alternative and Complementary Medicine.* 3rd ed. Oxford: Oxford University Press.

General Medical Council. 1992. *General Medical Council Annual Report for the Year Ending 31 December 1991.* London: General Medical Council.

———. 1998. *Maintaining Good Medical Practice.* London: General Medical Council.

———. 2007. *Register of Medical Practitioners.* London: General Medical Council.

Generloos, P., et al. 1990. Influence of a Maharishi Ayur-Vedic herbal preparation on age-related visual discrimination. *International Journal of Psychosomatics* 37: 25–29.

Harley, Gill. 1989. AIDS victims discover the strength to fight through meditation. *The Sunday Times*, March 26. http://www.web.lexis-nexis.com/xchange-international, accessed February 22, 2004.

Harvey, Paul. 1988. Spring retreat with Paul Harvey. 1989. *Spectrum* (Autumn): 4.

Hatchard, Guy, Ashley J. Deans, Kenneth L. Cavanaugh, and David Orme-Johnson. 1996. The Maharishi effect: A model for social improvement. Time series analysis of a phase transition to reduced crime in Merseyside Metropolitan area. *Psychology, Crime, and Law* 2: 165–74.

Hempsons, Solicitors. 1991. London: Wellcome Library Western Manuscripts and Archives. MS 7967.

Herbal Medicine Regulatory Working Group (HMRWG). 2003. *Key Recommendations on the Regulation of Herbal Practitioners in the UK*. London: HMRWG. http://www.advisorybodies.doh.gov.uk/herbalmedicinerwg/INDEX.HTM, accessed October 21, 2004.

House of Lords Select Committee on Science and Technology. 2000. *Complementary and Alternative Medicine (CAM)*. Sixth Report. London: HMSO. http://www.parliament.the-stationery-office.co.uk/pa/ld199900/ldselect/ldsctech/123/12301.htm, accessed October 8, 2004.

Hubbers, Nigel. 2007. Founder-member of the Ayurvedic Practitioners Association. Personal interview, February 1.

Hughes, C. E. 1997. Prayer and healing. A case study. *Journal of Holistic Nursing* 15: 318–24; discussion 325–26.

Iyengar Yoga Jubilee with Geeta Iyengar. 2002. London: Jubilee Committee.

Jeannotat, Françoise. 1996. De la quête de la santé à la quête du salut. Réflexion sur le recours aux pratiques thérapeutiques alternatives: L'exemple de l'Ayurvéda. *Equinoxe* 15, numéro special "Sacré(s)": 71–80.

Jenkins, Anna. 1989. AIDS need not be a death sentence. *Southern Evening Echo*. In Campbell 1990a: 38.

Khanum, Sultana Mustafa. 1994. We just buy illness in exchange for hunger: Experiences of health care, health, and illness among Bangladeshi women in Britain." Dissertation, University of Keele.

Law, Ric. c.1990. *The Centre Reference Manual*. Skelmersdale: Ayur-Veda Products Centre.

Le Brasseurs, Solicitors. 1991. London: Wellcome Library Western Manuscripts and Archives. MS 7967.

Leland, John, and Carla Power. 1997. Deepak's instant karma. *Newsweek (US)* (October 20): 44–51.

Letters. 1991. *Journal of the American Medical Association* 266: 1769–74

———. 1992. *Journal of the American Medical Association* 267: 1337–40.

Letters: Ayur-Vedic medicine. 1990. *The Lancet* 336: 1260

Lines, David (national director of Transcendental Meditation). 1992. Letter to Inform. Comments on Reports in the Guardian and the Evening Standard Relating to the General Medical Council Hearing in October 1991. In the files of Inform, Houghton Street, London WC2A 2AE.

Malnak vs. Yogi, 440F. Supp. 1284, 1322 (NJ 1977).

Mackinnon, Ian. 1991. Doctor defends AIDS therapy treatment. *The Independent* (July 24): 6.

Maharishi European Sidhaland News/Transcendental Meditation News. 1990–1998. Skelmersdale: TM.

Maharishi International University. 1990. *The Maharishi Effect: Creating Coherence in World Consciousness—Promoting Positive and Evolutionary Trends throughout the World—Results of Scientific Research 1974–1990*. Fairfield, IA: Maharishi International University Press.

———. 1998. *Scientific Research on the Maharishi Technology of the Unified Field: The Transcendental Meditation and TM-Sidhi Program—One Program to Develop All Areas of Life*. Fairfield, IA: Maharishi International University Press.

Mahomet, Dean. c.1997. *The Travels of Dean Mahomet: An Eighteenth-Century Journey through India*. Edited by Michael H. Fisher. Berkeley: University of California Press.

Mason, David. 1995. *Race and Ethnicity in Modern Britain*. Oxford: Oxford University Press.

McNaught, Allan. 1990. Organization and delivery of care. In *Health Care for Asians*, ed. Brian AcAvoy and Liam Donaldson, 31–39. Oxford: Oxford University Press.

Medical Act. 1983. (As amended by the Professional Performance Act 1995, the European Primary Medical Qualifications Regulations 1996, the NHS (Primary Care Act 1997, the Medical Act (Amendment) Order 2000, the Medical Act 1983 (Provisional Registration) Regulations 2000, the Medical Act 1983 (Amendment) Order 2002) and the National Health Service Reform and Health Care Professionals Act 2002). http://www.gmc-uk.org/about/legislation/medical_act.htm, accessed October 22, 2004.

Medicines Control Agency. 1996. Medicines Act 1968. London: HMSO.

———. 2001a. *Review of Herbal Ingredients for Use in Unlicensed Herbal Medicinal Products*. London: MCA.

———. 2001b. *Traditional Ethnic Medicines: Public Health and Compliance with Medicines Law*. London: MCA.

Medicines and Healthcare Products Regulatory Agency (MHRA). 2004. *Licensing of Medicines: Policy on Herbal Medicines*. London: MHRA. http://www.medicines.mhra.gov.uk/ourwork/licensingmeds/herbalmeds/herbalmeds.htm, accessed October 8, 2004.

Mehta, Mira. 2002. *Health through Yoga: Simple Practice Routines and a Guide to the Ancient Teachings*. London: Thorsons.

Nader, Tony A., et al. 2001. A double-blind randomized controlled trial of Maharishi Vedic Vibration Technology in subjects with arthritis. *Frontiers in Bioscience* 6: 7–17.

Orme-Johnson, D. W., and J. T. Farrow, eds. 1977. *Scientific Research on the Transcendental Meditation Program: Collected Papers Volume I*. Zurich, Switzerland: Maharishi European Research University Press.

Perfect Health News. 1991. Skelmersdale: TM.

Porter, Roy. 1999. *The Greatest Benefit to Mankind: A Medical History of Humanity from Antiquity to the Present*. London: HarperCollins.

———. 2000. *Quacks: Fakers & Charlatans in English Medicine.* Stroud, Gloucestershire: Tempus.

Power, R. N. 1991. The Whole Idea of Medicine: A Critical Evaluation of the Emergence of "Holistic Medicine" in Britain in the Early 1980s. PhD diss., Polytechnic of the South Bank.

Qureshi, Bashir. 1990. Alternative/Complementary medicine. In: *Health Care for Asians,* ed. Brian McAvoy and Liam Donaldson, 93–116. Oxford: Oxford University Press.

Richman, D. D., et al. 1987. The toxicity of azidothymidine (AZT) in the treatment of patients with AIDS and AIDS-related complex—A double-blind, placebo-controlled trial. *New England Journal of Medicine* 317: 192–97.

Ross, Deborah. 1997. Interview: Deepak Chopra. *The Independent (London),* March 3, p. 13.

Saks, Mike. 2003. *Complementary and Alternative Medicine.* London: Continuum.

Sharma, Hari, and Christopher Clark. 1998. *Contemporary Ayurveda: Medicine and Research in Maharishi Ayur-Veda. (Medical Guides to Complementary and Alternative Medicine).* London: Churchill Livingstone.

Sharma, Hari, Brihaspati Dev Triguna, and Deepak Chopra. 1991. Letter from New Delhi. *Journal of the American Medical Association* 265: 2633–37.

Skelcey, Graham (principal of the School of Economic Science). 2003. Personal interview, November 17.

Skolnick, Andrew A. 1991. Maharishi Ayur-Veda: Guru's marketing scheme promises the world eternal "Perfect Health." *Journal of the American Medical Association* 266: 1741–50.

Spectrum: Journal of the British Wheel of Yoga. 1979–1993.

Stone, Julie, and Joan Matthews. 1996. *Complementary Medicine and the Law.* Oxford: Oxford University Press.

UK: Ayur-Vedic medicine. 1990. *The Lancet* 336: 1060–61.

Wainwright, Martin. 1986. Healthy mind plea/Doctors call for NHS adoption of system of natural medicine associated with Transcendental Meditation. *The Guardian (London),* December 29. http://www.web.lexis-nexis.com/xchange-international, accessed February 22, 2004.

Walker, Martin. 1993. *Dirty Medicine: Science, Big Business and the Assault on Natural Health Care.* London: Slingshot.

Warrier, Gopi. 2003. Personal interview, November 14.

Watchdogs in "gay plague" blood probe. 1983. *The Sun,* May 2. http://www.web.lexis-nexis.com/xchange-international, accessed February 22, 2004.

Waters, Jo. 1989. AIDS relief from old cures claim. *Southern Evening Echo* (September 23): 15ff.

Webster, Charles. 2002. *The National Health Service: A Political History.* Oxford: Oxford University Press.

Weeks, Jeffrey. 1988. Love in a cold climate. In *Social Aspects of AIDS,* ed. Peter Aggleton and Hilary Homans, 10–19. London: The Falmer Press.

Wellings, Kaye. 1988. Perceptions of risk—Media treatment of AIDS. In *Social Aspects of AIDS,* ed. Peter Aggleton and Hilary Homans, 83–105. London: The Falmer Press.

Whitley, David (manager of the Ayur-Veda products in Skelmersdale). 2004. Personal interview, February 14.

World Health Organization (WHO). 1978. *The Promotion and Development of Traditional Medicine: Report of a WHO Meeting.* Geneva: WHO.

Wujastyk, Dominik. 2003. *The Roots of Ayurveda: Selections from Sanskrit Medical Writings.* London: Penguin.

———. 2007. Personal interview, February 1.

Yoga: Journal of the British Wheel of Yoga. 1969–1979.

Zamarra, John W. 1989. Book review: Quantum Healing by Deepak Chopra. *The New England Journal of Medicine* 321: 1688.

Zimmerman, Francis. 1992. The gentle purge: The flower power of Ayurveda. In *Paths to Asian Medical Knowledge,* ed. Charles Leslie and Allan Young, 209–23. Berkeley: University of California Press.

Zysk, Kenneth Gregory. 2001. New Age Ayurveda, or what happens to Indian medicine when it comes to America. *Traditional South Asian Medicine* 6: 10–12.

CHAPTER 16

Maharishi Ayur-Ved

A Controversial Model of Global Ayurveda

FRANÇOISE JEANNOTAT

Ayurveda came to public notice in the West, particularly in Europe and the United States, in the 1980s. In Europe, interest in Ayurveda developed first within the circles of yoga practitioners and naturopaths. For example, toward the end of the 1970s, T. K. Shribhashyam, one of the sons of the Indian *yogācārya* T. Krishnamacharya, settled in the South of France and began teaching Ayurveda to a small group of French and Swiss yoga teachers. Another organization, the International Association of Ayurveda and Naturopathy (IAAN), promoted Ayurveda in 1985 at the 1st World Congress of Yoga and Ayurveda (which I attended). But in its initial phases, Ayurveda was principally popularized by Maharishi Mahesh Yogi, founder of the Transcendental Meditation (TM) movement. In 1985, Maharishi introduced in his teaching what he called Maharishi Ayur-Ved (MAV), a form of Ayurveda he tried to spread beyond the borders of India.

Today, however, MAV is only one of many forms of Ayurveda in the West. In Switzerland, for example, other forms of ayurvedic treatment are available that consist mainly of wellness and body care approaches. They are practiced by allopathic doctors or nonbiomedical practitioners who are trained in various places in India in special courses for foreigners[1] or at various ayurvedic training centers in the West, such as the Ayurvedic Institute in Albuquerque, New Mexico. In India, it is now common for luxury (and even semi-luxury) hotels and alternative health centers to also offer "ayurvedic massage" and diets. However, the first Ayurveda clinic in Switzerland was opened by Maharishi Mahesh Yogi (Maharishi Ayurveda Gesundheitszentrum, Seelisberg) in January 1987 (SIMS/IMS 1987:4: 14–15).

At first sight, the many forms of Ayurveda seem primarily defined by their commercial aspects. The case of MAV, however, is somewhat different. Without denying the importance of MAV as an independent commodity, it is important to point out that it belongs to the wider and more complex ideological system of the TM movement. To date, MAV is among the most successful models of a globalized Ayurveda, and as such it is likely to provide essential elements to the understanding of this phenomenon.

Considering the dearth of academic research on MAV, the aim of this chapter is to introduce its main concepts to highlight issues that could contribute to more general reflections on global Ayurveda. The perspective here will be that of religious studies, using TM and MAV publications as primary sources. It should be pointed out that most of these publications were written by Maharishi's followers. Maharishi Mahesh Yogi himself only gave talks on MAV, some of which have been transcribed. I refer to these transcriptions and also to the writings of TM followers who are well placed in the movement (scientists, teachers, etc.) and as such can be considered spokespersons of MAV. I also refer to fieldwork data obtained during a panchakarma treatment and a course on MAV in Switzerland, as well as during meetings with one person in charge of a MAV center in Delhi. One of the classical texts of Ayurveda, the *Caraka-Saṃhitā*, is used especially when discussing panchakarma. For the development of Maharishi's teaching, I use more general sources on TM published by the TM movement. Finally, the secondary literature includes anthropological, sociological, and religious studies analyses of New Age or new religious movements.

After a brief introduction to Maharishi Mahesh Yogi and his movement, I outline how MAV presents itself and point out some of the issues raised by MAV's reinterpretation.[2] The point here will not be to resolve these issues but to highlight certain aspects of MAV that are likely to contribute to a better understanding of global Ayurveda. I then examine some of the cultural conditions that enabled MAV to establish itself in the West. Finally, I share some reflections regarding the more general contribution of MAV to the study of global Ayurveda.

MAHARISHI MAHESH YOGI AND HIS TEACHING

There is no completely reliable information available on the life of Maharishi Mahesh Yogi before he arrived in the West. We can find some information on this period in his own writings (Maharishi 1986: 184–200) as well as those of a few other researchers (e.g., Mitchiner 1992: 99–100, Finger 1987: 198–202). We can state, however, that

Maharishi Mahesh Yogi was born as Mahesh Prasad Srivastava sometime between 1911 and 1920, though most people cite January 12, 1917 as his date of birth, in Jabalpur, in the present state of Madhya Pradesh. He took a degree in physics at Allahabad University, at that time one of the premier universities in India, in 1939 or 1940. During that period he met his spiritual teacher, Brahmananda Saraswati, who was then the Śaṅkarācārya of Jyotir Math in North India.

The main centers of this Vedantic institution established in the eighth century by philosopher Śaṅkarācārya were in Joshimath (on the road to Badrinath in Himalayas) and, importantly, in Allahabad itself. He remained with Brahmananda Saraswati as one of his chief aides until the latter's death in December 1953. After the passing of his master, Maharishi spent several months in seclusion or semi-seclusion in Uttarkashi, in the lower Himalayas. He then traveled to South India, where he slowly developed a meditation practice, a technique inspired by his guru, which later became known as Transcendental Meditation. In 1958, Maharishi founded the "Spiritual Regeneration Movement" in Madras (now Chennai), which eventually evolved into the Transcendental Meditation movement. At the end of 1958, he left India to spread his technique and to "spiritually regenerate" the whole world.

Over the years, Maharishi's teaching underwent various refinements, as he adapted it to the values and concerns of his Western audience. Maharishi himself defined TM as a process of leading the mind inward toward the subtle nature of creation, until the innermost, subtlest level of creation is reached. This, then, also is transcended, giving rise within one's conscious awareness to the source of creation beyond relativity—the blissful field of the Absolute (Maharishi 1986: 262).

The first paper published on TM in the United States was entitled "Non-Medicinal Tranquilizer," and it described TM as a way to cure insomnia. Maharishi reports that he was so shocked that his first thought was to run away from this country, but on second thought he realized that:

> [. . .] for whatever reason people may start Transcendental Meditation, they are going to get the total effect that it produces, and the goal that they will arrive at will be full enlightenment. Therefore, I should not mind the angles with which people will approach. They will enjoy much more than for what they begin. (Maharishi 1986: 242)

Thus the spiritual purpose of TM was gradually relegated to the background, and its effects on stress or personal development were increasingly emphasized. Generally, Maharishi presents his teaching as a combination of modern science with what he calls "Vedic tradition." His main concepts remained the same in the course of the succeeding years, but their formulation and, to a certain extent, their direction transformed themselves. I have identified three different stages in his teaching, defined by the terminology that he has used, as well as by a few well-known references to some of the sources of the Indian philosophico-religious tradition:

1. Ca. 1960–1970:
   In 1960, Maharishi established a link between what he called "Pure Being" (which he equates to "the Self" and "the Absolute") and science (Maharishi 1986: 299). But he really systematized and formulated his teaching as the "Science of Being" in 1962, when he wrote *The Science of Being and Art of Living*, which was first published in 1963 (see Maharishi 1986: 459–85, 1995).

2. 1970–1980:
   During the early 1970s, Maharishi redefined his teaching as the "Science of Creative Intelligence" (see Maharishi 1995: 328; Forem 1976: 16–18, 122–44), which is explained "in terms of the principles of different disciplines of modern science" (Maharishi 1997, vol. 1: II). This stage of Maharishi's teaching was characterized by a great amount of scientific research conducted on TM, and in the late 1970s by the introduction of an advanced series of meditation practices called the "TM-Sidhi Program," based on Maharishi's notion of the way the third chapter, "Vibhūti-pāda," of Patañjali's *Yogasūtra* should be practiced (Maharishi 1995: 331–32). The aim of the TM-Sidhi Program is to develop consciousness through the concomitant development of paranormal powers (*siddhis* or *vibhūtis*), levitation or "yogic flying," as he calls it, in particular (cf. *Yogasūtra* 3.42).[3]

3. 1980—present:
   Since 1980, Maharishi's teaching refers increasingly to the sources of the Indian philosophico-religious and cultural traditions, and it has been redefined as "Vedic Science" (see Maharishi 1995: 335–36; 1988: 4–67). With this Vedic Science, "Maharishi wanted to support and give authenticity to the knowledge of life that he was teaching from the subjective approach of consciousness available in the Vedic Literature. For this purpose, he organized the centuries-old scattered Vedic Literature as the literature of a perfect science" (Maharishi 1997, vol. 1: III).

MAHARISHI AYUR-VED (MAV)

As mentioned earlier, Maharishi began promoting MAV—the "holistic approach to life" (Maharishi 1988: 113)—in the mid-1980s. This practice has gradually taken an essential place in his teaching, and the movement has published numerous books on the subject, none of them, as noted, written by Maharishi. From him we only find transcriptions of talks (see Maharishi 1988: 46–47, 108–15; 1996a: 304–14; 1997, vol. 4: 161–81). In these talks, he sometimes uses the term *Ayurveda* instead of *Maharishi Ayur-Ved*. The identification of Ayurveda with MAV also is documented in the publications of other authors within the movement (e.g., Baierlé 2002: 135–47).

In this section, I examine more closely the characteristics of MAV as presented by the movement. According to Maharishi, "(J)ust as the Veda has been misinterpreted for thousands of years in the past, so Ayurveda has also been misunderstood" (1988: 47). R. Keith Wallace, founding president of Maharishi International University (now Maharishi University of Management), Fairfield, Iowa, and now professor of physiology there, one of the movement's leading researchers, adds that

> particularly due to India's history of political turbulence, over hundreds of years, this knowledge became fragmented, much of it was forgotten, and the rest was known to just a few experts. In the 1980s, the complete and holistic value of Ayur-Ved was brought to light by Maharishi Mahesh Yogi from the Vedic literature as part of his revitalization of the ancient Vedic wisdom. One of his first contributions to Ayur-Ved was the restoration of mental techniques, such as TM, to unfold the full potential of the physiology of consciousness. Originally, these were an integral part of Ayur-Ved, but they had become deemphasized or abandoned. Maharishi's next step was to work with the leading remaining experts of traditional Ayur-Ved to restore the completeness of this knowledge. (Wallace 1993: 64–65)

The assertion that Indian traditions have been misinterpreted by others is a recurring theme in publications by Maharishi and his followers (cf. Maharishi 1986: 341, 549; 1971: 12–17; Tourenne 1981: 45), and Maharishi's claim that these misinterpretations are one of the main causes of the past and present spiritual degeneration is central to the movement's proclaimed raison-d'être.

Accordingly, Maharishi has not only saved Ayurveda from further decline, he also has restored its true sense and value by reintroducing knowledge that has been lost, namely, TM and the TM-Sidhi Program. Thus Maharishi's major techniques—TM and the TM-Sidhi Program—were not eclipsed by MAV. This attempt to rescue Ayurveda from continued misinterpretation was fulfilled with the help—I would even say the *guarantee*—of prominent figures of Ayurveda. The choice of experts is interesting and will be examined further here.

THE SOURCES OF MAV

Maharishi and his followers rarely cite their sources, and when they do their references are vague. They merely mention the *Caraka-Saṃhitā* and the *Suśruta-Saṃhitā* as the major texts of classical Ayurveda, without defining precisely MAV's concepts in relation to the statements in these texts.

Moreover, MAV is presented as part of Vedic Science. This latter is said to result from Maharishi's efforts "to restore this Vedic Science in all its purity and to establish a bridge between itself and modern science to formulate an integral science of life, combining the latest discoveries of modern physics with the timeless wisdom of the Veda" (Baierlé 2002: 53, my translation).

Vedic Science is said to be based on three realms of theoretical and practical knowledge (Baierlé 2002: 53): (1) traditional Vedic literature;[4] (2) principles of modern science; and (3) the technology of consciousness, meaning Vedic techniques of meditation. In spite of this, interpretations of Vedic Science remain vague with respect to both "Vedic" literary sources and modern science. Thus without ever becoming specific, Maharishi says, rather tautologically, "Vedic science is the science of Veda. 'Veda' means pure knowledge and the infinite organizing power that is inherent in the structure of pure knowledge" (1988: 26). Vedic Science describes both the structure of this "pure knowledge," considered the unmanifest basis of all creation, and the manner in which, by its own power, it reveals itself and organizes itself to give rise to creation. Vedic Science's methods of investigation are TM and the TM-Sidhi Program, while its practical application is MAV.[5]

DEFINITION AND PURPOSE OF MAV

Wallace defines MAV more closely as follows:

> Ayur-Ved comes from two Sanskrit words, *ayus*, meaning "life" or "lifespan," and *Ved*, meaning "knowledge" or "science." Ayur-Ved may be translated as "the science of life or, more

> specifically, "the science of lifespan." Ayur-Ved includes knowledge about every aspect of life and health (1993: 64). Maharishi Ayur-Ved is a complete approach to health care which emphasizes prevention rather than cure, the patient rather than the disease. The physician focuses not only on the symptoms of illness in a patient, but on creating a complete state of balance in the mind, physiology, and behavior. Maharishi Ayur-Ved emphasizes the proper interaction of—and the balance between—mind and body, consciousness and matter. (1993: 94)

The emphasis on prevention rather than treatment and on the patient rather than the disease is reminiscent of some of the criticism of Western biomedicine since the 1970s.

MAV has a distinctive definition of health that relates more to the philosophico-religious aspects of life than to physiological ones. Some authors present it as the supreme value of life, as a state of total and ultimate perfection that eventually relates back to the Hindu conception of salvation. Thus according to Baierlé, one of the French-speaking spokespersons of MAV:

> In Sanskrit, the language of Vedic science, the word health is called *swasthya*. *Swa* means the Self, and *sthya* what is established. Thus, health is the state of being established in the Self, in pure consciousness, the absolute and unchanging value of life. "*Yogasthah kuru karmani*" says *Bhagavad Gita*: "established in *yoga*—the union with the Self—perform action." (Baierlé 2002: 102, my translation)[6]

This shift toward a more philosophico-religious sense must be related to the fact that MAV is said to be a system "that has its basis in consciousness" (Sharma 1993: 236). It follows that MAV's central approach is TM, which enables one to experience pure consciousness, "the Self," "the unmanifest basis of creation" (Wallace 1993: 23). Although Maharishi and his followers evade the question of the link between TM and "Hindu religion" (see Maharishi 1986: 558), their formulations, descriptions, or quotations constantly refer to it. For example, they often use concepts such as "ātman," "brahman," "self-realization," and "enlightenment," or quotations such as "aham brahmāsmi," "aham vishwam," and so on (their own transcription of Sanskrit). But, according to them, TM is not a religion but a simple and natural practice that can be scientifically verified (Maharishi 1986: 502, 515; Sharma and Chopra 1991: 1774). In the same way, for the TM movement authors, there is no connection between Vedic Science and the Hindu religion or religion in general (Wallace 1993:220; Baierlé 2002: 31–34).

BASIC CONCEPTS

Wallace writes:

> One of the central concepts described in classical Ayurvedic texts is known as Panchamahabhuta. This describes how matter arises from consciousness. . . . In this theory, the universe's origin is *avyakt*, "unmanifest"—the unmanifest unified field of pure consciousness. Arising from this field (the Self) are the various levels of the physiology of consciousness . . . : ego, intellect, mind and senses. . . . They are broad principles and structures of natural law at the foundation of everything in creation. (Wallace 1993: 70)

Without entering into details of the "physiology of consciousness," it must be underlined here that the process of manifestation mentioned earlier, in which ego is the first principle emerging from the unmanifest, deviates from the view of the classical texts. At first sight, Maharishi's conception of cosmology seems to align with Sāṃkhya—for example, *avyakt* (Skt. *avyakta*) can correspond to *prakṛti*, primordial materiality—even if it is not clearly expressed. But he and his followers would rather refer to "Vedic Science," that is, to a more vague category that allows any type of reinterpretation.[7] As I suggested elsewhere (Jeannotat 1997: 1111), this reversal of the perspective could be explained by the objectives of Maharishi in general and of TM in particular. If TM's ultimate goal is frequently mentioned in terms of self-realization or enlightenment, then it is in the worldly sense of maximization of one's own capacities and potential, of self-confidence, and so on. Such a goal can only be achieved thanks to the acknowledgment or even the preeminence of ego.

According to MAV, as in classical Ayurveda, material creation is described on the basis of the *panchamahābhūta* theory, with its five basic constituents. On the level of the body, the *panchamahābhūtas*, or five great elements (earth, water, fire, air, and ether), combine to form the three *doṣas*. These principles, which are in perpetual interaction, govern all functions of the body, and it is their imbalance that causes disease. The three *doṣas* are present in each person in different proportions, with one or two predominating, to constitute the basic psycho-physiological body type (*prakṛti*). To maintain health, one must adapt one's lifestyle to one's own body type. Because it is the imbalance of the three *doṣas* that produces disease, the treatment depends on the aggravated *doṣa(s)*.

If the disease is caused by the imbalance of the *doṣas*, then the cause of this imbalance lies in the way in which the intellect functions:

> The intellect has the ability to shift our attention in one of two directions: either toward the diversity of life, or inward, toward the unity of consciousness. Maharishi's Vedic Science refers to a condition known as *pragyaparadh*, the "mistake of the intellect." In this condition, the intellect becomes so absorbed in the diversified value of creation that it cannot perceive the underlying unity of life. (Wallace 1993: 95)

To escape from this disease-producing situation, "[t]he intellect, lost in its own discriminations, must remember its source once again—the undifferentiated unity of pure consciousness (Sharma 1993: 259). And the means to achieve this is TM. TM is once again highlighted, even if the different authors acknowledge that it is not the only approach to recover health. These quotations demonstrate the major place of TM in MAV as a practice that not only restores health but above all prevents the emergence of disease. When the intellect is constantly connected to its source—pure consciousness—it will be less inclined to become disturbed.

THERAPEUTICS OR MAV'S APPROACHES

The list that follows is a reproduction of one distributed by the Seelisberg Health Center. The twenty approaches are not always presented in the same way by the different TM movement authors, but these are the most commonly quoted.[8]

THE TWENTY APPROACHES OF MAHARISHI AYUR-VED TO CREATE PERFECT HEALTH

1. Consciousness—Development of higher states of consciousness through Maharishi's Transcendental Meditation, its advanced techniques, and the TM-Sidhi programme.
2. Primordial Sound—Use of the primordial sounds of the Samhita of the four aspects of the Ved and their Ved-Angas and Up-Angas to eliminate imbalances in the functioning of human nature as a whole.

3. Intellect—To correct the habit of the intellect to make mistakes—pragyaparadh [sic. *prajñāparādha*]—so that the totality of the unified structure of life is perceived while one is perceiving the diversified structure. In this state of knowledge of the Self, disease cannot flourish because life is intimately connected with the source of natural law.

4. Emotions—Strengthening of the finest level of feeling to develop the emotions fully.

5. Language—Using Vedic principles of the structure of language to promote balance and integrity in the mind and body.

6. Gandharva-Ved—Traditional music therapy using sound and melody to restore harmony in the physiology and eliminate the imbalances responsible for disease.

7. Senses—Vedic procedures to enliven through all five senses, perfect balance in psycho-physiology.

8. Pulse Diagnosis—Detecting any existing or forthcoming imbalance simply by feeling the pulse.

9. Psycho-physiological Integration—Restoration of homeostatic balance and acceleration of neuromuscular co-ordination and balance in the physiology and psychology.

10. Neuromuscular Integration—Vedic exercises to restore mind-body coordination and the integrated functioning of all levels of life.

11. Neuro-respiratory Integration—Vedic exercises pertaining to the physiology of breathing to restore integrated functioning to all levels of mind and body.

12. Physiological Purification—Sophisticated purification procedures applied at regular intervals to eliminate and prevent the accumulation of physiological impurities due to faulty dietary and behavioural patterns.

13. Diet—Appropriate dietary measures to support the restoration of physiological balance in the prevention and treatment of disease.

14. Herbs and Minerals—Use of medicinal flora and minerals from every country to bring perfect balance to the functioning of mind and body.

15. Rasayana—Sophisticated herbal and mineral preparations formulated for the prevention and cure of disease and the promotion of longevity.

16. Behaviour—Bringing behaviour into accord with natural law through daily and seasonal routines.

17. Jyotish—Securing perfect health for the future; mathematical prediction of environmental influences on health.

18. Yagya—Vedic performances to restore environmental balance and promote individual and collective health.

19. Environment—Creating collective health through the Transcendental Meditation and TM-Sidhi programme so that society provides a nourishing and strengthening environment for the individual to rise to perfect health.

20. World Health/World Peace—Group performance by 7,000 experts in Maharishi's Transcendental Meditation and TM-Sidhi programme to create coherence in world consciousness, the basis of world peace and collective health on a global scale.

Thus it appears obvious that MAV is a generic concept referring to a mixture of these twenty different practices or approaches. But only some of them can be found in the classical ayurvedic texts; these are (16) Behavior, (13) Diet, (14) Herbs and Minerals, (15) *Rasāyaṇa*, and (12) Physiological purification (*panchakarma*). (8) Pulse diagnosis appears in later ayurvedic sources. (10 and 11) Neuromuscular and Neuro-respiratory integrations refer to *āsanas* and *prāṇāyāma*, respectively, that is, to yoga. As far as the other approaches are concerned, they cannot be considered part of a generally recognized ayurvedic medical practice, even if they are sometimes mentioned in the medical texts. Furthermore, among these latter, seven refer to TM, techniques associated with it, or the results that are supposed to result from their practice: (1) Consciousness, (2) Primordial sound (though this also refers to an ancillary form of sound-based healing that Maharishi has since developed), (3) Intellect, (4) Emotions, (9) Psycho-physiological integration, (19) Environment, and (20) World Health/World Peace. The practice of (18) Yagya (Sanskrit: *yajña*) refers, in this context, to ritual offerings of rice, ghee, and other substances into fires, as gifts to various deities such as Śiva and the Goddess. These are performed on auspicious dates by "pundits" in India. The movement sells them to its members for prices ranging from $3,000 to $11,000 and it has become a relatively popular (and fashionable) thing to do by the well-heeled meditating public in Fairfield, Iowa, and elsewhere. The sponsor is not expected to attend but is said to receive spiritual benefit and cures for mental and physical disorders as a result of the sponsorship. The movement apparently includes it as a part of MAV because of its supposed healing benefits.[9]

Next to TM, the most prominent MAV practice is panchakarma, which "includes sophisticated massages with medicated oil, heat treatments with herbalized steam, inhalation therapy to cleanse sinuses and lungs, and a variety of purgative and eliminative therapies. The experience is both relaxing and invigorating" (Sharma 1993: 286).

In classical Ayurveda, panchakarma (Skt. *pañcakarma*) is a strong purificatory treatment that consists of a succession of five (*pañca*) actions (*karma*) or procedures forming a whole. Historically these procedures were drastic, presenting risks and requiring precautions. The medical texts spend several chapters on the accidents that could happen during treatment (see *Caraka-Saṃhitā, Siddhisthāna*, chs. 4 and 6). The five actions or procedures are vomiting, purgation, evacuative enema, purgation of head, and oil enema. The first four are purgative, and the last one is repletive. Each of these procedures is preceded by oleative and sudative sequences (see, in particular, *Caraka-Saṃhitā, Sūtrasthāna,* chs. 2, 13–16; *Siddhisthāna,* chs. 2, 4, 6). The two types of enema are sometimes considered a single procedure, the fifth one being bloodletting.

In a promotional booklet published by the Centre de Santé par l'Ayur-Ved Maharishi (Maharishi Ayur-Ved Health Center), Seelisberg, panchakarma is presented as a purificatory and rejuvenative treatment, which is "pleasant and relaxing . . . creating the basis for greatly improved vitality, performance, and joy in life." With respect to the procedures, vomiting has been discarded, so the treatment usually begins with the oleative and sudative sequences, followed by the purgative, as in classical Ayurveda. The other procedures are chosen according to the condition of the patient, but also according to their desires. From then on, the oleative and sudative sequences are treated as separate procedures, whereas they should precede each evacuative procedure. As noted by Zimmermann, "Instead of a fixed sequence, from oil to heat to catharsis, culminating in the final process of discharging unwanted excreta—which is the traditional method of *pañcakarma*—we now have a panoply of alternative actions: massages, heat treatments, and/or internal cleansing. . . . Catharsis has changed into a kind of physical therapy" (1993: 215).

In fact, the promotional leaflets emphasize the oil massages, their gentle and healing properties, and the fact that they enable one to experience true bliss.[10] The risks and, even more so, the violence inherent in this treatment in its traditional version are here completely concealed in order to conform to the gentleness claimed by practitioners of natural medicine. Yet this way of representing panchakarma is not specific to MAV. Zimmermann states that

> in contemporary practice in South Asia, as well as in Ayurvedic therapies exported to the West, practitioners avoid using emetics or drastic purgatives. All violence has disappeared from medications aiming to cleanse the patient's humoral system. Neither red (the red of bloodletting), nor black (the black or chemical oxides), but green—the green of herbs freshly gathered, a symbol of nonviolence: this is the new motto of Ayurveda's flower children. (1993: 210)

The TM techniques, panchakarma, and the *rasāyaṇas* have been and continue to be the object of scientific research into their effectiveness. However, the research has been conducted solely by TM followers in laboratories created by the movement for that purpose. The fact that most of the scientific studies on TM and MAV are conducted by members of the movement, with their vested interest in a positive outcome, induces an evident and problematic bias. Finally, the different approaches of MAV practiced in the health centers of the movement are administered only by practitioners trained in its Vedic universities. These practitioners are not always trained in biomedicine, and this can be a problem. In my experience, these practitioners are very cautious with their sick patients, but they clearly prefer the healthy ones.

WHY MAV?

We have seen that the distinctive feature of MAV is that it is presented as a restored version of classical Ayurveda by Maharishi Mahesh Yogi, who reintroduced into it certain mental techniques, in particular TM and the TM-Sidhi Program, which he claims were abandoned over time. The problem is that although the classical medical texts mention certain mental techniques, they do not describe them in detail, as this is not their purpose (see, for example, *Caraka-Saṃhitā, Śārīrasthāna* 1.130–155). The TM movement authors do not mention any other relevant source for this supposed original Ayurveda, except "Vedic Science" or the "Veda," concepts that are dealt with vaguely or obscurely. With this in view, namely, the dominant position of the TM techniques within the practice of MAV, I would say that Maharishi Mahesh Yogi, contrary to what he asserts, extracted the data and techniques from the classical medical texts and included them in the service of his own teaching of TM. He finally appropriated the whole, giving it his name and trademark.

Although the concepts and approaches of MAV that are reflected in historical Ayurveda roughly correspond to what is found in the medical texts, they are presented in a modern and simplified form, adapted to the expectations of the Western public. This brings us to ask why Maharishi deemed it necessary at the time to introduce in his teaching a medical practice with a "focus on prevention" (Sharma 1993: 272). Since 1970, Maharishi has increasingly emphasized the beneficial effects of TM on health and on the prevention of disease. He has legitimized these claims through numerous experiments conducted in the laboratories of the movement, which consistently offer scientific proof of the positive physiological benefits of TM. In 1979, the movement published a *Mémoire sur la promotion d'une santé parfaite grâce au progamme de Méditation Transcendantale et de MT-Sidhi*, (Memorandum on the Promotion of Perfect Health Bestowed by the Transcendental Meditation and TM-Sidhi Programs) addressed to Mrs. Simone Weil, the French Minister of Health and Family Welfare. This booklet was signed by thirty-seven doctors and health workers and supported by more than thirty other doctors and health workers. One of the measures proposed in this booklet is "to include TM teacher's training in the curriculum of medical studies and other medical professions" (Association Française pour la Promotion . . . 1979: 5, my translation). The booklet also invited the French minister to take the techniques of TM into account, because "the responsibility of the medical authorities is to promote every new technology in order to establish a state of perfect health for every citizen and the whole nation" (1979: 4, my translation).

If the TM techniques were already presented as a scientifically proved, ideal tool for prevention or even for treatment, then why was it necessary to wrap it up in a medical system such as Ayurveda? MAV could be seen as an attempt to provide the appearance of medical backing for Maharishi's claims about TM. In fact, in the late 1970s, the movement had to cope with criticism and controversy over the question of whether TM was a scientific or a religious practice. This question was taken into the U.S. court, which ruled in 1978 that TM was a religion (Melton 1986: 188). In Europe, the TM movement also began to appear in studies on sects (for example, in France and Germany: see Gibon and Vernette 1987: 47; Haack 1980: 81–96). Thus the focus on MAV both diverted the attention from TM and provided a medical, which is to say scientific, basis for TM. Admittedly, MAV referred more to alternative medical practices that were not considered scientific. But in the mid-1980s, this was no longer an obstacle, with the rising tide of claims to success of various types of similar alternative and complementary practices.

It is tempting to suggest that the introduction of MAV into Maharishi's teaching has its primary origins in commercial interests. Indeed, the teaching of TM is not a well-paid professional option in the long run—the initiation of TM is given or sold only once—in spite of the different courses offered in TM centers. In order to survive, the movement must continually find new meditators, without knowing for sure if it will attract enough people. According to Melton, "[a]round 1976, the number of new people taking the basic TM course dropped dramatically" (1986: 188), and by 2005, the number of new meditators had dropped to practically zero. The introduction of MAV ensured, along with the clinical treatments, the commercialization of numerous products under its label, such as cosmetics, essential oils, complementary food products, herbal teas, spices, and so on. These products are mainly sold in MAV centers or by mail order, but they also can be bought beyond the boundaries of the movement, in shops selling natural products. It is clear that MAV has become a significant source of income for the movement.

Finally, it appears that with MAV and Vedic Science, Maharishi had found a more effective way to fulfill his mission. In fact, MAV's twenty approaches aim to work on the individual (mind, intellect, body, behavior, daily routine, lifestyle) as well as on the collective levels (environment, collective consciousness). As such, MAV and primarily TM aim to shape human life in order to create a new, neo-Vedic civilization. As Maharishi states:

> The Technology of the Unified Field is a purely scientific procedure for the total development of the human race. This is the time when objective, science-based progress in the world is being enriched by the possibility of total development of human life on earth, and that is the reason why we anticipate the creation of a unified field based ideal civilization. (1988: 35)[11]

The advent of this ideal civilization will depend on the time it takes for the people to know MAV and other aspects of Vedic Science and to introduce them in their daily lives.

CONDITIONS OF MAV'S ESTABLISHMENT IN THE WEST

With the introduction of MAV into his teaching, Maharishi started up a huge business of clinics, health centers, remedies, cosmetics laboratories, and so on. MAV also was integrated into the curriculum of the movement's Vedic universities and its effects investigated in its research laboratories. Books on the beneficial effects of MAV multiplied, as well as conferences where Indian doctors demonstrated pulse diagnosis, all backed by major publicity initiatives and articles in the media. In short, everything was done to make MAV known to a large public. The establishment and, above all, the development of MAV essentially depended on both the sociocultural context into which its practice was introduced and the strategies elaborated by the movement.

Maharishi introduced MAV in the West at the beginning of the 1980s. That particular moment coincided, on the one hand, with a more generalized public criticism of scientific medicine, together with increasing interest in alternative medical practices (such as acupuncture, shiatsu, etc.) and, on the other hand, with the emergence of a new type of spiritual quest and a corresponding worldview entering into all realms of life. This phenomenon has been identified by Champion as *nébuleuse mystique-ésotérique* (1990: 17–69), including the New Age, and it consists of groups and networks of various trends, influenced in particular by Oriental religions, esotericism, and transpersonal psychology (see also Heelas 1996: 15–132; Jeannotat 1996: 71–80, 2000: 150–52). Without going into detail about this broad and complex phenomenon with many facets and diverse practices, it must nevertheless be added that these different groups and movements have a number of common features, in particular:

- an approach of "mystical self-improvement" whose aim is the quest and realization of a certain state of being leading to salvation, the latter being seen as innerworldly. The emphasis will be put on the pursuit of happiness as a state of fulfilment and harmony, implying a particular concern for one's health and body (well-being, vitality, beauty, and so on).

- inner and personal experience prevailing on belief in order to find one's own spiritual path; the conceptions and dogmas particular to the official institutions are rejected, especially those of scientific medicine, churches, official science, and so on.

- a holistic view establishing the unity of all things, of man with God and the world, and leading to the wish for a global approach of health—taking into account its physical, mental, and spiritual aspects—as well as to various aspirations such as world peace and global consciousness.

- a sense of personal responsibility toward one's own life and the possibility to reach a state of global well-being, and consequently a desire for personal transformation through corporal and mental techniques or exercises, diet, astrology, and other divinatory practices, belief in karma, and so on.

- experimenting with nonordinary realities or modified states of consciousness, including astral travel, visions, or mystical experiences.

Such representations and concerns also are to be found in many other alternative medical practices in which the search for health appears as a true spiritual path. The different techniques they advocate (for example, mind-body techniques, massage, yoga, etc.) are presented as the means to arrive at an ultimate or a transcendent dimension, or to spiritual realization. Thus, the very concepts of MAV and its worldview found in the context of the 1970s and 1980s a favorable ground to establish itself in the West.

We also should recall that when Maharishi created his movement in the late 1950s and early 1960s, his primary aim was to establish TM on a global scale. He could only realize this ambition if there was a sufficient demand for TM, which required an organization sufficiently savvy and efficient to make TM known to the general public. To maintain and perpetuate its achievements, the organization not only had to ensure the development and sanctity of its operations, policies, and procedures, as well as its spiritual teachings, but also to find the financial and political means to support the whole structure.

Over the years, Maharishi structured and organized his movement one step at a time in order to spin a network of TM centers and educational institutions through the six populated continents.[12] His network included prominent public figures occupying key positions in society. For example, in 1967 and 1968, the Beatles and Mia Farrow frequented Maharishi's ashram in Rishikesh. This was widely noted in the media, to the great benefit of the movement (Melton 1986: 188). Other notable public figures included Buckminster Fuller, who spoke at a symposium sponsored by Maharishi in Amherst, Massachusetts, in 1971, a number of prominent scientists, including Nobel Prize-winning physicist Brian Josephson in the mid-1970s and, most notoriously, Ferdinand Marcos, the brutal dictator from the Philippines, in the late 1970s. Thus Maharishi had in his hands a powerful tool that provided him the financial means and channels necessary to enable him to spread his ideas. This network has been one of the key elements in the establishment of MAV in the West.

Organized on international and national levels in a "World Plan for Perfect Health," MAV was, at least initially, publicized and marketed through the TM centers, which organized courses and conferences on MAV and sold books and MAV products manufactured in the laboratories of the movement. Some centers also became health centers, where practitioners trained by the movement were consulted.

Having found its first users among the followers and other regular customers of the TM centers, MAV gradually began to reach a larger public due to the promotion in the media by the local TM centers, by movement advertising in popular yoga and New Age periodicals, and by movement initiatives to market its products in health food stores.

Furthermore, to introduce MAV in the West, Maharishi surrounded himself with prominent figures who gave him, at least on a symbolic level, significant support. These include, in particular, three prominent Indian ayurvedic doctors: B. D. Triguna, V. M. Dwivedi, and Balraj Maharshi, who took part in many conferences on MAV and who agreed to allow their pictures to be printed on the labels of MAV products. Triguna was president of the All India Ayurveda Congress for more than twenty years, and was granted by his peers the title "Raj Vaidya" (Baierlé 2002: 128). To show in public one of the Indian experts on Ayurveda together with other representatives of this medicine—all of them wearing the traditional dress—is designed to guarantee MAV's reliability and faithfulness to the tradition. In the same way, Maharishi conferred on MAV an aura of credibility and respectability by appointing Dr. Deepak Chopra, a practitioner trained in scientific medicine who has practiced in the United States, its main spokesperson, a position he retained until about 1993. In 1991, Chopra was embroiled in a controversy after the publication of a paper in the *Journal of the American Medical Association* (Sharma, Triguna, and Chopra 1991: 2633–37). As the *JAMA* required of all its authors, Chopra and his coauthors signed a statement attesting to the fact that they were in no way implicated in any organization that could benefit financially by the publication of their article. When the *JAMA* editors discovered that they had been misled, they immediately published a corrective as well as a paper on the TM movement and its practices (see Skolnick 1991: 1741–50).

Maharishi and his followers had excellent organizational and communication skills, as well as a remarkable capacity for anticipation. As we saw earlier, MAV was introduced in the West at the right moment, and the "product" also was ready for the flourishing alternative medicine market. When Maharishi arrived in the United States, he was willing to listen to his potential audience and ready to adapt his message to its needs. The different ways in which he formulated his ideas proved instrumental in enabling his teaching to take root in the West. The adaptive process that Maharishi's teaching in "Vedic Science" underwent stands in complete contradiction to its characterization as a "return" to the Indian philosophico-religious tradition, whether in the use of Sanskrit terms, in the frequent references to "Vedic texts," or in its general concepts.

CONTRIBUTION OF MAV TO THE UNDERSTANDING OF GLOBAL AYURVEDA

The sectarian aspect of the TM movement and the commercial interests of TM and MAV and their questionable reinterpretations of the medical and philosophical traditions have proven to be barriers to serious study of this important movement. Nevertheless, any attempt to better understand the phenomenon of global Ayurveda must inevitably consider the case of MAV, as it has played a major role in making Ayurveda known in the West. In fact, MAV was one of the most important early participants in the globalization of Ayurveda. It represents the first adaptation of Ayurveda intended for the Western public, and it has contributed to the shape, representations, and practices of the different groups that eventually became engaged with Ayurveda. MAV also popularized the practice of panchakarma in the West, as well as ayurvedic herbal teas and cosmetics, even if it has been overtaken by other ayurvedic initiatives in the last fifteen years. In this sense, comparing MAV's practices with those of other forms of Ayurveda in the West could provide significant information for the understanding of global Ayurveda.

We also have seen that *āsanas* (or Neuromuscular integration) and *prāṇāyāma* (or Neurorespiratory integration) were two of MAV's approaches. The integration of these practices as well as TM and the TM-Sidhi Program into MAV corresponds to the relationship that has been established between yoga and Ayurveda, especially in the West. The study of MAV can greatly contribute to current research on modern yoga, and vice versa.

Finally, the study of MAV raises a number of methodological problems, mainly because of the sectarian aspect of the TM movement. While there are numerous sources on MAV, most of them are of general rather than scientific interest, being intended for a large public. There are also sources intended for the training of MAV teachers and practitioners, but they are not available to outsiders. It also would be necessary to explore and discuss some of the concepts of Vedic Science with insiders. Such meetings are problematic, as the more specialized or detailed information is restricted to advanced teachings for which one has to pay considerable sums.[13] Another issue concerns the numerous structures surrounding the teaching and practice of MAV, including associations, foundations, corporations, companies, societies, TM health centers, schools, universities, and so on. Here also, the information that not only identifies but also distinguishes these structures and provides an understanding of their real function is almost impossible to obtain. The movement has blurred the distinction between spiritual or esoteric knowledge and trade secrets. In fact, in refusing to provide information, Maharishi contradicts his claim that his secularized knowledge, based on a historical outlook and scientific standards, is accessible to all.

To sum up, the greatest difficulty related to the study of MAV is access to information. Yet this also is characteristic of any research on practices of a spiritual nature that are taught within the context of contemporary movements. Thus the study of such practices also should lead to further methodological reflections, taking into account their particular configuration and background. The study of MAV is a good example of the problems found in such research, and in this sense it could greatly contribute to a wider reflection on how to develop a methodology better suited to the study of such practices.

NOTES

1. For example, the Banaras Hindu University, Varanasi (http://www.bhu.ac.in/ayurveda/course.htm), and the Arya Vaidya Pharmacy, Coimbatore (http://www.avpayurveda.com/educational_program.html), offer such special courses for foreigners.

2. Classical Ayurveda refers to the classical period in the history of Ayurveda, which "is marked by the advent of the first Sanskrit medical treatises, the *Caraka* and *Sushruta* Samhitas, which probably date from a few centuries before to several centuries after the start of the common era" (Zysk n.d.).

3. As far as Maharishi's concepts are concerned, I kept his own transcription of Sanskrit words (for example *dosha*, *yagya*, etc.). They appear italicized except in the term "TM-Sidhi," which is a registered name.

4. On the movement's conceptions of Vedic literature, see, for example, Wallace (1993: 217–50). For a brief discussion of the link between Ayurveda and Vedic literature, see Wujastyk (1998: 16–18).

5. This paragraph reproduces some elements of my paper on Vedic Science. See Jeannotat (1997: 1107–1108).

6. For a discussion of the term *svasthya*, see Halbfass (1991: 249–57). This phrase from *Bhagavad Gita* 2.48 is one of the most important passages from that text for Maharishi; see Maharishi (1971: 135 ff).

7. On the link between Maharishi's conceptions of the cosmology and Sāṃkhya, see Jeannotat (1997: 1108–11).

8. Maharishi Ayur-Ved Foundation (1991, Chart 30).

9. The movement publishes leaflets entitled "Maharishi Jyotish and Yagya Programmes," listing the dates in the month and the combination of days particularly favorable for the performance of *Yagyas*. See Maharishi (1996b).

10. In 1996, I personally experienced a "Maharishi panchakarma" in the Health Center of Seelisberg in Switzerland. See Jeannotat (2000: 153–61).

11. The "Technology of the Unified Field" is another title for TM.

12. The location of the different national health or TM centers can be found on the numerous Web sites of the movement. See, for example, http://www.tm.org; http://www.alltm.org; http://www.francemedicale.com.

13. I personally tried to establish contact at one of the movement's centers in Switzerland to discuss the approach of MAV. I was immediately directed to the paying courses proposed by the center. In India, on three occasions, I met one of the persons in charge of a MAV center in Delhi. I had not only to pay for the information given to me, but it also was impossible to go beyond the general information that can be found in the books published by the movement.

REFERENCES

Association Française pour la Promotion d'une Santé Parfaite. 1979. *Mémoire sur la promotion d'une santé parfaite grâce au programme de Méditation Transcendantale et de TM-Sidhi à Madame Simone Veil, ministre de la Santé et de la Famille, Gouvernement de la République Française*. West-Germany: MERU Press.

Baierlé, Pierre. 2002. *Ayur-Véda. Science de la joie*. Romont: Recto-Verso.

Champion, Françoise. 1990. La nébuleuse mystique-ésotérique. In *De l'émotion en religion. Renouveaux et traditions*, ed. Françoise Champion and Danièle Hervieu-Léger, 17–69. Paris: Centurion.

Chopra, Deepak. 1992. *La Santé Parfaite. Guide complet pour le corps et l'esprit*. Paris: A.L.T.E.S.S.

Esnoul, Anne-Marie. 1964. *Les strophes du Sāṃkhya. Texte sanscrit et traduction annotée*. Paris: Les Belles Lettres.

Finger, Joachim. 1987. *Gurus, Ashrams und der Westen. Eine religionswissenschaftliche Untersuchung zu den Hintergründen der Internationalisierung des Hinduismus*. Frankfurt am Main: Peter Lang.

Forem, Jack. 1976. *La méditation transcendantale*. Montréal: Les Editions de l'Homme.

Gibon, Yves de, and Jean Vernette. 1987. *Des sectes à notre porte*. Paris: Ed. du Chalet.

Haack, Friedrich-Wilhelm. 1980. *Des sectes pour les jeunes*. Paris: Mame.

Halbfass, Wilhelm. 1991. *Tradition and Reflection*. Albany: State University of New York Press.

Heelas, Paul. 1996. *The New Age Movement*. Oxford: Blackwell.

Jeannotat, Françoise. 1996. *De la quête de la santé à la quête du salut. Réflexion sur le recours aux pratiques thérapeutiques alternatives: L'exemple de l'ayurvéda. Equinoxe* 15: 71–80.

———. 1997. *La science védique Maharishi. Etudes Asiatiques* LI.4: 1105–12.

———. 2000. *Ayurvéda: Massages à l'huile, bains de vapeur et petites plantes. Les dessous d'une douceur annoncée*. In *Religions et violences. Sources et interactions*, ed. Anand Nayak, 149–61. Fribourg: Editions universitaires.

Maharishi Ayur-Ved. n.d. *Centre de santé par l'Ayur-Ved Maharishi*. Seelisberg, Suisse: Promotional Booklet.

Maharishi Ayur-Ved Foundation. 1991. *Maharishi Ayur-Ved: The Twenty Approaches of Maharishi Ayur-Ved to Create Perfect Health*. Chart 30.

Maharishi Mahesh Yogi. 1971. *On The Bhagavad-Gita. A New Translation and Commentary with Sanskrit Text. Chapter 1 to 6*. Harmondsworth: Penguin Books.

———. 1986. *Thirty Years around the World: Dawn of the Age of Enlightenment. Volume 1 1957–1964*. The Netherlands: MVU Press.

———. 1988. *World Assembly on Vedic Science: Life Supported By Natural Law. Lectures by His Holiness Maharishi Mahesh Yogi*. Fairfield, IA: Maharishi International University Press.

———. 1995. *The Science of Being and Art of Living: Transcendental Meditation*. New York: Meridian.

———. 1996a. *Maharishi Forum of Natural Law and National Law for Doctors*. India: Age of Enlightenment Publications.

———. 1996b. *Maharishi Jyotish and Yagya Programmes*. Valkenburg, the Netherlands: Leaflet.

———. 1997. *Maharishi Speaks to Students, vols. 1 and 4*. India: Age of Enlightenment Publications.

Melton, J. Gordon. 1986. *Encyclopedic Handbook of Cults in America*. New York: Garland.

Mitchiner, John. 1992. *Guru: The Search for Enlightenment*. New Delhi: Viking.

Sharma, Hari. 1993. *Freedom from Disease: How to Control Free Radicals, a Major Cause of Aging and Disease*. Toronto: Veda Publishing.

Sharma, Hari M., and Deepak Chopra. 1991. Letters: Maharishi Ayur-Veda: In reply. *JAMA* 266: 1774.

Sharma, Hari M., Brihaspati Dev Triguna, and Deepak Chopra. 1991. Maharishi Ayur-Ved: Modern insights into ancient medicine. *Journal of the American Medical Association* 265: 2633–37.

Sharma, P. V. 1981, 1983. *Carakasaṃhitā vol. I, II. Text with English Translation*. Varanasi: Chaukhambha Orientalia.

Sharma, Ram Karan, and Bhagwan Dash. 1977, 1983. *Carakasaṃhitā. Vol. I, II. Text with English Translation and Critical Exposition Based on Cakrapāṇi Datta's Ayurveda Dīpikā*. Varanasi: Chowkhamba Sanskrit Series Office.

SIMS/IMS. 1987. *TM aktuell. Informationsmagazin der SIMS/IMS-Internationale Meditationsgesellschaft Schweiz* 4: 14–15.

Skolnick, Andrew A. 1991. Maharishi Ayur-Veda: Guru's marketing scheme promises the world eternal "perfect health." *JAMA* 266: 1741–50.

Tourenne, Christian. 1981. *Vers une science de la conscience*. Paris: Les Editions de l'Age de l'Illumination.

Wallace, Robert Keith. 1993. *The Physiology of Consciousness: How Maharishi's Vedic Physiology and Its Practical Application, Maharishi Ayur-Ved, Can Solve the Problems of Individual and Collective Health and Raise Life to a New Level of Fulfillment*. Fairfield, IA: Maharishi International University Press.

Wujastyk, Dominik. 1998. *The Roots of Ayurveda: Selection from Sanskrit Medical Writings*. New Delhi: Penguin Books.

Zimmermann, Francis. 1993. Gentle purge: The flower power of Ayurveda. In *Paths to Asian Medical Knowledge*, ed. Charles Leslie and Allan Young, 209–23. New Delhi: Munshiram Manoharlal.

Zysk, Kenneth G. n.d. *Traditional Ayurveda*. http://www.hindu.dk, accessed October 2004.

CHAPTER 17

Maharishi Ayur-Veda™

Perfect Health™ through Enlightened Marketing in America

Cynthia Ann Humes

Through the development of Maharishi Ayur-Veda (MAV),[1] Maharishi Mahesh Yogi, founder of the Transcendental Meditation™ (TM) movement, became enormously influential in the 1980s and 1990s in popularizing Ayurveda in American culture. I here will primarily discuss the philosophical and business aspects of Maharishi's influential ayurvedic health system and note certain historical developments as they pertain to the American context.[2]

I proceed by organizing my arguments around distinctive features that make Maharishi's alternative health empire unique. The first aspect I explore is Maharishi's consistent privileging of a specific philosophy. Ananda Chopra notes that ayurvedic physicians throughout India have for centuries tended to be pragmatists with little interest in formulating a theoretical or philosophical system (Chopra 2003: 81). It is commonly regarded, however, that there are deep historical connections between early Ayurveda and the Sāṃkhya philosophical system. In contrast, Maharishi Ayur-Veda emerges from and consistently reflects Advaita Vedānta, the nondualistic system formulated by the eighth-century philosopher Śaṅkara.

I next turn to the practice of Transcendental Meditation, Maharishi's trademarked form of mantra meditation, whose purported benefits have been the subject of over 600 studies (*Scientific Research* 2000). A unique feature of Maharishi Ayur-Veda is its claim that the first (and most essential) step toward "Perfect Health" is the practice of TM.

The third section treats the unique way that Maharishi Ayur-Veda explains how the health system "works." Maharishi fuses his nondual philosophy with terms from Western science, particularly physics—for example, "quantum" healing and the "Unified Field." Yet this use of Western scientific terminology is merely a way of narrating a far earlier system: Vedic Science, the knowledge locked inside the ancient scriptures of Hindu India.

The fourth section centers on how Maharishi has set up an organization to support MAV. I sketch out the basic structures and programs, as well as some of his many offerings, and I indicate where his organization accords with other Ayurveda programs and where it differs. For example, I argue that these are marketed to maximize pampering and minimize potentially unattractive aspects of traditional Ayurveda. "Stressed" Westerners enjoy the products' exoticism, diversity, and aesthetic appeal, and their feel-good, enjoyable health regimen simultaneously caters to their desire to attain perfect health, despite glum prognoses from the standard medical establishment. Less attractive aspects of traditional Ayurveda are conveniently omitted. This method of spalike treatment, while privileging its essential Indian-ness, is not, however, simply to maximize MAV's exoticism; indeed, this method allows Maharishi and his ayurvedic practitioners to walk a fine line between medicine and religion in highly litigious America, following an unresolved but a potentially dangerous lawsuit filed in 1995 naming Maharishi Ayurveda Products International (MAPI) and various officials of MAV. Simply put, benign consumerism is safe, because it applies to everybody, avoids medical counseling, and situates religious participation in a protected context.

While American law prohibits the actual corporate licensing of herbs and plants, Maharishi is keenly aware of Western business practices and, indeed, many books that support the TM program employ the language of business to sell TM to people *in* business. I explore in the fifth section Maharishi's marketing model for his products and service franchising, that is, the authorization to conduct business to individuals using his name and his operating methods. I consider how this business model contributes to the creation of a positive product differentiation for his concoctions in a competitive alternative health market, even as it supports the preservation of the purity of Maharishi's teaching. By virtue of the many scientific tests purporting to demonstrate the value of Transcendental Meditation, the simple appendage of Maharishi's name to the products helps legitimate dozens of his remedies to the mass market and confirms their linkage to Vedic knowledge.

In the sixth and final section, I note that in Maharishi's universe, MAV has been rolled out as another complex service pack. Maharishi's philosophy and programming functions like an ERP (enterprise resource planning). It is an amalgamation of information systems and function-specific modules designed to bind more closely together all of his movement's functions.[3] As with all successful ERPs, literally hundreds of other potential products may be deployed in the future to fulfill the promise of a full-blown "enterprise" solution written in Maharishi's flavor of cosmic code.[4] The full Maharishi "Enlightenment Suite" offers the savvy consumer spiritual release while simultaneously exploiting new spiritual "technologies" to create ideal relationships, love, health, wealth, management, music, architecture, beauty, and more. I conclude with comments on Maharishi's profound influence on the development of Ayurveda in the West.

MAHARISHI MAHESH YOGI AND NONDUALISM

To understand the Maharishi conglomerate, one must begin with his philosophy, for it serves as the interpretive lens through which Maharishi explains how his entire operating system works. Maharishi was a disciple of Brahmananda Saraswati. Known in the TM movement simply as Guru Dev, he served in the mid-twentieth century as the Śaṅkarācārya, or chief pontiff, of the Jyotir Maṭh hermitage, said to be established by Śaṅkara in the late eighth century CE. Advaita Vedānta as systematized by Śaṅkara posits (among other things) that human beings suffer in *samsāra*, the endless cycle of birth and death. The ultimate goal of human endeavor, then, is to find release (*mokṣa*) from this bondage to *saṃsāra*. The principal means of liberation for the proponent of Advaita is knowledge (*jñāna*) of one's true nature, for one's bondage is due to ignorance of one's true self (*avidyā*). Liberation is none other than realizing this true nature, which is *ātman*, the Cosmic Self, precisely equated with *brahman*, or the ultimate abstract absolute.

Perhaps the most distinguishing feature of Advaita Vedānta is its concept of *māyā*, or cosmic illusion. *Māyā* operates as a filter between the world as we conventionally know it, rendering it inherently false (*mithya*) and obscuring the true perception (*satya*) of the identity of *brahman* and *ātman*. Maharishi has not emphasized *māyā* in his teachings, possibly because the modern world has little use for the idea that the world is unreal. His emphasis, instead, has been that liberating knowledge of *brahman* is obtained through direct experience of the Cosmic Self, mediated exclusively by his own oral teachings rather than through the study of texts. In this understanding, *māyā* is presented as a type of *jñāna*. Advaita, presented by Śaṅkara and acceded to by Maharishi, promises that through knowledge, a person can become liberated even while living. The enlightened person who experiences himself as *brahman* does not return to *samsāra*, the cycle of rebirth. For Maharishi, Transcendental Meditation is his guru's rediscovered means for directly experiencing *brahman*; it is distinctly unlike other forms of meditation; and it is intended for householders rather than renunciates.

In 1955, Maharishi experienced a revelation that he had a divine mission to spread spiritual regeneration to the entire world (Humes 2005: 62). Conspicuously, he taught his master's advaitic message through metaphors and analogies rooted in Western scientific concepts, even as he invoked a "science of the soul":

> The spirit or soul is the basic motive force of our existence and spirituality is the science of that motive force. The material science of today speaks highly of atomic power. Today the political power of a nation depends upon its resources of atomic energy. But we in India know that the atomic energy is not the basic motive power of our existence. It can only be called the basic motive force of material existence, because it is found to be very gross when compared with the powers of our mental and spiritual existence. That is the reason why India laid more importance on the field of the soul which is the ultimate motive power behind our life in all its aspects; spiritual, mental and physical. That is the reason why India always regarded the science of the soul as the best and most useful of all sciences. This is the reason why His Holiness has called spirituality as the backbone of India.[5]

Since 1955, Maharishi has not wavered in his view that the world is best understood through the superior Indian science of the soul, whose subject is *brahman*, a field of knowledge even more subtle and fine than the smallest atom. Maharishi's special gift, his core intellectual property, is his ability to transmute Western science into his vision of Advaita Vedānta that he calls "Vedic Science." And all human beings, because we can all become enlightened, are potential proponents of Vedic Science, and by no accident consumers of his products.

"PERFECT HEALTH" AND THE PRACTICE OF TRANSCENDENTAL MEDITATION

Maharishi claimed that his simple technique of mantra meditation was the gift of Guru Dev, and its practice allowed anyone to access the true self, or *ātman*, which was none other than *brahman*: being, consciousness, and bliss (*saccidānanda*).

> Although nothing is new in the realm of the soul the experience of it which was thought to be very difficult has now

> become very easy under the grace of Guru Deva. . . . Kerala Maha Sammelam is raising a voice that under the universal benevolence of Shri Guru Deva, MIND CONTROL IS EASY, PEACE IN DAILY LIFE IS EASY AND EXPERIENCE OF ATMANANDAM (Bliss of the Self) IS EASY. (Mahesh 1955)

The promise that his form of meditation was uniquely open to everyone and easier to adopt than other approaches to enlightenment eventually translated to terrific success. But even more significant than the claim that meditation could lead to enlightenment was Maharishi's claim that meditation relieved "stress." Indeed, Jerry Jarvis, the most successful TM teacher in America (and perhaps the world) in the 1960s and 1970s,[6] once told me that Maharishi joked to him that of the two outcomes of TM, people preferred release from stress over release from bondage. According to TM literature, millions have eventually lined up to be taught the simple technique.[7] TMers were told to meditate for twenty minutes twice a day and to go about their normal routine, assured that their chosen path to a "stress-free" life and enlightenment involved no change in lifestyle beyond whatever they might choose for themselves.

Beginning early in 1971, Maharishi asked his "initiators," teachers of his technique, to speak to the public exclusively using the new terminology set forth in a series of thirty-three videotapes called the "Science of Creative Intelligence™" (SCI). SCI was an encompassing term for Maharishi's advaitic teachings. This new mode of discourse was important for TM in America because it represented another step toward substituting Western terms for Brahmanical theological notions in an attempt to garner Western scientific support for the value of Maharishi's teachings. True to his Advaita heritage, Maharishi advocated a spiritual ideal that could be experienced here, in this world, within this lifetime. Enlightenment, he taught, is experienced within the context of the mind and body, and thus contacting the *ātman* through meditation results in measurable effects on a person's physiology. Scientific research in support of TM's health benefits helped clinch the movement's new respectability and attracted academics, researchers, and intellectuals. Virtually all scientific study of the Transcendental Meditation technique concerns its effect on physiology and potential health disorders.[8]

Although Maharishi insisted that the benefits of TM were scientifically verifiable, the TM technique itself was soon deemed religious. In 1977, the judge in a New Jersey court case (*Malnak v. Yogi*) decided in favor of the plaintiffs' claim that Transcendental Meditation was a religious practice.[9] As initiators anxiously awaited the judgment, memos came down from national TM headquarters urging them to take caution to appear nonreligious. Teachers and meditators alike were asked to refrain from saying "Jai Guru Dev," their usual term of greeting in public, and to put away their devotional pictures of Guru Dev and Maharishi. TM teachers were implored to avoid spiritual terms in their lectures and courses.[10] The court's finding that TM was religious presaged the later 1995 lawsuit that had a similarly formative effect on the movement's development.

After the decision was eventually confirmed to all TMers, Maharishi accepted the court's determination and made it clear publicly to all TMers in America that to start the TM program no lifestyle change was required, but to continue along the path to cosmic consciousness, numerous new commitments and product consumption were recommended, if not expected. According to Maharishi's voluminous literature, in 1978, he inaugurated the "Ideal Society Campaign in 108 Countries" and created the World Peace Project, which consisted of sending teams of "Yogic Flyers" to the most disturbed parts of the world to calm the violence through meditation. These were meditators, mostly TM teachers—by now called "Governors of the Age of Enlightenment," or simply "Governors," who were taught a new, additional technique called "yogic flying." These techniques were based on Maharishi's practical interpretation of Chapter 3 of Patañjali's *Yoga Sūtras*. That same year, he also formulated his "Absolute Theories of Government, Education, Health, Defense, Economy, Management, and Law and Order" so that all would know what an Ideal Society would look like. And the Ideal Society looked, at least to the general public, like Hinduism.

Of course, one was not to abandon the original practice of TM. Supplemental packages were delivered in yearly upgrades. Specifically, the standard SCI program popularized in the late sixties and early seventies was repackaged as a more high-tech platform, complete with new explanations and products supposedly based on the Vedas, the earliest, and at least mythically central, core of Sanskrit scriptures.[11] Dedicated Western disciples of Maharishi were taught to adopt traditionally Hindu cultural warrants, religious markers, and the philosophy of Advaita to secure the highest promises of TM. And one of these upgrades was Maharishi Ayur-Veda, which emerged in 1985, when Maharishi brought out complete expositions not only of Ayur-Veda but also Gandharva-Veda, Dhanur-Veda, Sthapatya-Veda, and Jyotish, all with the combined purpose to create a disease-free, problem-free world.[12]

In Maharishi Ayur-Veda literature, readers are informed that classical ayurvedic texts caution that to treat a patient effectively, the physician must act holistically. Each of us has three aspects—consciousness, mind, and body—and it is the attention to consciousness that "distinguishes Maharishi Ayur-Veda™."[13] Most non-TM/-MAV ayurvedic physicians or *vaidyas* do not prescribe meditation. Somewhat more often, but by no means as a general practice, they prescribe *yajñas* (always spelled in the Hindi-ized form "*yagya*" in TM circles), or Sanskrit-based rituals performed by Brahman priests. Though Maharishi has increasingly emphasized the benefits of these in the last two decades, often at a hefty cost to the meditator (for this, too, has been institutionalized in the TM Movement), his primary emphasis has continued to be on meditation and the development of consciousness. When all is said and done, ill health is caused due to our own "mistake of the intellect"—*Pragya Aparadh* (Sanskrit: *prajñāparādha*), forgetting the underlying unity, leading to faulty judgment of how to act with regard to health, thus acting out of accordance with natural law.[14] By failing to understand our true nature, we become estranged from the ultimate source of universal consciousness, and we fall ill.

In describing this unique approach to Ayurveda, Hari Sharma and Christopher Clark explain that Maharishi consistently privileges his belief that "the basis of health is consciousness." They note, "In the last few years, Maharishi has placed MAV into a larger context, Maharishi's Vedic Approach to Health," and they quote Maharishi:

> There is an inseparable, very intimate relationship between the unmanifest field of consciousness and all the manifest levels of the physiology: that is why Maharishi's Vedic Approach to Health handles the field of health primarily from the most basic area of health—the field of consciousness—through the natural approach of consciousness, Transcendental Meditation.[15]

One must adopt the "technologies of consciousness of MAV" to reboot one's system, if you will, and thereby "overcome pragya-aparadh—to 'restore memory' of the unified field."[16]

The concept of *pragya-aparadh* in MAV mirrors Maharishi's basic advaitic interpretation of *avidyā*. Just as *avidyā,* or ignorance, of our true self is the cause of bondage, with *jñāna,* or knowledge, as its antidote, so *pragya-apradh* is the cause of ill health, and *jñāna,* through tapping the field of consciousness by TM, is its antidote. To communicate to Americans how *pragya-aparadh* can be overcome by *jñāna,* Maharishi employs the more familiar language of science.

PHYSICS, MAHARISHI AYUR-VEDA, AND "QUANTUM HEALING"

Maharishi holds an undergraduate degree in physics from the University of Allahabad. To formulate his theoretical system for Maharishi

Ayur-Veda, he has fused Advaita philosophy with Indian medicine as well as with Western physics. In particular, Maharishi's understanding of *brahman*, or Ultimate Reality, functions as the linchpin between both.

All Advaitins agree that *brahman* is the sole cause of the universe. That is, all hold that *brahman* is both the instrumental and material cause of the universe. Creation proceeds out of *brahman*, even as all believe that *brahman* is eternal and changeless. *Brahman* is pure Being itself. At a 1971 conference held by Maharishi in Amherst, Massachusetts, physicist Lawrence Domash affirmed,

> I'm proposing that what we're doing in meditation is actually consciously experiencing the quantum mechanical level of the mind. Maharishi has said that science is destined to discover pure Being; it is possible that science has already discovered pure Being in the form of the so-called "vacuum state" of the quantum theory, which has within it all the possible excited states of particles, but in an unrealized, ever-fluctuating form.[17]

After Domash finished his comments, Maharishi enthusiastically continued,

> It is interesting to hear that the vacuum state of the quantum theory draws upon the fullness of Being, and Transcendental Meditation gives the direct experience of it. These are, I believe, the first significant expressions in the history of science to connect the principles of physical phenomena with the experience of non-physical nature. The turning point in the history of physics has begun, and it has begun well with the recognition of the subjective experience from the objective viewpoint. In this realization, what we find is the fulfillment of physics in its quest for the ultimate Reality. Dr. Domash's unique interpretation of the quantum field theory has erected a bridge between physics and metaphysics.[18]

Maharishi was not the first thinker to promote direct connections between quantum theory and religion.[19] His unique contribution was to promote the belief that all Western sciences were merely branches of his Science of Creative Intelligence, which is a cultural and linguistic refinement of the same Science of the Soul he mentioned as early as 1955. All Western sciences except physics are simply analyses of phenomenal things in and of themselves. Quantum physics is an exception because it centers on basic cosmic structures, thus Maharishi's claim that it bridges physics and metaphysics. And so, since the 1971 symposium, Maharishi has publicly pushed the relationship between physics and SCI above all others—often even borrowing terms from the former to explain the latter.[20] And Deepak Chopra, another Maharishi protegé, would attempt to extend the nonlocal model from physics to physiology, using it as a basis to explain the value of traditional Indian medicine in his 1989 book *Quantum Healing*.

Maharishi's theory of the "quantum mechanical body" rests on his view that all particles and subparticles of reality are infused with consciousness, an assertion he made as early as 1965 in his commentary on *Bhagavad Gita* 3.11: "Through yagya you sustain the gods and those gods will sustain you. By sustaining one another, you will attain the highest good." Maharishi comments,

> The "gods" mentioned here are the deities presiding over the innumerable laws of nature, which are present everywhere throughout relative life. They are the powers governing different impulses of intelligence and energy, working out the evolution of everything in creation. The existence of gods may be understood by an analogy: each of the myriad cells in the human body has its own level of life, energy and intelligence; together, these innumerable lives produce human life. A human being is like a god to all these small impulses of energy and intelligence, each with its own form, tendencies, sphere of activity and influence, working for the purpose of evolution.[21]

By understanding the powers governing different impulses of intelligence and energy as "gods," Maharishi translates Hindu concepts of divinizing material components into the language of science, which preserves another product line, Maharishi Yagya, as pointed out earlier, rituals dedicated to influencing these eponymous "laws of nature."

In modern physics, the unified field is the objective reality of nature; consciousness is understood to be a subjective experience. Maharishi's "Vedic Science" rejects this fundamental principle. Maharishi says that the ground state of physics and the ground state of consciousness are the same. When he uses the term *Unified Field*, he means the Unified Field as amplified by Vedic Science, and therefore it includes both objective and subjective aspects. Thus "objective and subjective aspects of nature are seen as but two manifest modes of this unified field at the unmanifest basis of existence." Accepting his "Unified Field" theory that all of creation is infused with intelligence at the "quantum" level, no part of the body lives apart from the rest; each molecule has consciousness and can be transformed, since all coexist in webs of relation. Thus as higher frames of consciousness shift, so will the body. For this reason, by healing the consciousness, Maharishi insists, the entire body can be healed.

Yet a lot is required to heal one's consciousness. For instance, MAV constitutes a whole complex of approaches to health that may include meditation, pulse diagnosis, diets keyed to body type and personality, purification techniques, yoga, music therapy, aromatherapy and, of course, herbal remedies. Each packaged product is available for the asking price to anyone, whether or not they meditate, although persons are strongly advised to begin meditation if they have not yet done so. Attractive color catalogs and brochures display the varying products and services for sale. The panchakarma purification techniques include massage and stimulation of *marmas* (energy points in the body), healing oils, and cleansing enemas. Health is achieved when the forces of the body and mind are in balance.

Balance can be achieved only after diagnosing the patient's mind and body type. The three fundamental principles of physical manifestation (*doṣa*) influence health and govern all the activities of one's mind and body, and in MAV their description does not stray from fairly common interpretations. *Vāta* is associated with an enthusiastic nature, a restless mind, anxiousness, a tendency toward overexertion, and occasional insomnia. *Pitta* is characterized by a sharp intellect, orderliness, a tendency to anger quickly and be demanding. *Kapha* appears as an easygoing disposition, lethargy, and tendency to gain weight easily. *Marmas*, however, are understood in a unique sense. They are connecting points between the mind and body, "where consciousness becomes the material structure of the quantum mechanical body."[22] By gently stimulating the 107 classical *marma* points, with the appropriate Maharishi approved, *doṣa*-specific oil, energy blockages can be reduced, and the flow of energy and "intelligence" or proper consciousness can be reestablished throughout the body.[23]

A final philosophical innovation in MAV occurred at the hand of Dr. Anthony (Tony) Nader, who is credited on Maharishi Web sites as "the world's foremost neuroscientist, who discovered that the human physiology is a direct, material reflection of the field of consciousness, the field traditionally known as Veda, which in the language of modern physics is the Unified Field of all the Laws of Nature."[24] The significance of Nader's discovery is that "through proper education, every individual can have direct access to the Unified Field—the source of all the laws of nature governing the Universe—in the simplest form of human awareness."[25] And most crucially, "Access to this Unified Field brings mastery over Natural Law," Nader has been credited with saying, remarkably in unison with Maharishi's original theses in South India over forty years earlier.[26] Nader has painstakingly linked forty aspects of the Vedic corpus to forty qualities of Natural Law, and to forty expressions of human physiology. Thus, for example, the *Sāma Veda* has the quality of the natural law of flowing wakefulness, and its expression in physiology is the sensory systems.[27] We are all "living, breathing, talking embodiment of Veda—a storehouse of pure knowledge, pure intelligence, pure orderliness, happiness, and organizing power. Every person has a blueprint for living perfect health and a perfect life within his or her own body."[28]

Tony Nader's *Human Physiology: Expression of Veda and the Vedic Literature* has been rolled out as a culminating element in a panoply of products whose greatest promise is their function within a full-blown "enterprise" solution. His research is surely the capstone, for it was the scientific discovery that "offers the full disclosure of the Total Knowledge of Natural Law—Unity in diversity and diversity in Unity. It raises the status of every individual to Cosmic dimensions, bringing to light the secrets of the peaceful, problem-free administration of the universe through Natural Law."[29]

This discovery is at the base of one of the newest services in MAV: Maharishi Vedic Vibration Technology or MVVT, a service that promises "to awaken the body's own intelligence" to relieve chronic disorders. MVVT consists of a trained professional softly uttering in a patient's ears select mantras from Vedic texts that are "targeted" for specific physiological problems or areas in keeping with Dr. Nader's discoveries on linkages between the body and the Vedas. The underlying belief is that the body is rooted in physics wave/particle theory. The body is itself a vibration, so when the MVVT practitioner blows softly over the patient's body, she or he provides the proper "vibrations" to enliven the powers resident in the body to counteract disease.

BUILDING MAV IN AMERICA

Maharishi inaugurated the Program for Chronic Disorders in 1994, because "nearly half the [American] population suffers from chronic disease, and in many ways our modern medical system has failed them."[30] However, Maharishi assures us that the "Maharishi Vedic Approach to Health is destined to create a disease-free, healthy, enlightened society."[31]

Prior to announcing this ambitious new program, Maharishi had begun to set up an organization to accomplish it. He abandoned the more traditional mode of ayurvedic training and education conducted through apprenticeships in nonhospital settings. Instead, he followed the strategy of leaders of the ayurvedic revivalist movement in early twentieth-century India, who adopted what was understood as "modern" biomedical technology, pairing that technology with European institutional forms. They founded ayurvedic pharmaceutical companies, colleges, and professional associations.[32] Over the last two centuries "these revivalists used the ideology of medical revivalism to create parallel institutions, parallel medicine, a 'professionalized' system of ayurvedic knowledge for the modern Indian state."[33] Also like these same revivalists, Maharishi located authentic Ayurveda in the ancient texts. However, Maharishi was quite unlike the revivalists in one respect:

> [T]hey sought to cleanse Ayurveda of the ritual esoterica and magical practices that had always existed side by side with rational therapies in early practice. In doing so, they recast Ayurveda as a great tradition that had to be differentiated from the "folk" or little traditions that were a sign of Indian backwardness.[34]

Maharishi would continue his rituals (*yagya*) and what might be characterized as "magical practices" by virtue of reinterpreting them in light of his Vedic Science.

Chronic disease does not just happen. Indeed, "much chronic disease begins with the choices a person makes every day—the choice to eat healthy or unhealthy foods, to avoid or to court stress, to listen to the body when it cries for rest or to force it to function even when fatigued. We call these wrong choices 'violations of Natural Law,' and such violations, over the long run, create disease."[35] I explained earlier how the belief that the "mistake of the intellect"—*pragya aparadh*—can be alleviated in part through meditation. Meditation naturally helps instill better choices in practitioners. But there are many other questions of behavior, and Maharishi is prepared to provide answers to all realms of activity for the mistaken individual, as he has discovered the Natural Laws and how to countermand those violations.

Just as he accomplished with meditation, wherein he introduced the practice of the initiator, eliminating the need for a "guru-to-student" transmission of the mantra, Maharishi has created a simplified system of body typing presided over by his core of *vaidyas*, who are trained at his ayurvedic instructional centers. All Western MAV physicians are allopathic doctors who have received special MAV training with qualified *vaidyas* from India who work for Maharishi. The patient is urged to travel to special centers for professional guidance, and thereby to improve his or her quality of life by adoption of Maharishi's many services and specialized products.[36]

MAV has reacted to the American context not just in terms of its potential consumer appeal but also in terms of potential legal challenge.

In the Flint case, two issues emerged: fraud and consent. Jonie Flint filed suit against the famous Dr. Deepak Chopra, Dr. Brihaspati Dev Triguna (a renowned expert in pulse diagnosis from New Delhi), the Sharp Institute, and MAPI. Flint's husband David had consulted Triguna in 1993 while suffering from leukemia. After David Flint died, his wife filed suit, charging that the defendants had fraudulently obtained $10,000 for useless ayurvedic services and products, and according to Jonie Flint's complaint, Triguna was represented as a licensed health professional, when in fact he was not. Jonie Flint did not have the resources to pursue her suit, so the case was never resolved. The questions the case posed, however, reveal a problem regarding the position of Ayurveda as practice or business in America. Are *vaidyas* to be understood in American medical regulatory schemes as "licensed medical physicians" with wide professional privileges and responsibilities, or should they be legally defined as "religious healers," with constitutional exemptions from medical licensing laws? If the former, then informed consent and the potential legal, structural, and cultural problems of their enforcement would pertain. If the latter, then the efforts to revolutionize modern medicine are compromised.[37]

Parallel to the outcome of *Malnak v. Yogi*, Maharishi seems to have moved forward in a similar trajectory. After the Flint case, MAV has continued to provide scientific-sounding interpretations of what most people interpret to be religious phenomena, thus walking a fine line between religion and medicine. He has kept distant from elaborate prescriptive and herbal remedies that could be found legally fraudulent, and only in the case of panchakarma has he instituted the practice of requiring consent forms. He has developed his connections with ayurvedic practitioners carefully, often privileging established *vaidyas* of Indian origin or ethnicity.[38] He also has built into the client's range of expectations some personal responsibility for the treatment's success.

Maharishi has institutionalized a new paradigm of Ayurveda—it is a traditional science, yet verifiable under the test of allopathic methodology. It is simultaneously "authentic" and cutting edge. Yet much of MAV does not look like what most Indian Ayurveda practitioners would recognize as authentic, nor mainstream, allopathic doctors as science. Maharishi adopted New Age institutional frameworks such as seminars and retreats under the rubric of holistic healing. Customers were encouraged to come to luxury spas to be treated and pampered with individualized attention, particularly for panchakarma. Yet the panchakarma Maharishi taught was pruned of the more unappealing aspects, such as emetics. The Raj, located in Maharishi Vedic City,[39] exemplifies this kinder, gentler new entrepreneurial approach to MAV offerings—oil treatments, massages, body typing, MVVT sound treatments, and more—among those who find such pampering appealing, and not necessarily among those who accept Maharishi's philosophy and spiritual program. In this sense, MAV has found a larger audience than most of Maharishi's other products, leading to issues of branding and product quality control.

BRANDING THE MAHARISHI

During the *Malnak v. Yogi* crisis, a two-page memorandum was sent to "All Departments" by Lenny Goldman, one of the chief lawyers for the TM movement in Fairfield, Iowa, regarding the "Proper use of term: "Transcendental Meditation." Goldman describes how the World Plan Executive Council (WPEC) was in the process of seeking to register as "service marks" in all countries around the world all terms identifying movement activities, such as Transcendental Meditation (TM) and Science of Creative Intelligence (SCI). The success of registration applications depended on their proper use; accordingly, he describes a service mark as "a word, phrase, or design which distinguishes the source of a particular service from other sources." By associating these terms with WPEC's services, he continues, people enrolling in programs can be assured they come from the same source. This recognition, he explains, serves the following important functions: "(1) It helps and protects the public: (a) by distinguishing our services from others so that people make easy and accurate choices; and (b) by serving as a guarantee of consistent quality. (2) It helps us to advertise our services."[40]

Maharishi's way to take advantage of an avid consumer base while preserving his unique mode of Ayurveda is to develop a service marked and franchised model of branding by appending his own name to each and every constituent in his product line, and acting to ensure quality control. Architects can learn Maharishi's style of proper building design, for example, and then construct homes according to his Maharishi Sthapatya-Veda, having been granted the right, that is, the franchise, to carry on that certain line of business as controlled by Maharishi, that is, the franchiser.[41]

Kevin McFarlane comments about a similar style of marketing adopted in the corporate world: "A former soap salesman, Rowland Hanson, hired by Microsoft in its early days, came up with the idea of including the Microsoft name in every product. Hence, not just Windows, Word, Excel but Microsoft Windows, Microsoft Word, Microsoft Excel. Simple, but effective. A glance at the IT press provides an indication of how often Microsoft products are referred to by their full names."[42] The appendage of Maharishi's name to his product line helps introduce and legitimize dozens of his remedies, just as the Microsoft name helps introduce and legitimize new software products. The perception among technology end users, that "Microsoft is more likely than others to produce better-designed applications for its own operating system,"[43] is equally true for adherents of Maharishi's system, who are primed to be open to his new services and products. These I will address in turn.

Whereas the traditional *vaidya* or ayurvedic physician treated his patients individually, diagnosing and then formulating concoctions to treat all of the complexity of the patient's symptoms or describing how patients could create appropriate mixtures themselves, Maharishi has created many common blends of ingredients to treat common problems for his large flock.[44]

The Maharishi Ayur-Veda product line employs a mass-market approach to reach out beyond TMers, and one need not go to a Maharishi *vaidya* to take advantage of many of his products. Once people are typed according to problem/*doṣa*/gender, or by their own self-diagnosis through helpful explanations in MAV advertisements, customers are free to purchase products at their own discretion. Since one needs to keep purchasing herbs, and since anyone is free to purchase them, these products are potentially more profitable than one-time initiation fees for meditation. Although non-TMers may not be able to enlighten themselves, they may still improve through use of the concoctions, and if the products help, they may even encourage consumers to look at the other products in Maharishi's line.

The urge to control his product line is shown forcefully in the example of Maharishi's one-time protégé, Deepak Chopra. Encouraged and supported by Maharishi himself, endocrinologist Chopra began to study with Maharishi's head Ayurveda specialist, Brihaspati Dev Triguna. Subsequently, Chopra established the Maharishi Vedic Health Center in Lancaster, Massachusetts. Chopra possessed an unusual ability to explain complex Ayurveda teachings in simple language, providing great exposure and credibility to Maharishi's medical programs. Chopra was elevated first to the presidency of the newly minted American Association of Ayur-Vedic Medicine. Shortly thereafter, Maharishi referred to him publicly as "Dhanvantari of Heaven on Earth," a richly symbolic title, evocative of Vedic mythology's Dhanvantari: the physician to the gods themselves.

Chopra could speak with health care professionals or a television audience with equal ease, and he was as much at home in the West as he was in his native Delhi. He was—and continues to be—charismatic and intellectually compelling. Soon he was establishing Maharishi Ayur-Veda as the most successful of Maharishi's new programs, and while doing so, gaining fame of his own. This led to conflict among the TM ranks.

Eventually, Chopra left Maharishi. According to one reporter, Chopra believed his association with the TM was compromising his credibility.[45] He says Chopra told him that he was rejected for a television show with Bill Moyers for fear of his association with TM. And in 1991 he was roundly attacked by his professional colleagues for an article he wrote for the *Journal of the American Medical Association.*

Chopra was drawing so much heat and so little reward, "Right after the *JAMA* thing, I left the movement. . . . I said, 'Who needs this?' " He continued, "I didn't want to be restricted by being TM's representative. I felt that if I confined myself to just this, a whole body of knowledge [Ayur-Vedic medicine] that could find legitimacy would never do it."[46]

As a result of Chopra's departure, on July 16, 1993, the "Maharishi National Council of the Age of Enlightenment" wrote to all TM centers in America. Not only had Deepak Chopra left the movement, the National Council affirmed, but "Dr. Chopra has said that the Centers, Governors, Teachers, Sidhas and Meditators 'should ignore him and not try to contact him or promote him in any way.' " The council went on to say,

> Accordingly, we should discontinue promoting him, his courses, tapes and books (including *Creating Health, Return of the Rishi, Perfect Health, Quantum Healing, Unconditional Life,* etc.). Since he is no longer affiliated with our Movement in any way, if you happen to hear that Dr. Chopra is coming to your area to lecture you should in no way try to contact him or organize for him. This is extremely important for the purity of the teaching.

No matter which position you take on who owns the intellectual property to "quantum healing," Chopra offers an extremely user-friendly flavor of the advaitic Ayurveda operating system. By providing more accessible explanations, he remains an industry leader, offering an array of alternatives competing both with his former rishi as well as with the Western medical establishment for consumer health dollars.

Maharishi's effort to control the message and content of spiritual services among his adherents mirrors a commercial tradition most Americans would recognize: supposed "quality control issues" in a franchiser/franchisee relationship. McDonald's, for example, requires its franchises to stick to the corporate agenda, as well as to order food products and paper goods solely through their parent company. Maharishi also expects his franchisees—teachers, meditators, *vaidyas*, and so on—to use his products, and, preferably, his alone.[47]

Might Maharishi's strategies function as a kind of "product differentiation"—that is, does his insistence on only Maharishi-approved products help his line of wares be perceived as higher quality, even if no real difference exists? In their literature, Maharishi's companies make explicit claims that only his products are truly superior and can meet the needs of the spiritual consumer. Are competing products capable of achieving similar effects? Are these measures to assure quality—the purity of the Teaching or the Big Mac or Maharishi Amrit Kalash—or is it a marketing ploy to make an additional profit selling the goods that are prescribed as necessary components?

While it is tempting to ascribe a mundane and cynical motive to this, a philosophical warrant exists in support of this strategy. One cannot simply heed the Self and one's own assessment of goods and services in lieu of a Master's discretion. Whereas before the mid-seventies "Guru Dev" was on every TMer's lips, the emphasis shifted so that virtually everything Maharishi touched bore his name: it is Maharishi who would determine appropriate goods and services.[48]

THE ENTERPRISE SOLUTION: THE MICROCOSM AND MACROCOSM

Maharishi gained the interest of Americans with a simple technique that promised to relieve stress. Decades later, he had found the nondual blueprints for perfection in every realm of life, embodied—literally—within every individual. Throughout, he has continued to act on his 1955 pronouncement that India is the source of a superior "science of the soul," which must be communicated to the world. For Maharishi, the first step one must take is connecting with Pure Consciousness through the practice of TM. But atop this foundation, he has rolled out a number of new forms of ancient "sciences" based on his understanding of the Vedas: political science based on "natural law," food supplements and Ayurveda treatments, strict diets according to diagnosed body types, "life supporting" music (*Gandharva Veda*), dwellings built in accordance with natural law (*Sthapatya Veda*), astrological consultations (*jyotish*), postural yoga, and rituals (*yagyas*) performed out of one's purview by priests to avoid natural calamity.

The Maharishi enterprise solution has continued to find an audience for many good business reasons. He has been persistent and not complacent, always seeking improvements and additions, never content to stand still. To "ensure the purity of the teaching," Maharishi acts to offer approved products that he discovers to be in accordance with Natural Law should competitive teachings or spiritual products arise.

Yet as Chopra intimated, selling Maharishi's entire Ayurveda package (much less his full rack of programs) to Americans is still a challenge. For one, his explanations—although consistent—are complicated and unappealing to most Americans. The movement also clearly privileges the supremacy of Maharishi's version of thought about Ayurveda. By situating itself as rediscovered "truth," MAV represents itself as the entirety of the Ayurveda tradition, thus ignoring and even rejecting diversity in Ayurveda, which is an exclusionary tendency anathema to many Americans who are interested in Ayurveda. Finally, those people that Maharishi places in positions of leadership bear titles that some find outlandish and peculiar, leading to public skepticism about the entirety of MAV and Maharishi's movement in general. The reader will recall that at one time Chopra was the "Dhanvantari of Medicine" before he resigned from Maharishi's universe. Subsequent to Chopra's departure (and consequent ostracism), Maharishi appointed Tony Nader as his chief protégé. "Dr. Raja Raam Nader" is the new "sovereign ruler," "King," or "Raja" of Maharishi's utopia. Protected by an "invincible shield" created by the sustained protective meditation of thousands of "yogic flyers,"[49] this new world order exists by virtue of Maharishi's decree and is maintained by his followers through their shared willingness to believe and participate.

Deepak Chopra took pains not to chain himself just to the Hindu tradition, and especially just to Maharishi Ayur-Veda, because he wanted to broaden his appeal to a more diverse America, and potentially, the world. In contrast, Dr. Nader—King Nader, who underwent a Vedic coronation ceremony—resolved to link quantum healing firmly to the Vedas, underscoring Maharishi's system as his own brand of Vedic Science, albeit a system global in application.

This outcome is a long way from the 1960s, when Maharishi declared his method of TM to be perennial, transcultural. He argued that anyone, espousing any religion, would benefit from his mantra "technology." TM was supported by personal experience and, since the early seventies, empiricism and numerous scientific studies. As Maharishi gradually incorporated many facets commonly understood as "Hinduism," distinguished from the old, unimproved Vedic wisdom by his unique spellings and his name-brand recognition, all individual experience and even one's body came to be interpreted through the advaitic belief system Maharishi provides. Thus despite declaring his insights to be "perennial," "primordial," timeless truth accessible to each person, for Maharishi, the perennial truth is fundamentally Vedic.

While those who adopt the full Maharishi enterprise solution in America may be few, Maharishi can nevertheless take considerable credit for the popular success of the advaitic interpretive model of Ayurveda cast in the terms of physics. He shares those laurels with his former disciple Deepak Chopra, who popularized his master's enterprise by removing many of the Hindu encumbrances necessitated by the TM movement's self-selected Vedic provenance. Also, taking a page from Maharishi's playbook, numerous rivals have entered the field, seeking to find their own market in America for their own versions of Ayurveda. Some deliberately eschew typically Maharishi-style adaptations, whereas others see some benefits to his style. Further, ayurvedic pampering at spas is now so commonplace that many upscale hotels now incorporate new Ayurveda treatments in their spas. Thanks in part to Maharishi, like Gideon's Bible, Ayurveda can be found in one's upscale hotel home away from home; it is up to individual customers whether they choose to use it.

NOTES

1. By "Maharishi Ayur-Veda," or MAV, I refer to Maharishi's interpretation and line of products and services, and "Ayurveda" to the general complex of theories and health services deriving from the indigenous Indic health tradition. For a good introduction to the primacy of MAV in introducing Ayurveda in America, see Reddy (2000: 5 ff).

2. Reddy suggests that "Maharishi Ayur-Veda not only changed the way Ayurveda presented itself to the public, but was also positioned as the fulcrum around which other sub-traditions aligned themselves. From this time on, definitions of each of the ayurvedic sub-traditions were marked either by their alignment with Maharishi Ayur-Veda or their distance from it as a measure of their true cultural authenticity" (Reddy 2000: 38).

3. In my position as an information technology professional, I find strong parallels to the interconnected products of the computing world with Maharishi Ayur-Veda. The example has sufficient currency that I use it as a touchstone from time to time in my analysis.

4. "Physicists speak of the 'cosmic code,' the mathematically describable laws of nature that structure creation. In Maharishi's explanation, the complex sound patterns in the Rk [*sic*] Veda and other central Vedic texts are this cosmic code" (Sharma and Clark 1998: 145).

5. Mahesh (1955). This unnumbered pamphlet is the transcription of Maharishi's speeches in English at a festival that took place October 23–26, 1955.

6. Jerry once commented to me that he "had stopped counting" how many initiations he had done after having taught TM to 5,000 people. At one point, people were literally lined up around a city block, waiting to accept initiation.

7. Marcus (1977: 8).

8. Keith Wallace conducted the earliest research on the physiological effects of Transcendental Meditation,™ publishing his results in articles for *Science*, *American Journal of Physiology*, and *Scientific American* during the period 1970–1972. He concluded that the TM technique produces a physiological state of restful alertness, with benefits for the release of stress. A near professionally organized anti-TM movement called "TM-EX" has attempted to establish that many of these hundreds of studies—usually conducted by TM proponents—are flawed, as are most aspects of the TM movement. My point here is not to evaluate that literature but to note its use in creating and sustaining Maharishi's enterprise.

9. The case was argued before the court at the end of 1976, but a decision was not issued until a year later, on December 12, 1977. *Alan B. Malnak et al. v. Maharishi Mahesh Yogi et al.*, United States District Court, District of New Jersey, in Civil Action No. 76–341. The complete text of the federal court's opinion in this case is provided in a booklet published by a Christian group, *TM in Court* (Berkeley: Spiritual Counterfeits Project, 1978).

10. Jerry Jarvis, the national leader, told me in an interview that once he requested during a national conference call that initiators refer to their *pūjā* sets (the brass bowls, etc., used during the initiation ceremony) as "portable SCI laboratories."

11. To extend the computer analogy, TM can be seen as a sufficiently robust operating system on its own, but the new TM-Sidhi Program drawn from the *Yoga Sūtras* was an upgrade that provided greater potential for interoperability. This analogy is sustained by insider terminology. The *Sidhis*, whose unique spelling signaled the distinctiveness of Maharishi's technique, were called by practitioners the "Maharishi Technology of the Unified Field."

12. Gandharva-Veda is the science of music. In TM, the focus is on discovering the properties of healing sounds. In fact, however, Gandharva-Veda amounted to North Indian classical music, especially as practiced by Hindus. The Islamic roots of this music were conveniently ignored by Maharishi and the rest of the TM movement. Dhanur-Veda is the science of weaponry, which has become a remarkably important arena of concern in TM. Maharishi claims that groups of meditators can, through the power of their shared positive effects on their surroundings, reduce tension and crime, creating an "Invincible Defense" perimeter around an area. Meditation becomes an alternative to military violence and fear-based deterrence. Dr. David R. Leffler, who "received his Ph.D. on the topic of Invincible Defense Technology," writes with his wife Lee Leffler, "Maharishi's Vedic Technology of Invincible Defense is a scientifically validated means to maintain homeland security without the need for killing or destruction. It has its origins in an ancient branch of Vedic literature called Dhanur-Veda. Maharishi Mahesh Yogi, along with other Vedic scholars and leading defense experts, are reviving and reconstructing the preventive aspects of this ancient military science to end terrorism and war." Sthapatya-Veda is the science of (Vedic) building design, leading to a new growth industry for meditating architects. And Jyotish is the science of identifying astrological forces and determining proper *yagyas* or rituals to expiate potential dangers.

13. Sharma and Clark (1998: 7). *Caraka-Saṃhitā, Sūtrasthāna* 1.46 asserts that humans are made of the imperishable self (*ātman*), mind (*citta*), and body (*śārīra*).

14. Sharma and Clark (1998: 14).

15. Ibid., 6.

16. Ibid., 14.

17. Quoted in *International Symposium on the Science of Creative Intelligence* (1971: 42). Domash was president of Maharishi International University in Fairfield, Iowa, for a few years in the 1970s. Since then, Domash has disappeared from the TM movement.

18. Maharishi quoted in *International Symposium on the Science of Creative Intelligence* (1971: 42).

19. See the brief overview in Albanese (1992: 68–84). Albanese discusses nineteenth-century American authors who employ quantum discourse to promote theosophy.

20. Maharishi would later equate *brahman* with the phrases "vacuum state," "state of least excitation," the "self-referral state" and, his personal favorite, the "Unified Field." In the late 1970s and throughout the 1980s, he would fund the research of John Hagelin, a young and gifted Harvard-trained physicist, who attempted to develop a "unified-field-based" quantum theory in the professional physics community. In addition to running for president on the Natural Law Party ticket in 2000, Hagelin was one of the physicists featured in the 2004 film *What the Bleep Do We Know!?*, which blended physics, biology, consciousness, and mysticism.

21. Maharishi Mahesh Yogi (1984: 143–44).

22. Sharma and Clark (1998: 121).

23. The unbalancing of the *doṣas* according to MAV, is explained in Reddy and Egenes (2002: 46–47). "Our consciousness is three-in-one—the knower, known, and the link between them. These three are analogically connected to conceptual features of Vedic mantras: rishi, devata, and chhandas, respectively. Our three-in-one consciousness precipitates into matter, and within human physiology, this appears as the three doshas. The experience of perfect health is the experience of the three doshas in true unity, or samhita. Pragya-aparadh, or the error of the intellect, occurs when the intellect loses connection to samhita, or wholeness, and the three doshas become unbalanced."

24. *Parliaments of World Peace to be Inaugurated on June 14, 2001.* See http://www.global-country.org/press/2001_06_12.html, accessed July 3, 2003.

25. Ibid.

26. Ibid.

27. Reddy and Egenes (2002: 25).

28. Ibid., 26.

29. "His Majesty Raja Nader Raam: Professor Tony Nader M.D., Ph.D." See http://www.maharishitm.org/en/tonynaderen.htm, accessed January 7, 2006.

30. Reddy and Egenes (2002: 3).

31. Ibid., 5.

32. Reddy (2000: 2).

33. Ibid., 3.

34. Ibid.

35. Reddy and Egenes (2002: 11).

36. For example, a client may be initiated into Transcendental Meditation, undergo panchakarma purification processes at a spa, receive a diet consultation, be prescribed a list of proper Ayurveda remedies, be informed that he or she must sponsor a ritual to ward off dangerous effects, and be sold a house properly designed to enhance the environment.

37. For a detailed examination of the Flint case, and the question of identity for all Ayurveda healers in America in general, see Reddy (2000).

38. This may be easily surmised from pictures on various Maharishi Web sites. Perhaps this is a strategy for infusing his cadre of *vaidyas* with an air of authenticity within the precincts of Maharishi's movement.

39. Vedic City is two miles north of Fairfield, Iowa, and it is the capital of Vishwa Shanti Rashtra, the Global Country of World Peace, which Maharishi proclaimed into existence.

40. Two-page undated memorandum from Lenny Goldman to "All departments." Private collection.

41. The term *franchise* is used to depict this specific relationship in MAV by Reddy (2000, especially 89 ff., 153 ff.).

42. McFarlane (2004). http://www.la-articles.org.uk/gates.htm, accessed November 10, 2004.

43. Ibid.

44. This has been true at large in India for several decades. Ayurveda "has evolved over the years, with a move toward standardized compound medications and away from the practice of preparing a medication specific to a particular patient, as the original texts dictated" (Tucker 2003: 375, citing Dominik Wujastyk 1996: 19–37).

45. Dennis (1994).

46. Ibid.

47. For several examples of what she describes as the franchising of panchakarma centers, for example, see Reddy (2000 passim).

48. For an excellent early essay on TM and the relation between the movement and its "consumers," see Johnston (1980 [1988]). Many of his explanations remain on target, even twenty years later.

49. See my discussion of Dhanur-Veda, supra.

REFERENCES

Albanese, Catherine. 1992. The magical staff: Quantum healing in the new age. In *Perspectives on the New Age*, ed. James R. Lewis and J. Gordon Melton, 68–84. Albany: State University of New York Press.

Chopra, Ananda S. 2003. Ayurveda. In *Medicine across Cultures: History and Practice of Medicine in Non-Western Cultures*, ed. Helaine Selin, 75–84. Dordrecht, the Netherlands: Kluwer Academic Publishers.

Dennis, Gregory. 1994. What's Deepak Chopra's secret? *New Age Journal* (January–February). Article available at http://mionet.org/TM-EX/news 94sp.dtp.0.html.

Humes, Cynthia Ann. 2005. Maharishi Mahesh Yogi: Beyond the TM technique. In *Gurus in America*, ed. Thomas A. Forsthoefel and Cynthia Ann Humes, 55–80. Albany: State University of New York Press.

International Symposium on the Science of Creative Intelligence. 1971. Seelisberg, Switzerland: MIU Press.

Johnston, Hank. 1980. The marketed social movement: A case study of the rapid growth of TM. *Pacific Sociological Review* 23: 333–54. Repr. in *Money and Power in the New Religions*, ed. James Richardson. Lewiston, NY: Edwin Mellen Press, 1988; pp. 163–83.

Maharishi Mahesh Yogi. 1984. *Maharishi Mahesh Yogi on the Bhagavad Gita: A New Translation and Commentary, Chapters 1–6.* Washington, DC: Age of Enlightenment Press.

Mahesh, Bal Brahmachari. 1955. *The Beacon Light of the Himalayas—The Dawn of the Happy New Era*. Kerala: Adhyatmic Vikas Mandal.

Marcus, Jay B. 1977. *TM and Business: Personal and Corporate Benefits of Inner Development*. New York: McGraw Hill.

McFarlane. 2004. Hanging, drawing and quartering—American style: The brutal dissection of Microsoft. http://www.la-articles.org.uk/gates.htm, accessed November 10, 2004.

Parliaments of World Peace to be Inaugurated on June 14, 2001. Available at http://www.global-country.org/press/2001_06_12.html, accessed July 3, 2003.

Reddy, Kumuda, and Linda Egenes. 2002. *Conquering Chronic Disease through Maharishi Vedic Medicine*. Schenectady, NY: Samhita Productions.

Reddy, Sita. 2000. *Reinventing Medical Traditions: The Professionalization of Ayurveda in Contemporary America*. Ph.D. diss. University of Pennsylvania.

Richardson, James, ed. 1988. *Money and Power in the New Religions*. Lewiston, NY: Edwin Mellon Press.

Scientific Research on the Maharishi Transcendental Meditation and TM-Sidhi Programs: A Brief Summary of 600 Studies. 2000. Fairfield, IA: Maharishi University of Management Press.

Sharma, Hari, and Christopher Clark. 1998. *Contemporary Ayurveda: Medicine and Research in Maharishi Ayur-Veda*. New York: Churchill Livingstone.

TM in Court. 1978. Berkeley, CA: Spiritual Counterfeits Project.

Tucker, Jim B. 2003. Religion and medicine. In *Medicine across Cultures: History and Practice of Medicine in Non-Western Cultures*, ed. Helaine Selin, 373–84. Dordrecht, the Netherlands: Kluwer Academic Publishers.

Wujastyk, Dominik. 1996. Medicine in India. In *Oriental Medicine*, ed. Jan Alphen and Anthony Aris, 19–37. Boston, MA: Shambhala Publications.

Contributors

Joseph S. Alter teaches anthropology at the University of Pittsburgh. He is the author of a number of books, including *Asian Medicine and Globalization* (University of Pennsylvania Press, 2005) and *Yoga in Modern India: The Body between Philosophy and Science* (Princeton University Press, 2004). His research interests include the history and philosophy of science and medicine in Asia, broadly defined.

Madhulika Banerjee currently is a reader at the Department of Political Science, University of Delhi. Her research interest is the politics of knowledge, particularly the contention between traditional and modern knowledge. Her PhD thesis (University of Delhi, 1996) focused on the development of Ayurveda from the vantage points of policy, research, and the market in the postcolonial period. Banerjee has published papers on related subjects in Indian academic journals, and her book on the same, *Power, Knowledge, Medicine: Ayurveda at Home and in the World*, was published in 2007 by Orient Longman.

Rachel Berger is assistant professor of history at Concordia University in Montreal. Her doctoral work addressed the history of ayurvedic medicine in colonial North India, comparing political discourses of public health and development with popular discussions of health, medicine, gender, and sexuality.

Ananda Samir Chopra was born to Indian parents and raised in Germany. He studied medicine and Indology at the University of Heidelberg, Germany, and worked as a physician in Germany before studying Ayurveda in Kolkata, India. Since 1996 he has headed the Ayurveda section of the Habichtswaldklinik AYURVEDA in Kassel, Germany. This is a clinical Ayurveda section within a larger German hospital, with a ward of approximately thirty beds and a large ambulatory. It is a unique feature of this Ayurveda section that authentic ayurvedic medicine (especially panchakarma therapy) is practiced there in a constant dialogue with modern biomedicine. In March 1998, Chopra was honored by the Ayurveda Board of Karnataka with a plate and a shawl. His research interests include diachronic developments of ayurvedic concepts and clinical application of Ayurveda in Germany. Chopra has been learning classical north Indian music on the sitar since his childhood and has served as director of studies at the Tagore-Institute, Bonn, Germany.

Elizabeth De Michelis's areas of expertise and current research are history, philosophy, and texts relating to Indic forms of yoga and meditation; the Hindu and Buddhist contexts within which these practices developed and continue to develop and their spread East and West; and Indic-inspired aspects of Western esotericism.

De Michelis completed her bachelor's degree in modern languages at Milan, Italy, then worked for several years in business at the management level. Eventually, her wish for a career change, and ongoing questions regarding the nature and history of modern forms of yoga, led her to return to academia. She obtained a master's degree in religious studies at School of Oriental and African Studies (SOAS), University of London, then her Ph.D. from the Faculty of Divinity, University of Cambridge. Her doctoral work, now published under the title *A History of Modern Yoga: Patañjali and Western Esotericism*, was on the modernization of Hinduism and more particularly on the modernization of yoga and its transmission to the West.

De Michelis currently holds the Gordon Milburn Research Fellowship at the University of Oxford (Theology Faculty and Oriel College). She was previously at the Faculty of Divinity, University of Cambridge, where she worked as director of the Dharam Hinduja Institute of Indic Research, promoting and carrying out innovative research on the modernization of yoga and Ayurveda.

Cynthia Ann Humes is associate professor of religious studies as well as chief technology officer and executive director of information technology services at Claremont McKenna College. When not conducting administrative tasks, she devotes time to her research interests. Her publications concern the contemporary use of Sanskrit literature, modern ritual in North Indian goddess worship, the political and economic dimensions of modern Hinduism, women's roles and experience in world religions and, more recently, the phenomenon of the guru in Western forms of Hinduism. She is coeditor of *Living Banaras: Hindu Religion in Cultural Context* (State University of New York Press, 1993, and Manohar Publications, 1998) and coeditor of *Gurus in America* (State University of New York Press, 2005). *Gurus in America* brings together the work of ten scholars focusing on nine important Hindu gurus and is the result of a panel discussion with gurus that was organized by Humes in 2001. She recently cowrote with Dana Sawyer a book on the history of the Transcendental Meditation movement in the United States, and she translated an annotated the popular discourse of Shankaracharya Swami Brahmananda Saraswati.

Françoise Jeannotat received her bachelor's degree in sociology and anthropology in 1992 and her master's degree in social sciences in 1993 from the University of Lausanne. She then worked as an assistant in Science of Religions and Hinduism (1995 to 1999) and coordinated the Département Interfacultaire d'Histoire et de Sciences des Religions of the University of Lausanne (1998 to 1999). Her fields of interest are modern and global Ayurveda as well as classical and modern Hinduism.

G. Jan Meulenbeld was born in 1928, in Borne (the Netherlands). He studied medicine and Sanskrit at the State University of Utrecht from 1946 to 1954 and specialized in psychiatry and psychotherapy from 1956 to 1961. He was a member of the psychiatric staff of two psychiatric hospitals until the year of his retirement, 1988. He is the author of a doctoral thesis on the Madhavanidāna, published in 1974, taught Sanskrit at the State University of Groningen from 1978 to 1986, and wrote the three-volume *History of Indian Medical Literature*, published in 1999, 2000, and 2002. He continues writing articles on various aspects of Indian medicine.

Suzanne Newcombe is completing her doctorate in the history faculty at the University of Cambridge. Her dissertation is a social history of yoga and Ayurveda in postwar Britain. She has an MSc in the sociology of religion and has taught on courses in this field at the London School of Economics and Cambridge University. She is employed as an assistant research officer for Inform, a registered charity based at the London School of Economics, which provides inquirers with balanced and up-to-date information on new and alternative religions.

Unnikrishnan Payyappallimana studied at the Ayurveda College, Coimbatore, India (Bharathiar University), and graduated in 1992 as an ayurvedic physician. After graduation, he worked as a Research Fellow at the famous Amala Cancer Hospital and Research Center in Kerala, and he was also in 1998 a Visiting Research Fellow at the Toyama Medical and Pharmaceutical University, Toyama, Japan. He worked as well as a visiting associate professor at the same university from 2003 to 2004.

Unnikrishnan completed in 2000 his postgraduation studies in medical anthropology at the University of Amsterdam. He has been working since 1995 with the Foundation for the Revitalization of Local Health Traditions in Bangalore. He spent his initial years there building up a database of medicinal plants used in Ayurveda. He is currently coordinating the Endogenous Development and Local Health Traditions program at the Traditional Systems of Medicine unit of the Foundation. His professional interests include intercultural medical research and the role of traditional medicine in public health.

Sebastian Pole is an ayurvedic and Chinese medicine practitioner registered with the Ayurvedic Practitioners Association, the Register of Chinese Herbal Medicine, and the Unified Register of Herbal Practitioners. He has studied at the East West College of Herbalism, the London College of Oriental Medicine, and the College of Ayurveda, and he has also completed a clinical internship in India. In line with traditional medicine principles, Pole focuses on bringing revitalized health to the whole mind-body-spirit system using herbs, diet, and yogic breathing practices. He has a special interest in treating skin and digestive problems. He also is a passionate conservationist involved in the organic movement to help promote the supply of sustainably grown ayurvedic herbs. Pole is herbal director of Pukka Herbs, specializing in organic ayurvedic herbs, teas, capsules, and tinctures. See http://www.pukkaherbs.com for further information on his work.

Mike Saks is currently pro vice chancellor (Research and Academic Affairs) at the University of Lincoln. He studied at the University of Lancaster, University of Kent, and London School of Economics and obtained at the latter a PhD in sociology. He was formerly dean of the Faculty of Health and Community Studies at De Montfort University in Leicester. He has published extensively on professionalization and health care and has given many keynote presentations at national and international conferences.

Saks has been a member and chair of many NHS and other health committees at the local, regional, and national levels, covering a number of areas from the changing health care workforce and complementary medicine to research and development. In addition, he has frequently acted as an advisor at all levels of the National Health Service, most recently on health professional regulation in the wake of the Shipman Inquiry.

Internationally he is involved in several research projects, including collaborations with the Russian Academy of Sciences and the University of Toronto. He also is a member and president-elect of the Executive of the International Sociological Association Research Committee on Professional Groups and part of the editorial team for the international journal *Knowledge, Work, and Society,* produced by Parisian publisher L'Harmattan.

Frederick M. Smith teaches Sanskrit and Indian religion at the University of Iowa. His most recent book is *The Self Possessed: Deity and Spirit Possession in South Asian Literature and Civilization* (Columbia University Press, 2006). His primary academic interest, into which the current project falls, is to understand the history, development, and mechanics of South Asian cultural and religious traditions. He has examined these from a variety of synchronic and diachronic perspectives in his writings for the last twenty-five years.

Robert E. Svoboda is the first Westerner ever to graduate from a college of Ayurveda and be licensed to practice Ayurveda in India. The winner of all but one of the University of Poona's awards for academic excellence in Ayurveda, including the Ram Narayan Sharma Gold Metal, he was tutored by his mentor, the Aghori Vimalananda, in Ayurveda, Yoga, Jyotish, Tantra, and other forms of classical Indian lore during and after his formal ayurvedic training. Svoboda also served as Viomalananda's Authorized Racing Agent at the Royal Western India Turf Club in Bombay and Poona between 1975 and 1985.

After extensive travel in Europe, Asia, and Africa (where he was ritually initiated into the Pokot tribe of northern Kenya as its first white member), Svoboda moved to India in 1974 and lived there for more than a decade. Since 1985, he has continued to spend many months of each year in India when he is not lecturing, consulting, or teaching in other lands. The author of more than a dozen books and numerous articles, including the entry on Ayurveda for *Encyclopedia Britannica,* 2000, he serves as an adjunct member for the Ayurvedic Institute in Albuquerque, New Mexico, for Bastyr University in Seattle, Washington, and for the Institute for Religion and Health in Houston, Texas.

Manasi Tirodkar is a postdoctoral Research Fellow at the Institute for Healthcare Studies, Northwestern University, Chicago. She graduated in 2005 from the University of Chicago with a doctorate in human development and a specialization in cultural psychology and medical anthropology. She has two primary areas of research interest: the utilization of complementary, alternative, and traditional medicines, and disparities in health status and access to health care. She has researched caste and gender differences in health status and concepts of health as well as the cultural meanings of obesity among the African American population in Chicago. Her dissertation described the impact of globalization on the contemporary practice of ayurvedic medicine in India. Her current research projects examine conceptual models of heart disease in South Asians and differences in health outcomes based on acculturation in immigrant populations.

Richard S. Weiss is a lecturer in South Asian religions at Victoria University in Wellington, New Zealand. His research focuses on South Indian religion, culture, and history. He is currently finishing a book that examines the strategies through which Siddha medical practitioners attract patronage in modern Tamil Nadu. His newest research focuses on representations of religious community in Tamil Shaiva literature. He has published articles on tradition, Siddha medicine, Sai Baba, and Tamil revivalism.

Claudia Welch began studying ayurvedic medicine in 1987 under the personal supervision of Dr. Robert Svoboda. She pursued her interest throughout three years in India and continued her education for many years while working with Dr. Vasant Lad at the Ayurvedic Institute in Albuquerque, New Mexico. She has studied Sanskrit and Jyotish and graduated from Hart De Fouw's Advanced Jyotish course. She frequently spends time in India. She is currently on the teaching faculty at the Kripalu School of Ayurveda in Lenox, Massachusetts, the RISHI Center in Newport, Rhode Island, where she is on the board of advisors, the Ayurvedic Institute, and Southwest Acupuncture College in Albuquerque, New Mexico, from where she obtained in 1997 her master of science degree in oriental medicine.

Welch has authored the e-book *Secrets of the Mind: The Ten Channels Revealed,* which describes little-known aspects of the Manovahasrotas, and a beginning online ayurvedic learning course, both offered through http://www.Bigshakt.com. She also has been a contributing author to various other publications. Welch, who has lectured on Ayurveda internationally, maintains a private practice in Albuquerque, New Mexico, where she specializes in women's health.

Dagmar Wujastyk is completing her doctorate at the Faculty of Indology at the University of Bonn, Germany. Her dissertation surveys and analyzes concepts of medical ethics in the Sanskrit medical classics, with special reference to the doctor-patient relationship. From 2002 to 2004, Wujastyk was research assistant at the Dharam Hinduja Institute of Indic Research, Cambridge University, where she developed and organized a two-year research project on modern and global Ayurveda. The present volume is partly based on the outcomes of this research project.

Dominik Wujastyk was educated in the exact sciences (physics, London University) and in Asian studies (Sanskrit and Pali, Oxford University). His professional career began with curatorial work on the Indic manuscript collection at the Wellcome Library in London, which holds one of the largest and most important collections of Sanskrit manuscripts outside of India. He took up in 2002 a Senior Research Fellowship at University College, London, where he has been researching the history of Ayurveda in the precolonial period, from 1550 to 1750, working chiefly from Sanskrit sources of the time. His publications include *Metarules of Pāṇinian Grammar* (2 vols., 1993) and *A Handlist of the Sanskrit and Prakrit Manuscripts in the Wellcome Library* (2 vols., 1985, 1998), *The Roots of Ayurveda* (Penguin Classics, 1998, 2nd ed., 2001, 3rd ed., 2003), *Studies in Indian Medical History* (ed. with G. J. Meulenbeld, 1987, 2nd ed., 2001), *Contagion in Pre-Modern Societies* (ed. with L. I. Conrad, 2000), *Mathematics and Medicine in Sanskrit* (ed., in press), and numerous articles and chapters on the history of manuscript illustration, Ayurveda, vyākaraṇa, the history of science in India, and Sanskrit literature and culture.

Index

Note: Page numbers with a *t* indicate tables.